# UNDERSTANDING Human Behavior

## A Guide for Health Care Providers

### EIGHTH EDITION

Alyson Honeycut, M.A., N.C.C.

and

Mary Elizabeth Milliken, B.S.N., M.S., Ed.D.
Certified Healing Touch Practitioner

Australia • Brazil • Japan • Korea • Mexico • Singapore • Spain • United Kingdom • United States

**Understanding Human Behavior: A Guide for Health Care Providers, Eighth Edition**
Alyson Honeycutt, M.A., N.C.C. and Mary Elizabeth Milliken, B.S.N., M.S., Ed.D.

Vice President, Career and Professional Editorial: Dave Garza

Director of Learning Solutions: Matthew Kane

Acquisitions Editor: Matt Seeley

Managing Editor: Marah Bellegarde

Product Manager: Laura J. Wood

Editorial Assistant: Samantha Zullo

Vice President, Career and Professional Marketing: Jennifer Baker

Marketing Director: Wendy E. Mapstone

Senior Marketing Manager: Kristin McNary

Marketing Coordinator: Jonathan Sheehan

Production Director: Carolyn Miller

Content Project Manager: Anne Sherman

Senior Art Director: Jack Pendleton

© 2012, 2004, 1998, 1993, 1987 Delmar, Cengage Learning

ALL RIGHTS RESERVED. No part of this work covered by the copyright herein may be reproduced, transmitted, stored, or used in any form or by any means graphic, electronic, or mechanical, including but not limited to photocopying, recording, scanning, digitizing, taping, Web distribution, information networks, or information storage and retrieval systems, except as permitted under Section 107 or 108 of the 1976 United States Copyright Act, without the prior written permission of the publisher.

For product information and technology assistance, contact us at
**Cengage Learning Customer & Sales Support, 1-800-354-9706**
For permission to use material from this text or product,
submit all requests online at **www.cengage.com/permissions.**
Further permissions questions can be e-mailed to
**permissionrequest@cengage.com**

Library of Congress Control Number: 2010930403

ISBN-13: 978-1-4354-8660-7
ISBN-10: 1-4354-8660-9

**Delmar**
5 Maxwell Drive
Clifton Park, NY 12065-2919
USA

Cengage Learning is a leading provider of customized learning solutions with office locations around the globe, including Singapore, the United Kingdom, Australia, Mexico, Brazil, and Japan. Locate your local office at:
**international.cengage.com/region**

Cengage Learning products are represented in Canada by Nelson Education, Ltd.

To learn more about Delmar, visit **www.cengage.com/delmar**
Purchase any of our products at your local college store or at our preferred online store **www.CengageBrain.com**

**NOTICE TO THE READER**

Publisher does not warrant or guarantee any of the products described herein or perform any independent analysis in connection with any of the product information contained herein. Publisher does not assume, and expressly disclaims, any obligation to obtain and include information other than that provided to it by the manufacturer. The reader is expressly warned to consider and adopt all safety precautions that might be indicated by the activities described herein and to avoid all potential hazards. By following the instructions contained herein, the reader willingly assumes all risks in connection with such instructions. The publisher makes no representations or warranties of any kind, including but not limited to, the warranties of fitness for particular purpose or merchantability, nor are any such representations implied with respect to the material set forth herein, and the publisher takes no responsibility with respect to such material. The publisher shall not be liable for any special, consequential, or exemplary damages resulting, in whole or part, from the readers' use of, or reliance upon, this material.

Printed in the United States of America
2 3 4 5 6 7 12

# Contents

Preface .................................................... xi

**SECTION I    ON BECOMING A HEALTH CARE PROVIDER** .................... 1

**UNIT 1    Challenges and Responsibilities of Health Care Providers** .............. 3

    Satisfactions ................................................ 4
    Challenges ................................................. 4
    Responsibilities .............................................. 6
    Achievement as Progress ....................................... 8
    Attitudes and Interests ........................................ 10
    Empowerment ............................................... 10
    Making a Decision ........................................... 11

**Unit 2    The Philosophy of Individual Worth** ............................ 21

    Meaning of Individual Worth ................................... 21
    The Health Care Provider and Cultural Bias ....................... 22
    Implications for Health Care Providers ........................... 25
    Practicing a Philosophy of Individual Worth ....................... 25

**UNIT 3    Striving for Self-Understanding** ............................... 31

    You, the Student ............................................ 31
    Taking a New Look at Yourself ................................. 32
    You, a Person with Several Life Roles ........................... 35
    Guidelines for Growth ........................................ 36

**SECTION II    STRIVING TO UNDERSTAND HUMAN BEHAVIOR** ................ 43

**UNIT 4    Influences on Behavior** ..................................... 45

    How People Are Alike ........................................ 45
    How People Are Different ..................................... 46
    Heredity .................................................... 46
    The Developmental Process .................................... 48
    Environment ................................................ 50
    Influences on Development During Childhood .................... 52
    Changing Influences During Life ............................... 54
    Assuming Responsibility for Behavior ........................... 56
    The Health Care Provider and the Patient ........................ 57

## UNIT 5 Physical Needs ... 63

Maslow's Hierarchy of Needs ... 63
Essential Physical Needs ... 64
The Sleep Cycle ... 66
Satisfaction of Physical Needs ... 67
Comfort and Safety Needs ... 67
Physical Needs and Behavior ... 68
Understanding Behavior in Terms of Physical Needs ... 69

## Unit 6 The Need for Self-Approval ... 73

Social Needs of People ... 73
The Self-Concept ... 75
Self-Esteem ... 78
Influence of Others on One's Sense of Self ... 79
Effects of Success and Failure ... 80
Success ... 82
Striving for Self-Approval ... 83

## Unit 7 The Need for Acceptance ... 89

The Importance of Acceptance ... 89
The Importance of Approval from Others ... 91
Conformity ... 92
The Need to Believe That Others Care ... 93
The Need for Appreciation ... 95
Social Needs and Behavior ... 95
Behavior and the Health Care Provider ... 96

## Unit 8 Emotions and Behavior ... 99

Meaning of Emotions ... 99
Importance of Emotions ... 100
Physiological Effects of Emotions ... 101
Stress ... 102
Positive Emotions ... 103
Negative Emotions ... 105
Formation of Emotional Patterns ... 108
Individual Differences in Emotional Patterns ... 108
Gender Differences in Emotions ... 110
Using Emotions Constructively ... 110
Emotions and Behavior ... 114

## Unit 9 Adjustment and Patterns of Behavior ... 121

Good Adjustment ... 121
Poor Adjustment ... 122
Effective Behavior Versus Ineffective Behavior ... 122

Emotions and Adjustment . . . . . . . . . . . . . . . . . . . . . . . . . . . . . . . . 124
Daily Hassles . . . . . . . . . . . . . . . . . . . . . . . . . . . . . . . . . . . . . . . . . 125
Improving Adjustment . . . . . . . . . . . . . . . . . . . . . . . . . . . . . . . . . . 125

**SECTION III  BEHAVIOR AND PROBLEMS IN LIVING . . . . . . . . . . . . . . . . . . . . . . . . . 135**

**Unit 10  Common Threats to Adjustment . . . . . . . . . . . . . . . . . . . . . . . . . . . . . . . 137**

Change as a Threat to Adjustment . . . . . . . . . . . . . . . . . . . . . . . . . 138
Life Stages and Change . . . . . . . . . . . . . . . . . . . . . . . . . . . . . . . . 138
Social and Cultural Stressors . . . . . . . . . . . . . . . . . . . . . . . . . . . . 141
Major Changes . . . . . . . . . . . . . . . . . . . . . . . . . . . . . . . . . . . . . . 145
Chronic Stressors . . . . . . . . . . . . . . . . . . . . . . . . . . . . . . . . . . . . 147
Coping Skills and Resilience . . . . . . . . . . . . . . . . . . . . . . . . . . . . . 150

**Unit 11  Effects of Traumatic Events . . . . . . . . . . . . . . . . . . . . . . . . . . . . . . . . . . 155**

What Is Trauma? . . . . . . . . . . . . . . . . . . . . . . . . . . . . . . . . . . . . . 156
Traumatic Experiences . . . . . . . . . . . . . . . . . . . . . . . . . . . . . . . . . 156
Domestic Violence . . . . . . . . . . . . . . . . . . . . . . . . . . . . . . . . . . . . 163
Reactions to Trauma . . . . . . . . . . . . . . . . . . . . . . . . . . . . . . . . . . 168
The Survivor Role . . . . . . . . . . . . . . . . . . . . . . . . . . . . . . . . . . . . 170
The Challenge . . . . . . . . . . . . . . . . . . . . . . . . . . . . . . . . . . . . . . 170

**Unit 12  Defense Mechanisms . . . . . . . . . . . . . . . . . . . . . . . . . . . . . . . . . . . . . . . . 175**

The Purpose of Defense Mechanisms . . . . . . . . . . . . . . . . . . . . . . 175
Rationalization . . . . . . . . . . . . . . . . . . . . . . . . . . . . . . . . . . . . . . 176
Projection . . . . . . . . . . . . . . . . . . . . . . . . . . . . . . . . . . . . . . . . . . 178
Displacement . . . . . . . . . . . . . . . . . . . . . . . . . . . . . . . . . . . . . . . 179
Daydreaming . . . . . . . . . . . . . . . . . . . . . . . . . . . . . . . . . . . . . . . 179
Escape into Illness . . . . . . . . . . . . . . . . . . . . . . . . . . . . . . . . . . . 181
Repression . . . . . . . . . . . . . . . . . . . . . . . . . . . . . . . . . . . . . . . . . 182
Withdrawal . . . . . . . . . . . . . . . . . . . . . . . . . . . . . . . . . . . . . . . . . 183
Substance Dependency . . . . . . . . . . . . . . . . . . . . . . . . . . . . . . . . 184
Codependency . . . . . . . . . . . . . . . . . . . . . . . . . . . . . . . . . . . . . . 189
Defense Mechanisms and Adjustment . . . . . . . . . . . . . . . . . . . . . . 190

**UNIT 13  Inner Conflict . . . . . . . . . . . . . . . . . . . . . . . . . . . . . . . . . . . . . . . . . . . . . 197**

The Meaning of Inner Conflict . . . . . . . . . . . . . . . . . . . . . . . . . . . 197
Types of Inner Conflict . . . . . . . . . . . . . . . . . . . . . . . . . . . . . . . . 199
How to Deal with Inner Conflict . . . . . . . . . . . . . . . . . . . . . . . . . 201
Inner Conflict and Adjustment . . . . . . . . . . . . . . . . . . . . . . . . . . . 203
Inner Conflict and the Health Care Provider . . . . . . . . . . . . . . . . . 204
Inner Conflict and the Patient . . . . . . . . . . . . . . . . . . . . . . . . . . . 205
Using Knowledge About Inner Conflict . . . . . . . . . . . . . . . . . . . . . 205

## UNIT 14  Frustration . . . . . . . . . . . . . . . . . . . . . . . . . . . . . . . . . . . . . . . . . . . . . . . . . . . 209

Degrees of Frustration. . . . . . . . . . . . . . . . . . . . . . . . . . . . . . . . . . . . . . . . . . . . 209
Cumulative Effects of Frustration . . . . . . . . . . . . . . . . . . . . . . . . . . . . . . . . . . 210
Sources of Frustration . . . . . . . . . . . . . . . . . . . . . . . . . . . . . . . . . . . . . . . . . . . 210
Effects of Frustration . . . . . . . . . . . . . . . . . . . . . . . . . . . . . . . . . . . . . . . . . . . . 214
Frustration and Behavior Patterns . . . . . . . . . . . . . . . . . . . . . . . . . . . . . . . . . 214
Perfectionism and Frustration . . . . . . . . . . . . . . . . . . . . . . . . . . . . . . . . . . . . 216
Coping with Frustration. . . . . . . . . . . . . . . . . . . . . . . . . . . . . . . . . . . . . . . . . 216

## SECTION IV  BECOMING AN EFFECTIVE HEALTH CARE PROVIDER . . . . . . . . . . . . . . . . . . . 223

## UNIT 15  Effects of Illness on Behavior . . . . . . . . . . . . . . . . . . . . . . . . . . . . . . . . . . . . . 225

Physical Effects of Illness. . . . . . . . . . . . . . . . . . . . . . . . . . . . . . . . . . . . . . . . 226
Emotional Effects of Illness . . . . . . . . . . . . . . . . . . . . . . . . . . . . . . . . . . . . . . 226
General Effects of Serious Illness. . . . . . . . . . . . . . . . . . . . . . . . . . . . . . . . . . 226
Influences on Patients' Reactions to Illness. . . . . . . . . . . . . . . . . . . . . . . . . . 227
The Challenge for Health Care Providers . . . . . . . . . . . . . . . . . . . . . . . . . . . 231

## UNIT 16  Coping with Patient Behavior . . . . . . . . . . . . . . . . . . . . . . . . . . . . . . . . . . . . 239

General Guidelines. . . . . . . . . . . . . . . . . . . . . . . . . . . . . . . . . . . . . . . . . . . . 239
Common Behavior Patterns of Patients . . . . . . . . . . . . . . . . . . . . . . . . . . . . 245

## UNIT 17  Human Relations and the Health Care Provider . . . . . . . . . . . . . . . . . . . . . . . . . . . . . . . . . . . . . . . . . . . . . . . . . . . . 257

Helping Patients Adjust to Illness. . . . . . . . . . . . . . . . . . . . . . . . . . . . . . . . . 258
Becoming a Member of the Health Team . . . . . . . . . . . . . . . . . . . . . . . . . . 260
Practicing Effective Patient Relations . . . . . . . . . . . . . . . . . . . . . . . . . . . . . . 264
The Challenge . . . . . . . . . . . . . . . . . . . . . . . . . . . . . . . . . . . . . . . . . . . . . . . 265

## SECTION V  PRACTICING EFFECTIVE COMMUNICATION. . . . . . . . . . . . . . . . . . . . . . . . . . . 269

## UNIT 18  Observing Nonverbal Behavior . . . . . . . . . . . . . . . . . . . . . . . . . . . . . . . . . . . 271

Observing and Interpreting Nonverbal Behavior. . . . . . . . . . . . . . . . . . . . . . 272
Setting the Stage for Practicing Interpersonal Skills. . . . . . . . . . . . . . . . . . . 275

## UNIT 19  Verbal Communication. . . . . . . . . . . . . . . . . . . . . . . . . . . . . . . . . . . . . . . . . . 281

Ambiguity. . . . . . . . . . . . . . . . . . . . . . . . . . . . . . . . . . . . . . . . . . . . . . . . . . . 282
Discrepancies in a Message . . . . . . . . . . . . . . . . . . . . . . . . . . . . . . . . . . . . . 283
Tone . . . . . . . . . . . . . . . . . . . . . . . . . . . . . . . . . . . . . . . . . . . . . . . . . . . . . . 283
Effective Listening. . . . . . . . . . . . . . . . . . . . . . . . . . . . . . . . . . . . . . . . . . . . . 284
Assumptions and Expectations. . . . . . . . . . . . . . . . . . . . . . . . . . . . . . . . . . . 284
Improving Communication Skills. . . . . . . . . . . . . . . . . . . . . . . . . . . . . . . . . 285
Opinion Statements to Serve as a Basis for Discussion . . . . . . . . . . . . . . . . 288
Class Challenge. . . . . . . . . . . . . . . . . . . . . . . . . . . . . . . . . . . . . . . . . . . . . . 288

| SECTION VI | **COPING WITH LOSS** .................................................. **291** |
|---|---|
| **UNIT 20** | **Gains and Losses throughout the Life Span** .................... **293** |

        Life Changes as Gains and Losses ............................... 293
        Learning to Cope with Loss ....................................... 294
        Significance of Loss ................................................. 294
        Losses Due to Death ................................................ 295
        Suicide .................................................................... 297
        Death of a Parent .................................................... 299
        Losses in Specific Periods of the Life Span ................... 300
        Striving for Readjustment Following Significant Loss ..... 305
        Guidelines for Using Loss and Grief as
           a Growth Experience ......................................... 305

| **UNIT 21** | **Death: Changing Attitudes and Practices** ........................ **311** |
|---|---|

        Past Attitudes and Practices ..................................... 312
        Changing Attitudes and Practices ............................... 312
        Current Attitudes and Practices ................................. 313
        The Emergence of Thanatology .................................. 314
        The Meaning of Death ............................................. 314
        Death with Dignity ................................................. 315
        Euthanasia .............................................................. 315
        Evolution of the Right-to-Die Movement ..................... 316
        Societal Issues Related to Care of the Dying ................ 318
        Legal Aspects of the Right to Die .............................. 320
        A Dilemma for Health Care Providers ........................ 324

| **UNIT 22** | **Grief and Bereavement** ................................................ **331** |
|---|---|

        Reactions to Loss and Bereavement ........................... 332
        Effects of Grief ....................................................... 332
        Importance of the Grief Process ................................ 333
        Influences on the Grief Process ................................. 334
        Grief Work ............................................................. 336
        Roles of Health Care Providers ................................. 338
        Guidelines for Assisting the Family of a Dying Patient ... 339

| **UNIT 23** | **Caring for the Dying Person** ......................................... **345** |
|---|---|

        Reactions to Diagnosis of a Terminal Illness ................ 345
        Stages of Dying ...................................................... 346
        Dying as a Growth Process ....................................... 348
        Personal and Family Issues Related to Care of the Dying ... 350
        Home Care ............................................................. 350
        Hospice Care .......................................................... 351
        Palliative Care ......................................................... 352
        Medical Issues Related to Care of the Dying ............... 353

Issues Related to Rights of the Dying Person . . . . . . . . . . . . . . . . . . . . . . 354
Roles of Health Care Providers . . . . . . . . . . . . . . . . . . . . . . . . . . . . . . . . 355
Guidelines for Care of a Dying Person. . . . . . . . . . . . . . . . . . . . . . . . . . . 356

## SECTION VII  TRENDS IN HEALTH CARE . . . . . . . . . . . . . . . . . . . . . . . . . . . . . . . . . . . 361

### Unit 24  Health Care through the Ages . . . . . . . . . . . . . . . . . . . . . . . . . . . . . . . 363

Definitions . . . . . . . . . . . . . . . . . . . . . . . . . . . . . . . . . . . . . . . . . . . . . . . . 363
Innovations in Science and Health Care . . . . . . . . . . . . . . . . . . . . . . . . . 364
Healing in Early Civilizations . . . . . . . . . . . . . . . . . . . . . . . . . . . . . . . . . 366
Evolution of Modern Health Care . . . . . . . . . . . . . . . . . . . . . . . . . . . . . 367
Beginnings of Holistic Medicine . . . . . . . . . . . . . . . . . . . . . . . . . . . . . . . 371
Innovators and Modern Medicine . . . . . . . . . . . . . . . . . . . . . . . . . . . . . 372
The Health Care System—Today and Tomorrow . . . . . . . . . . . . . . . . . 376
Scientific Study of Complementary Therapies . . . . . . . . . . . . . . . . . . . . 378
Issues in Health Care . . . . . . . . . . . . . . . . . . . . . . . . . . . . . . . . . . . . . . . 378
Staying Informed . . . . . . . . . . . . . . . . . . . . . . . . . . . . . . . . . . . . . . . . . . 382

### Unit 25  What Is Healing? Who Is the Healer? . . . . . . . . . . . . . . . . . . . . . . . . . 387

Placebo Effect . . . . . . . . . . . . . . . . . . . . . . . . . . . . . . . . . . . . . . . . . . . . . 387
The Immune System—Protector and Defender of the Body . . . . . . . . . 388
The Mind/Body Healing System . . . . . . . . . . . . . . . . . . . . . . . . . . . . . . 388
Who Gets Sick? Who Gets Well? . . . . . . . . . . . . . . . . . . . . . . . . . . . . . . 389
The Power of Love . . . . . . . . . . . . . . . . . . . . . . . . . . . . . . . . . . . . . . . . . 390
Healing Versus Curing . . . . . . . . . . . . . . . . . . . . . . . . . . . . . . . . . . . . . . 390
Intention . . . . . . . . . . . . . . . . . . . . . . . . . . . . . . . . . . . . . . . . . . . . . . . . 391
Who Survives? . . . . . . . . . . . . . . . . . . . . . . . . . . . . . . . . . . . . . . . . . . . . 391
The Holistic Approach to Health Care . . . . . . . . . . . . . . . . . . . . . . . . . 392
Future Health Care Systems . . . . . . . . . . . . . . . . . . . . . . . . . . . . . . . . . . 396

### Unit 26  Broadening Your View of Health Care . . . . . . . . . . . . . . . . . . . . . . . . 401

What Is Legitimate Therapy? . . . . . . . . . . . . . . . . . . . . . . . . . . . . . . . . . 402
Holistic Medicine . . . . . . . . . . . . . . . . . . . . . . . . . . . . . . . . . . . . . . . . . 403
Psychoneuroimmunology . . . . . . . . . . . . . . . . . . . . . . . . . . . . . . . . . . . 406
Energy Medicine . . . . . . . . . . . . . . . . . . . . . . . . . . . . . . . . . . . . . . . . . . 407
Osteopathy . . . . . . . . . . . . . . . . . . . . . . . . . . . . . . . . . . . . . . . . . . . . . . . 407
Chiropractic . . . . . . . . . . . . . . . . . . . . . . . . . . . . . . . . . . . . . . . . . . . . . 408
Naturopathy . . . . . . . . . . . . . . . . . . . . . . . . . . . . . . . . . . . . . . . . . . . . . 408
Psychotherapy/Counseling . . . . . . . . . . . . . . . . . . . . . . . . . . . . . . . . . . 409
Homeopathy . . . . . . . . . . . . . . . . . . . . . . . . . . . . . . . . . . . . . . . . . . . . . 411
Traditional Chinese Medicine . . . . . . . . . . . . . . . . . . . . . . . . . . . . . . . . 414
Ayurvedic Medicine . . . . . . . . . . . . . . . . . . . . . . . . . . . . . . . . . . . . . . . . 415
Complementary Therapies . . . . . . . . . . . . . . . . . . . . . . . . . . . . . . . . . . . 416
Healing Touch . . . . . . . . . . . . . . . . . . . . . . . . . . . . . . . . . . . . . . . . . . . . 416
Acupuncture . . . . . . . . . . . . . . . . . . . . . . . . . . . . . . . . . . . . . . . . . . . . . 418

|  | Acupressure and Shiatsu | 420 |
|---|---|---|
|  | Reflexology | 420 |
|  | Therapeutic Massage | 421 |
|  | The Self-Help Trend | 423 |
|  | Role of the Health Care Provider | 424 |

**UNIT 27  Managing Stress with Relaxation/Meditation** .......................... **429**

    Stress Management ........................................... 430
    Mind-Talk as a Source of Stress ............................... 430
    Mindfulness ................................................. 430
    Relaxation and Meditation .................................... 431
    Relaxation Techniques ....................................... 433
    Meditation Methods ......................................... 438
    Using Positive Affirmations .................................. 442

**Glossary** ............................................................ **447**

**Index** .............................................................. **455**

# Preface

## INTRODUCTION

*Understanding Human Behavior: A Guide for Health Care Providers* is designed to assist students in health occupations education programs to learn basic principles of human behavior. These principles provide a basis for increased self-understanding and improved interpersonal relationships. With technological advances in diagnostic and therapeutic procedures, it is easy for a health care provider to focus on procedures and routines. Patients, however, want personalized care that conveys respect for the patient as a person.

Patients' expectations are more likely to be met when health care providers strive for effective interaction with each patient. By consciously attending to each interaction with patients, the health care provider will experience greater job satisfaction.

## CONCEPTUAL APPROACH

In addition to basic principles of human behavior, several themes serve as unifying threads: effective communication, diversity of clients served by the health care system, effects of stress, physical and emotional needs in different life stages and as affected by illness, emotional responses to various life experiences, and specific emotions as they affect behavior. For example, grief is explained briefly as one of several emotions, discussed further when relevant to specific topics, and then discussed in depth in Unit 22, "Grief and Bereavement." Anger and fear are introduced as emotions that have powerful effects on behavior, then explored further in relation to specific topics, such as domestic violence.

## ORGANIZATION

*Understanding Human Behavior: A Guide for Health Care Providers,* Eighth Edition, is organized to proceed from relatively simple information to more complex concepts, from the known to the unknown, and from application to self to application in a variety of interpersonal situations. For that reason, Sections I through VI (Units 1 through 23) are designed for *sequential study*. Each section builds on the previous section, and each unit within a section builds on preceding units.

Section VII does not follow the sequential pattern. Although the first three units of Section VII proceed from historical content to current developments in health care, each unit is self-contained and can be studied independently. Ideally, instructors will assign Unit 27 early in the program, so students can start practicing stress management. Undertaking the role of a student, introduction to the clinical setting, and care of the sick all include stressful experiences. Preparing to become a health care provider includes learning the importance of self-care, and stress management is an essential component of self-care.

Section I provides an orientation to the role of health care provider, the importance of accepting each patient as a worthwhile human being, the challenge of striving for self-understanding, and guidelines for personal and professional growth. Section II presents information about various influences on human behavior: the role of heredity, basic physical and psychological needs, developmental factors, role of the social environment, emotions and their power to influence behavior, and adjustment as a composite of all these factors. Section III presents more complex concepts related to human behavior: stressful events that occur in the lives of most people, domestic violence and bullying, and the mental and emotional effects of traumatic experiences. Many victims of a traumatic event subsequently require health care. For both personal and professional reasons, health care providers need to be aware of the mental/emotional and physical effects of these traumatic experiences, as well as the potential for long-term adverse effects on the victim. The remainder of Section III covers other factors related to one's adjustment: common defense mechanisms, inner conflict, and frustration.

Section IV presents the effects of illness on patients' behavior and ways a health care provider can apply previous content to patient care. The emphasis is on effective interactions with patients and the role of health care providers in helping patients cope with the mental and emotional effects of illness or injury.

Section V contains expanded content on the components of effective communication. Practice exercises are designed to help students become better communicators by improving their skills in sending, receiving, and observing verbal and nonverbal exchanges. These exercises can involve all students and be accommodated readily within a class period. Unit 21 provides an overview of changing practices in relation to death and dying, the effect of these changes, and legislation related to the rights of patients to participate in health care decisions, especially those related to end-of-life care. In Unit 22, the grief process is discussed in detail, with guidelines for assisting the bereaved. Unit 23 is focused on ways the health care provider can assist terminally ill patients and their families during this period of crisis.

Section VII is designed to encourage advanced students to take pride in the role of health care provider and to accept the changes that inevitably will occur in the dynamic health care system. Unit 24 provides a historical overview that reflects the roots of current practices, including holistic health care. Unit 25 describes the emergence of the holistic emphasis and spotlights a number of modern-day innovators who have had an impact on medical and health care practices. Unit 26 describes several complementary healing modalities that have gained widespread acceptance with the public. The reader is encouraged to maintain an open mind in conjunction with a healthy skepticism in evaluating various treatment modalities. Unit 27 addresses stress management; it stands on its own merits as a component of a broadened view of health care and self-care.

## NEW TO THE EIGHTH EDITION

*Understanding Human Behavior*, Eighth Edition, includes the following updates and additions:

- **Unit 3** contains additional discussion of learning skills and time management.
- **Unit 4** includes an updated discussion of genetics; behavioral genetics is introduced. Culture and socioeconomics are discussed as influences on behavior.
- **Unit 8** describes ongoing research about gender differences in brain chemistry and emotions.
- **Unit 10** now includes information about autism spectrum disorders, including the current prevalence of autism.
- **Unit 11** provides information about two additional modern causes of trauma: cyberbullying and online sexual predators.

- In **Unit 12**, methamphetamine has been added to the discussion of drug abuse.
- **Unit 16** now includes HIPAA regulations in the discussion of confidentiality.
- In **Unit 20**, an updated discussion of suicide is provided.
- **Unit 21** includes an expanded discussion of euthanasia and the right-to-die movement, including the controversial Terri Schiavo case.
- **Unit 23** discusses end-of-life home care, as opposed to facility care, as an option for some patients.

## STUDENT SUPPLEMENTAL MATERIALS

### WebTUTOR™ Advantage

- *WebTUTOR™ Advantage on Blackboard- Printed Access Code* ISBN-10: 1-4354-8658-7
- *WebTUTOR™ Advantage on WebCT- Printed Access Code* ISBN-10: 0-8400-2081-3
- *WebTUTOR™ Advantage on Angel- Printed Access Code* ISBN-10: 0-8400-2082-1
- *Cengage-hosted WebTUTOR™ Advantage- Instant Access Code* ISBN-10: 0-8400-4084-8
- *Cengage-hosted WebTUTOR™ Advantage- Printed Access Code* ISBN-10: 0-8400-2085-6

This online course management tool provides study and assessment tools to enhance the classroom experience, whether learning in a hybrid or fully online course environment. Materials include the following items:

- *Advance Preparation guidelines* help students prepare for class.
- *Unit learning objectives* pulled from the book enhance student comprehension of materials.
- *Case studies* for each unit include *video clips* that help reinforce major concepts. *Discussion Questions* related to each case study appear in the Discussion Board forum to enhance classroom lectures and student involvement.
- *Media Links and Suggested Readings* offer outlets for additional information.
- *Quizzes*, including true/false and fill-in formats, provide a helpful study review tool for test preparation.
- *Slides created in Microsoft PowerPoint®* accompany each unit, allowing students to use these for unit review and test preparation and for in-class note taking.
- *Glossary flashcards* allow easy review of important terms and concepts from each unit.

## INSTRUCTOR SUPPLEMENTAL MATERIAL

### Instructor Resources CD-ROM to Accompany *Understanding Human Behavior*, Eighth Edition

ISBN-10: 1-4354-8659-5

With Delmar Cengage Learning's Instructor Resources to Accompany *Understanding Human Behavior*, Eighth Edition, preparing for class and evaluating students has never been easier! As an instructor, you will find that this CD-ROM offers invaluable assistance by giving you access to all of your resources–anywhere and at any time.

## Features

- Now in electronic format, the **Instructor's Manual** continues to offer suggested activities, topics for discussion, and teaching methods. Answers to the Review and Self-Check questions have been revised to coordinate with the changes made to the core textbook; it is available in Microsoft Word® format.
- The **Computerized Testbank in ExamView®** makes generating tests and quizzes a snap. The banks offer approximately 750 questions, including updated multiple choice, short answer, completion, and essay questions. New question types include true/false and matching formats. Matching questions offer scenarios that emphasize patient interaction and soft skills used while working as a health care provider. Instructors can create customized assessments for students with the click of a button. Add unique questions and print rationales for easy class preparation.
- New! Customizable **instructor support slide presentations in PowerPoint®** format focus on key points for each unit. Summary and Discussion Question slides prompt in-class discussion of concepts. "As a Health Care Provider" slides urge students to connect important themes from each unit to actual practice in the health professions. Use for lectures or for in-class handouts.

## Instructor Companion Website to Accompany Understanding Human Behavior, Eighth Edition

ISBN-10: 0-8400-2086-4

- Contains everything offered on the Instructor Resource's CD-ROM (listed above) in an online format available for downloading.
- To access this companion resource, please visit login.cengage.com.

## USING *UNDERSTANDING HUMAN BEHAVIOR*

The effectiveness of *Understanding Human Behavior* depends on the instructor's choice of activities: class time to clarify various concepts and specific activities to encourage student participation, especially the sharing of experiences, discussion of problem situations, and selection of effective behavior for real and hypothetical situations. The instructor's own creative use of the text material is the key to students' achievement.

No one ever fully masters human relations skills. Those who sincerely want to relate effectively to others must become lifelong students of human behavior. They must consciously practice human relations skills in order to improve their sensitivity to the possible meaning of observed behavior and select appropriate responses. The immediate challenge is to gain as much as possible from this course, as a foundation for the lifelong challenge of developing a high level of skill in human relations.

## ABOUT THE AUTHORS

Alyson Honeycutt, M.A., N.C.C., is a National Certified Counselor, holds a License in School Counseling from the North Carolina Department of Public Instruction, and has advanced degrees from North Carolina State University at Raleigh and Appalachian State University.

She has taught parenting and literacy classes, has been an instructor in English at the college level, has taught students with emotional and behavioral disabilities, and has served on the Board of Directors of the Piedmont Mediation Center. She has coordinated Positive Behavioral Support programs and has presented behavioral support strategies at professional conferences.

Mary Elizabeth Milliken, B.S.N., M.S., Ed.D., is a graduate of Duke University School of Nursing. Her graduate study at North Carolina State University at Raleigh concentrated on both education and psychology. She has practiced nursing in a variety of settings, served as instructor, then coordinator, of a practical nursing education program, was curriculum specialist for health occupations in the North Carolina Department of Community Colleges, and has been a consultant on curriculum and effective teaching. From 1971 to 1987 she served as Coordinator of Health Occupations Teacher Education at the University of Georgia in Athens. Dr. Milliken has followed the emerging holistic health movement since 1974, attending numerous workshops and conferences in which holistic concepts and complementary healing modalities were presented. She completed the curriculum sequence and certification requirements of Healing Touch International, Inc.

## ACKNOWLEDGMENTS

Instructors and students of various health care educational programs and reviewers selected by Delmar editors have contributed to the improvement of *Understanding Human Behavior* with each succeeding edition. Reviewers of proposed revisions for *Understanding Human Behavior* identified the need to clarify certain concepts and provided suggestions for making content relevant to current societal and health care issues. Nancy Mollett, Reference Librarian at Jefferson Community College, provided valuable assistance in updating reference lists and locating relevant Web sites. During the final stages of manuscript editing, Scott Milliken assisted in dealing with various computer problems and verified that all Web sites cited are current.

The cartoon drawings in Units 1 through 16 were the original work of the late Bill Pugh, whose talent for portraying human behavior through humor enriched *Understanding Human Behavior* through six editions. Early efforts to revise some of the original drawings proved that Bill's talent was indeed exceptional. The artist who accepted the task of updating these drawings, while retaining the original concept, is Chris Watkin. The authors acknowledge with gratitude this contribution to *Understanding Human Behavior*, Eighth Edition.

Other illustrations have evolved with expanding text content. Photographs were provided by Robert King, president, Chicago School of Massage Therapy, and Dr. C. Norman Shealy, Shealy Institute in Springfield, Missouri; Jo-Lynn Worley, business manager/agent for Dr. Harriet Lerner; and Judy Haskett, administrative assistant to Dr. Myss. Graphic illustrations were contributed by Project Safe in Athens, Georgia, and Coral McDonnell, administrator for the Minnesota Program Development, Inc., who reports that the diagrams "Power and Control" and "Equality" were developed by clients of the Domestic Abuse Intervention Project. The reflexology chart is reprinted with the permission of Dwight C. Byers, president, Ingham Publishing. Some photographs, tables, and charts have been borrowed from other Delmar authors to clarify or summarize a number of topics. The direction of editors and staff in the Health Care Division of Delmar Learning has been readily available, keeping the development of *Understanding Human Behavior*, Eighth Edition, on course. These many contributions are gratefully acknowledged.

## REVIEWERS OF THE EIGHTH EDITION

Diana Alagna, RN, RMA, CPT, AHI
    Medical Assisting Program Director
    Branford Hall Career Institute
    Southington, CT

Dr. Jessica Hanzel, RN, DNP
    Director of Nursing
    Herzing University
    Minneapolis, MN

Marsha Hemby, BA, RN, CMA (AAMA)
    Retired Department Chair, Medical Assisting
    Pitt Community College
    Greenville, NC

Margaret M. Nolan MEd, MA, LPC
    Director of Accreditation & Instructional Quality/ Counselor
    The College of Office Technology
    Chicago, IL

Mary White, MA, SPHR
    Co-Founder & Managing Director
    Mobile Technical Institute & MTI Business Solutions
    Mobile, AL

Section I

# On Becoming a Health Care Provider

This section introduces some of the challenges, responsibilities, problems, and satisfactions of being a health care provider. People from all walks of life have health problems. You, as a health care provider, will be challenged to learn how to serve each person effectively, within the role for which your course is preparing you. Section I is designed to help you become aware of the realities of a health career and also help you learn ways to succeed, both as a student and as a health care provider.

# UNIT 1

# Challenges and Responsibilities of Health Care Providers

## OBJECTIVES

Upon completion of this unit, you should be able to:

- List three challenges for health care providers.
- Explain the value of high standards for a health care provider.
- List two responsibilities of a student.
- Explain the relationship between your achievement standards as a student and your future performance standards as a health care provider.
- Use effective study habits to improve learning.
- Set personal standards for achievement as a student and for performance as a health care provider.
- Explain the meaning of empowerment.

## KEY TERMS

| | | |
|---|---|---|
| Empowerment | Mediocre | Self-reliant |
| Excellence | Self-confidence | Standards |

So you have decided to become a health care provider. Congratulations! Your decision will place you within a large group of people who are providing very important services to others. You will acquire new knowledge and develop new skills as you proceed through your educational program. Much satisfaction can be yours, both through your educational achievements and through your career as a health care provider. You will be able to take your place in the community as one who is making a significant contribution to society. You will be respected by your friends, especially those who do not have the benefit of your education and those who are not prepared, as you will be, to fulfill important responsibilities.

A career in the health field differs in many ways from careers in other fields. There are many satisfactions to be experienced and challenges to be met. There are heavy responsibilities to be fulfilled. The purpose of this unit is to help you be aware of these satisfactions, challenges, and responsibilities as they relate to you as a student and as a future health care provider.

## SATISFACTIONS

Your choice of career path indicates that you like people and have a strong desire to help others. Although you could possibly make more money in some other occupational field, a career that provides opportunities to help others may be very rewarding.

### Approval versus Inner Satisfaction

We all admire and envy those who can do something extremely well; each of us would like to be the kind of person who is admired by others. We get a lift from expressions of approval, yet this good feeling is only temporary. The athlete may enjoy hearing the cheers of the crowd when performing well, but the deepest satisfaction comes from the performance itself, from knowing that you performed with great skill. True satisfaction is an inner feeling of pride in doing something well, regardless of whether or not the performance is applauded by others.

As a health care provider, you will find your greatest satisfaction in trying to give each patient appropriate care. By striving to meet each patient's needs to the best of your ability, you will complete the day with an inner feeling of pride. The opposite approach—to view your work as a series of assigned procedures to be completed so that you can get off work or go on break—results in finishing the day by saying "Whew, I'm glad that's over!" Stop now and give a moment's thought to a very important question: How will you approach your work? As a challenge that may provide much satisfaction and a sense of accomplishment? Or, as work you have to do to get a paycheck?

### Setting Goals for Inner Satisfaction

Skillful performance can provide **self-confidence** and a deep sense of satisfaction that is not dependent on praise from others. Striving to improve one's performance, to do each task well, and to do better today than yesterday, is the means of achieving a high level of skill. Even though we would all like to be admired for our performance, many of us settle for mediocrity because it requires less effort to "just get by" than to do well. You have probably heard the saying, "If a job is worth doing at all, it is worth doing well." The time required to do a task sloppily is usually about the same as the time required to do it well, although doing the task correctly may require a little more effort. **Excellence** lies in that little bit of extra effort to achieve a superior performance. *In the health field, that little bit of extra effort may make the difference between safe and unsafe practice.*

Will the habits you form as a student carry over into your performance as a health care provider? You may be sure that they will! So, now is the time to set **standards**—the level of quality for your performance—and begin to establish the habits that will lead to skillful performance, self-confidence, and pride in your work.

## CHALLENGES

### Setting Standards of Performance

Only you can set the standards that will guide your performance over the coming years. Many times there will be the opportunity to take a shortcut. Sometimes a piece of equipment will be contaminated; obtaining sterile materials to complete the procedure will require extra effort and time. You are the only one who will know whether or not sterile technique was violated and the contaminated equipment was used—unless, of course, the patient develops a serious infection as a result of your poor technique. Your standards of performance serve as your conscience and determine whether or not you experience the inner satisfaction that comes from knowing the job was well done.

Your own standards should include accuracy in measurements, observations, and reporting. Time pressure may tempt you to take shortcuts, but erroneous reporting is not acceptable. Many health care facilities now utilize instrumentation for measurement of vital signs, but at times you will have to obtain vital signs without such aids. Suppose you are taking a patient's pulse and count for 15 seconds, then multiply by 4. If your count is off by 1 beat, your pulse count has an error of 4. If the patient's pulse skips two beats during that 15 seconds, the error in your count may be even greater than 4. By counting for a full minute, you obtain an accurate pulse rate. Which is more important—saving 45 seconds, or reporting the correct pulse rate?

Habits formed as a student will affect performance throughout your career. When making that little bit of extra effort to "do it right" has become a habit, doing it correctly no longer seems an effort; it becomes an essential part of your performance. Thus, excellence as a health care provider will depend upon setting high standards of performance for yourself and establishing the habit of making that extra bit of effort while still a student. Then, when someone takes a shortcut or settles for a mediocre performance, you can take pride in thinking, "I wouldn't do it that way, even though it does save a few steps."

## Excellence and Patient Safety

In the health field, all care providers should strive for excellence. Why? *Because anything less than excellence can endanger the patient.* The nurse should give the correct medicine to each patient 100% of the time. The medical assistant should use faultless technique in 100% of the situations that require asepsis. The laboratory assistant should report test results correctly 100% of the time. The dental assistant should sterilize instruments correctly 100% of the time. The ambulance attendant should move the accident victim correctly 100% of the time. *Performance that is less than 100% correct can have disastrous effects for the patient.* Should the patient benefit from health care or be the victim of it?

## Meeting Patient Needs

As a health care provider, you will work with many different people, each of whom is different as a person and as a patient. *The greatest challenge in the health field is to provide for each patient the health care that promotes the patient's well-being.* This requires concern about the patient as a person, rather than as someone for whom a specified procedure must be carried out as part of the physician's therapeutic plan.

Each of your patients is a unique individual—a physical, emotional, mental, and spiritual being (Figure 1-1). Each has a history of experiences, a life within the context of a specific family and community, beliefs and values that influence thoughts and expectations, and a unique genetic makeup.

Attending to each patient as a person is not only a challenge, it is also a responsibility—one that provides enrichment and opportunities to grow as a person and as a health care provider.

**FIGURE 1-1** Think of each patient as a person with specific needs, rather than a diagnosis. *Delmar/Cengage Learning*

## RESPONSIBILITIES

### As a Student

You are presently involved in activities designed to prepare you to function as a health care provider in some specific role. At the moment, your primary concern is with performance as a student; remind yourself frequently that your performance as a student *will* affect your performance as a health care provider.

Your first responsibility as a student, then, is to take full advantage of every opportunity to learn. Try to see the purpose in each assignment; look at it as an *opportunity to learn,* rather than as a chore to complete. With this attitude toward learning, you will not be tempted to "skip school" occasionally without good reason.

Your second responsibility is to decide what standards will guide your performance (Figure 1-2). This is related to the previous discussion about excellence, but now you should think about standards in relation to your performance as a student. Your school has set a certain grade as passing; let us say 70 is passing in your program. Suppose, through habit, you say to yourself, "I'll study this material until I know it well enough to make 75." In many courses of study, a grade of 75 is acceptable; in such courses, a deficiency in the student's knowledge of subject matter is not likely to cause harm to someone else.

### As a Health Care Provider

In a health occupations course, the implications of "just passing" are more serious. Any gaps in knowledge and performance skills can affect every patient served (Figure 1-3). Will your future services to patients be of "just passing" quality? Or do you wish to give the best service

**FIGURE 1-2** High performance standards ensure patient safety and effective care. *Delmar/Cengage Learning*

**FIGURE 1-3** Is "just passing" good enough for students in a health care preparatory program? *Delmar/Cengage Learning*

you are capable of giving? If your educational program is preparing you to provide health services, can you be content to learn only 70% of what your teachers expect you to learn? Can you be content to develop your skills just enough to get a passing grade in a laboratory course? Can you automatically change your standards and established habits after graduation?

## ACHIEVEMENT AS PROGRESS

If you set high standards for achievement now, then these high standards will carry over into performance as a health care provider. In setting standards for achievement, plan to *do your best,* rather than trying to be the best student in the class.

How can you do your best? Not by wasteful study procedures, such as putting in many hours of study when you are too tired to benefit or taking pages and pages of notes that mean nothing to you after they "get cold." Instead, work out a study routine and establish the habits that work best for you. This may take some experimenting, but you can establish a routine that enables you to learn with a minimum of time and effort. In order to get started, consider the following guidelines:

- Let your family and friends know that you have set aside a certain time of day as your study period. Do not allow them to violate your schedule by interrupting you. Phone calls can be returned when you have finished studying. Most family problems can wait until you are through studying. This is *your* time; do not let it become someone else's time.

- At the beginning of each study period, write out a list of specific things you need to complete; then, rank the items in order of importance. Complete task 1 (most important) first, and then move on to task 2. If one of the tasks is something you dislike but must get done, let it be task 1 so that you get it out of the way. Most of us tend to put off unpleasant tasks as long as possible; sometimes we never quite get around to them! "I didn't have time to do that" often means, "I didn't want to do that, so I kept putting it off."

- If your list of study assignments is too long to complete today, set up tomorrow's list; then put the items on that list out of your mind until tomorrow. Give your full attention to today's list.

- Set up a calendar or special notebook for assignments, due dates for projects or reports, and test dates. Note on your calendar the dates/times you will work on specific assignments or study for a test. By allocating time for these preparatory activities, you can avoid last-minute rushes to meet a deadline.

- Use the objectives stated by your instructor and in the textbook as guides to what you are expected to learn. Refer to the objectives of this text; note what you will *be able to do* after you have finished this chapter. How many of those objectives could you demonstrate at this time?

These guidelines will help you use an organized, systematic approach to studying. The following guidelines are specifically related to study habits. Practice applying two or more until they have become habit, then add one or two additional approaches. As you incorporate these learning principles into your studying, you will become more proficient at acquiring and retaining new information.

- Form the habit of testing yourself to decide whether or not you have achieved an objective. First, write out the ideas involved. For example, test your achievement of the objective, "Explain your responsibilities as a health care provider" by writing out, in your own words, a description of these responsibilities. Then check your description against the textbook. Add to or correct what you have written. With practice you will be able to test yourself by running the information through your mind rather than writing it out. Finally, use the Review and Self-Check at the end of each unit as a final check on whether or not you have learned the main ideas of the unit. By following these steps as you study each unit, you will soon develop study skills that increase learning and decrease the amount of study time required.

- When reading the text, note paragraph headings, as these help to set your mind for what you are about to read. Look up from the printed page at intervals and mentally run through the main ideas of the paragraphs you have just read. Take notes in the margins of your text or in a notebook to help you identify and remember these main ideas. Also, refer at intervals to the objectives so you can be alert for information that is related to specific objectives. Remember, the objectives can help you separate important ideas from those that are less important.

- When you have a lengthy assignment, pace yourself. Set a realistic goal for the first hour's effort; then spend an intensive 60 minutes completing that part of the assignment. Next, take about 15 minutes for a change of activity. By alternating study periods with physical activity, the effectiveness of each study period can be increased. In other words, an hour of study followed by 15 minutes of walking in the fresh air, followed by another 45 minutes of studying will be more productive for most people than a solid two hours of "plugging away" at the books.

- At intervals during your study period, take four very long, slow breaths; hold each for a count of four before exhaling. Then do several stretching exercises and two or three head rolls. You should return to your studying refreshed and with a clear mind.

- When you are studying material that includes totally new information, try to relate it to something you have already learned or to some past experience (e.g., Uncle Joe's broken leg that gave him such a bad time was a comminuted fracture of the tibia).

- Your nervous system can only handle a certain amount of new information at one time. When you begin to feel overwhelmed with new material, review about five to seven main ideas and think of ways to use the information. Then, do something else for a while to give your mind time to process the new information. After a lapse of time (maybe an hour, maybe a day or two), review those same ideas and try to think of new examples and other applications. By then the ideas will be very familiar—you will be comfortable with them—and you will be ready to study additional new information.

- If you tend to be "uptight" much of the time, learn a relaxation routine or meditation procedure (see Unit 27). By taking about 20 minutes a day to relax completely, you can avoid a buildup of tension that may interfere with your performance—and with your health if the tension persists over a period of time.

- As you acquire information or develop the performance skill described in a learning objective, consciously congratulate yourself. Recognize that you have reached a stepping-stone to becoming a health care provider. Enjoy a sense of achievement.

- Measure your achievement in terms of progress toward your goal of becoming a qualified practitioner in the health field. Take pride in each forward step. Avoid thinking of achievement as a "good grade." Avoid comparing your progress with the progress of others in your class. You are competing with the *you* of yesterday, not with your classmates. Where are you now as compared to last month? Last year? How much have you achieved since you entered this health care program?

- Take pride in your achievements, but also be honest with yourself about areas in which you need to improve. By investing additional effort in your areas of weakness, you can convert those, too, into achievements.

## ATTITUDES AND INTERESTS

The suggestions just discussed will help you form favorable attitudes toward your studies. Your attitudes influence the interest you have in your assignments and in various learning experiences. Your interest affects your achievement; that is, you learn more easily and perform better when you are interested in what you are doing.

There will be times of discouragement during your course of study. There will also be times when you experience the satisfaction that comes from doing well. You will have a sense of accomplishment as you draw on your knowledge to solve problems and use your skills to provide patient care that reflects the highest standards.

## EMPOWERMENT

All adults should control most aspects of their lives. During adolescence, learning to make decisions (i.e., take control) is an important developmental task; if this is not learned, the individual enters adulthood poorly equipped to cope with life problems. If you entered adulthood with a tendency to let your parents, spouse, friends, or anyone else make decisions for you, it is time to recognize that you are giving away your power—the power to be a **self-reliant, responsible** adult.

When you are planning to eat out with a friend, who decides which restaurant? Do you usually say, "Oh, I don't care. You choose." Does your spouse or boyfriend give you a choice? If you do not participate in small decisions that affect you, how can you expect others to include you in big decisions? For example:

> Kate is a dental hygienist whose earnings are about equal to her husband's. Each payday, she gives her check to her husband because "he handles our finances." They have only one car, so Kate usually waits as much as an hour for her husband to pick her up. She insists on keeping the car this week so she can do some errands after work. Yesterday her husband waited 45 minutes for her to pick him up. Today, he announces proudly, "Well, I bought you your own car." He has purchased a compact car with 125,000 miles on it. Kate has a strong dislike for compact cars, believing that a midsize car is safer. Buying a car is a major decision, yet Kate's husband did not see any need to involve her in that decision. Kate has given away her power; it will take much effort to renegotiate this relationship so that she is empowered to participate in decision making.

How does **empowerment** affect you? Suppose you have informed the family that your study hour will begin at 9 o'clock each evening. During the second day of this plan, your teenager calls you to the phone at 9:15; the caller is your sister-in-law who talks about her problems for a full half hour. Two days later, your 10-year-old opens the door at 9:30 and says, "I need a note for my teacher about the field trip next Monday." Each time you permit these violations of your study hour, you are giving away your power. You gave your two children the power to interrupt your study hour. You gave your sister-in-law the power to use 30 minutes of your study time for her own purposes. You probably responded to these requests because you are accustomed to meeting the needs of others, even if doing so interferes with your own needs.

Suppose you have completed eight months of your one-year program when your spouse complains that you are "spending too much time at that school." The complaints also include such things as not having homemade cakes any more and "You don't watch TV with me like you used to." Your spouse says you should quit the program and go back to your part-time job at the fast-food restaurant. You really hated that job! How will you handle this situation? If you quit the program, you *give your spouse the power* to control your occupational choice. *Your own empowerment* requires that *you make the decision, based on what you really want.* If you insist on completing the program, it may be necessary to negotiate a compromise. This might require you to find more time to be with the family, and family members to give you more help with homemaking tasks. If you leave the program in order to please your family, you are letting others control your life.

If you allow others to make decisions for you because you just do not like to make decisions, then you are *avoiding the adult task of taking responsibility for your life*. If this pattern applies to your life situation, you can start reclaiming your power by requiring others to respect your needs. For example, after informing all members of your family that a certain time period is your study time, do not permit any violations to occur. Remind those who interrupt you that you are not available during study hour. If you are consistent, the interruptions will eventually stop. Then you can use the same approach to another of your needs. You may choose to make the next decision about where to eat or which movie to see, instead of allowing someone else to make that decision. You may wish to inform your spouse or a friend that you are to be involved in any decisions that affect you. This type of change will not occur rapidly; be content with small changes initially. By persisting, you will eventually gain more control over your life. But do not be surprised if others reject your decision, especially if you are just beginning to participate in making decisions. Give your family and friends time to accept your change in behavior. Ideally, decision making is a give-and-take situation. Sometimes your decision is accepted, whereas at other times another person's decision prevails.

Empowerment may or may not be a problem in your own life. As a health care provider, however, be aware of the importance of empowerment to self-esteem and a sense of well-being. Patients who are dependent on others for their personal needs may express anger about their helplessness. Many patients need help in regaining some control over their life situations. By respecting their wishes and involving patients in decisions, *when appropriate,* you contribute to feelings of empowerment.

## MAKING A DECISION

A certain grade is necessary for passing a course, but it is your decision about the desired level of achievement that influences your performance. Even more important, the *standards that guide your performance as a student will carry over into your performance as a health care provider.*

Choosing to enter this educational program for the health field was an important decision in your life. Now, it is time to make another decision—what kind of health care provider will you be? Excellent? **Mediocre?** Or "just passing"? Remember, the standards of performance that will characterize you as a health care provider will be influenced by the standards you set for yourself now.

## REFERENCES AND SUGGESTED READINGS

Hewett, Les, Hewett, Andrew, d'Abadie, Luc, & Trump, Donald. (2005). *The power of focus for college students*. Deerfield Beach, FL: Health Communications.

Leland, Karen, & Bailey, Keith. (2008). *Time management in an instant*. Franklin Lakes, NJ: Career Press.

Siebert, Al, & Karr, Mary. (2008). *The adult student's guide to survival and success in college*. Portland, OR: Practical Psychology Press.

## REVIEW AND SELF-CHECK

1. List three challenges for a health care provider.

2. Explain why it is important that a health care provider have high performance standards.

3. List two of your responsibilities as a student.

4. Explain why your performance standards as a student are relevant to your future performance standards as a health care provider.

5. List five guidelines for improving the effectiveness of your study habits.

6. Write a statement about your personal standards for achievement as a student.

7. Write a statement about your personal standards for performance as a health care provider.

8. Explain the meaning of empowerment.

## ASSIGNMENTS

1. Use Worksheet A at the end of this unit to develop a tentative study plan. Try this plan for two weeks. Use a diary or journal to record your study habits during this time. If your plan seems to be effective, continue to use it. If it is not effective:

    a. List problems that interfered with the effectiveness of the plan.

    b. Modify the plan by changing the schedule, the place where you study, or any other details involved in "the problems." Try the modified plan for one week. If you continue to have problems, repeat steps a and b until you have a workable study plan.

    If other people are part of the problem, try to involve them in developing the "improved plan" to increase the probability of getting their cooperation. For example, a six-year-old may find numerous reasons for needing his mother's attention as soon as she disappears into her room for the study hour. By discussing mother's need to study so that she can become a health care provider, the six-year-old may begin to accept some responsibility for "helping" mother become a health care provider. The mother should negotiate so that "everybody is a winner."

    For example, she could agree to read to the six-year-old for 30 minutes in exchange for an hour of uninterrupted study. This could be done as a written contract: "If you (do this), then I will (do that)." Both of you would sign it. Shake on it to seal your agreement. The child gets the mother's attention, and mother gets to study. Needless to say, both parties must fulfill their parts of the agreement.

2. Complete each of the following using Worksheet B at the end of this unit.

    a. List the things you *have to do* each day.

    b. List the things you *have to do* each week, but not every day.

    c. List the things you *have to do* occasionally.

    d. Beside each item in a, b, and c, write the name of someone who could do that task for you, at least some of the time.

    e. Beside any items that have no names, write out the possible result of that task not getting done at all. (Be honest with yourself. What will *really* happen if the car doesn't get washed *today?*)

3. Revise the lists in Assignment 2 to include only those tasks that you, and you alone, must perform. Consider whether or not some of the daily tasks could be done on alternate days or perhaps weekly. Consider whether or not some of the weekly tasks could be done on alternate weeks or once a month.

4. Use Worksheet C at the end of this unit to plan your daily schedule for one week. Give your student role a high priority in this schedule, instead of letting it play "second fiddle" to all the responsibilities you fulfilled before becoming a student.

5. Try your schedule for one week, then:

   a. List the "time wasters" you experienced during the week.

   b. List the "energy wasters" you experienced during the week. Beside each, write out a justification; if you cannot justify the energy spent, resolve to eliminate that activity from your life.

   c. List three times you allowed someone else to control your time. (For example, a neighbor insisted that you go shopping with her. When you indicated that you needed to study, she responded, "You never spend time with me anymore." So, feeling guilty, you spent an entire afternoon doing what she wanted to do and came home too exhausted to study.) Consider how you could have controlled the situation.

> **Note:** Your instructor may schedule a group discussion to help members of the class share ideas on how to maintain control of your time without alienating your family and friends.

   d. Recheck your weekly schedule. Be sure you have given a reasonable balance of time to your various roles: as a member of the family; a student in a health occupations program; and an individual who requires activity, sleep, rest, and recreation and has various other needs to be met. Resolve to (1) give attention to each of these important aspects of your life and (2) hold to a minimum any time and energy wasters that interfere with your performance.

   e. After reviewing steps a through d, list three or more changes you can make to help yourself become more efficient at studying and managing your time.

   Stick to your plan. You are now taking control of your life. And becoming a *self-reliant person* is a major step toward becoming a *reliable health care provider!*

6. During the next week, note the times you have an opportunity to make a decision but delegate the decision-making power to someone else. List the types of situations where you give away your power.

7. Review the list you developed in Assignment 6. Consider ways you could regain your own power in each situation. How many of these situations merely require that you be more assertive? How many of these situations will require negotiating a different relationship with someone (spouse, significant other, parent, child) in order for you to regain your power?

8. Develop your own empowerment plan.

   a. List the types of situations in which you will insist on being involved in decisions.

   b. Number the items on the list according to priority. The simpler situations (e.g., where to eat, which television show to watch) should have high priorities. When you have gained confidence (are feeling somewhat empowered from making decisions in these situations), then you are ready to attempt the more difficult situations that involve someone who is accustomed to making decisions for you.

c. Select one type of situation for practicing decision making (experiencing empowerment).

d. Sometimes even a self-reliant person has an experience that arouses feelings of helplessness, or at least requires asking for help. For each situation below, list one or more actions that would indicate self-reliance rather than dependence on others:

   (1) You have a flat tire on the way to school.

   (2) You have locked your keys in the car.

   (3) You are going to lunch with two classmates and realize that you left your wallet at home.

9. You will hear the term "professionalism" during various courses that are preparing you for the role of health care provider.

   a. List three or more characteristics and behaviors that represent professionalism.

   b. List three or more behaviors of a health care provider that indicate a lack of professionalism.

   c. List three examples of how performing at 70% accuracy rather than 100% accuracy could endanger a patient.

## WORKSHEET A

### Study Plan

| Time | Monday | Tuesday | Wednesday | Thursday | Friday | Saturday | Sunday |
|---|---|---|---|---|---|---|---|
| 6 A.M. | | | | | | | |
| 7 | | | | | | | |
| 8 | | | | | | | |
| 9 | | | | | | | |
| 10 | | | | | | | |
| 11 | | | | | | | |
| 12 Noon | | | | | | | |
| 1 P.M. | | | | | | | |
| 2 | | | | | | | |
| 3 | | | | | | | |
| 4 | | | | | | | |
| 5 | | | | | | | |
| 6 | | | | | | | |
| 7 | | | | | | | |
| 8 | | | | | | | |
| 9 | | | | | | | |
| 10 | | | | | | | |
| 11 | | | | | | | |
| 12 Mn | | | | | | | |

## WORKSHEET B

### Tasks I Have to Do

Every day:

Once a week:

Occasionally:

## WORKSHEET C

### Daily Schedule for Week of _____

| Time | Monday | Tuesday | Wednesday | Thursday | Friday | Saturday | Sunday |
|---|---|---|---|---|---|---|---|
| 12:00 Mn | | | | | | | |
| 1:00 A.M. | | | | | | | |
| 2:00 | | | | | | | |
| 3:00 | | | | | | | |
| 4:00 | | | | | | | |
| 5:00 | | | | | | | |
| 6:00 | | | | | | | |
| 7:00 | | | | | | | |
| 7:30 | | | | | | | |
| 8:00 | | | | | | | |
| 8:30 | | | | | | | |
| 9:00 | | | | | | | |
| 9:30 | | | | | | | |
| 10:00 | | | | | | | |
| 10:30 | | | | | | | |
| 11:00 | | | | | | | |
| 11:30 | | | | | | | |
| 12:00 Noon | | | | | | | |

## Daily Schedule (Cont'd)

| Time | Monday | Tuesday | Wednesday | Thursday | Friday | Saturday | Sunday |
|---|---|---|---|---|---|---|---|
| 12:30 P.M. | | | | | | | |
| 1:00 | | | | | | | |
| 1:30 | | | | | | | |
| 2:00 | | | | | | | |
| 2:30 | | | | | | | |
| 3:00 | | | | | | | |
| 3:30 | | | | | | | |
| 4:00 | | | | | | | |
| 4:30 | | | | | | | |
| 5:00 | | | | | | | |
| 5:30 | | | | | | | |
| 6:00 | | | | | | | |
| 6:30 | | | | | | | |
| 7:00 | | | | | | | |
| 8:00 | | | | | | | |
| 9:00 | | | | | | | |
| 10:00 | | | | | | | |
| 11:00 | | | | | | | |

# UNIT 2

# The Philosophy of Individual Worth

## OBJECTIVES

Upon completion of this unit, you should be able to:

- Explain the philosophy of individual worth.
- Explain why cultural bias can affect the quality of patient care.
- List five examples of cultural differences that could contribute to misunderstandings between a patient and a health care provider.
- Apply the philosophy of individual worth to relationships with patients and their families.

## KEY TERMS

| | | |
|---|---|---|
| Affluent | Philosophy | Superstition |
| Cultural bias | Prejudice | Unique |
| Individual worth | Socioeconomic | Value system |

A health care provider comes in contact with people from many different backgrounds. Some patients have never known anything but poverty. Some have come from other countries or from homes in which the customs of other nationalities are followed. Some have been reared in a religious faith with beliefs very different from those of you and your friends.

If you have had little contact with people from other cultures or from other **socioeconomic** levels of society, your first reaction may be to view these people not only as "different" but also as less acceptable than people who are like you and your friends. However, it is not a health care provider's right to judge people or to vary the quality of services because the patient is "different."

## MEANING OF INDIVIDUAL WORTH

The philosophy of **individual worth** is the belief that *everyone, regardless of personal circumstances or personal qualities, has worth and is entitled to respect as a human being.* For health care providers, this means that the quality of service does not vary because of the patient's race, nationality, religion, sex, age, economic level, occupation, education, diagnosis, or any other characteristic.

Each patient is an individual. Each should receive health care that takes into consideration both the person's individuality and the specific health problem. The **philosophy** of individual

**FIGURE 2-1** Everyone has worth and is entitled to respect as a human being. *Delmar/Cengage Learning*

worth has many implications for patient care (Figure 2-1). Health care providers who do not accept the philosophy of individual worth may interact differently with patients from another culture than with patients from their own culture. Yet the health care providers would probably be unaware of any differences in care they are giving that patient.

## THE HEALTH CARE PROVIDER AND CULTURAL BIAS

Each of us represents a specific subclass within the larger society. The major subclasses are race, religion, national heritage, and socioeconomic level, each with its own beliefs, values, traditions, customs, and food preferences or prohibitions. In addition, one's occupational group is also a subclass that influences the thinking and behavior of its members.

As a health care provider, you will be developing a set of values and a sense of responsibility that your neighbor, who is a retail clerk, may not share. He may see nothing wrong with calling in sick, just to have a day off. But you will know that your absence would cause your co-workers to have extra assignments and the patients may not receive as much attention as they need. The health care provider's membership in a specific subgroup and socioeconomic level can be the basis for misunderstandings with patients who are from a different group. Your preparation for serving as a health care provider includes learning about cultural differences and respecting each patient's cultural heritage as you provide health care. The focus of the following discussion is on socioeconomic levels as a possible source of misunderstandings between patient and health care provider.

## Beliefs and Misinformation

Information about the human body, health practices, and modern methods of diagnosis and treatment are unknown to many people, in spite of widespread health education programs in the schools, on television and radio, and in the newspapers. People who do not have factual information are likely to believe the **superstitions** of their culture just as firmly as you believe the information in a textbook. In fact, their beliefs may be closely tied in with love and respect for their parents, since such beliefs are passed down from one generation to the next. The teachings of your parents are important to you; and so it is with others, even though those teachings may be different from what you think is "right."

## Socioeconomic Class

Each socioeconomic class within a society has its own customs, standards of living, **value system,** interests, expectations, and other characteristics that distinguish it from other socioeconomic classes. Members of one class generally do not understand the differences between their own class and other classes. The health care provider's expectations regarding patient behavior may be unrealistic for patients from a different cultural background or socioeconomic level. The tendency to make negative judgments about a person because of the culture or class from which that person comes is called **cultural bias.**

Most health care providers did not grow up as a member of an extremely wealthy family, nor did they live in poverty. Although there is great diversity within the middle class, members also have much in common. And one thing most of them have in common is a lack of understanding about poverty and about **affluence.** But the health care provider encounters patients from all socioeconomic groups. It is especially important that health care providers not allow their own beliefs and value systems to influence the care they give patients from other socioeconomic levels and other cultures.

## The Patient from the Poverty Class

People who have never lived in poverty find it difficult to understand those whose lives center around survival. People who live in poverty have a daily routine that is different from the daily activities of middle-class people. They may lack running water or electricity in the home. Badly decayed teeth may mean poor diet and lack of knowledge about oral hygiene. Deodorants are a luxury for those who do not know today where tomorrow's dinner will come from. The language of the poverty group may include words you regard as "bad," yet these words may be the patient's only means for expressing personal needs. Terminology used by health care providers may be unfamiliar to some patients, so you may need to provide additional explanation (Figure 2-2).

## The Patient from the Affluent Class

Consider a patient who is from the upper socioeconomic level. Perhaps this person is accustomed to the best of service and, through habit, expects to receive good service. Perhaps this person's wealth represents much hard work and successful competition in the business world. Perhaps it is inherited wealth, and this person has known a life of ease without having to struggle for material comforts.

FIGURE 2-2 The vocabulary of health care providers may be foreign to some patients. *Delmar/Cengage Learning*

Good health, freedom from pain, and escape from disabling accidents are not assured by wealth. Does a wealthy patient seem unwilling to put up with an inconvenient illness? Does the patient appear impatient when there is a delay in receiving an expected service or rebel against being a patient? Illness interrupts and alters patterns of living and does not respect the important matters that may await one's attention.

Even the wealthy have problems. Though different from those of the poverty group, their life problems may be very demanding. Therefore, the health care provider should not conclude that the wealthy patient should lie back and be a "good patient" because he does not have to worry about how to pay the medical bills.

## Expectations of Health Care Providers

Each patient, regardless of socioeconomic status, age, race, religion, or national origin, is entitled to the best care you can give. Each is a human being with feelings, hopes, problems, habits, and needs. All of these factors contribute to the uniqueness of each personality.

Can you, as a health care provider, expect people from other cultural groups to have the same beliefs, attitudes, hygienic habits, health practices, and understandings that you have? Are they either less worthy or more worthy as human beings because their lifestyles are different from yours?

## IMPLICATIONS FOR HEALTH CARE PROVIDERS

### Feelings about Patients

The degree to which you accept the philosophy of individual worth will influence your practice as a health care provider. You may need to overcome **prejudice** in order to apply this philosophy to your daily work. You may even have difficulty in understanding some patients, especially those whose cultural background is different from yours. Your responsibility as a health care provider is to *know your role and, within that role, to serve each patient effectively*. Avoid making value judgments about a patient or allowing your feelings to interfere with the quality of care you provide that person.

### The Challenge

It can be a challenge to provide health services to those who are from a different culture or economic level. Try to understand these patients in terms of their background; try to see situations as they see them. You can fulfill your role as a health care provider and at the same time adapt to the special needs of each patient. The example you set is important in teaching health habits. Your choice of words is important in helping the patient understand your meaning. Your sincerity and interest can influence a patient's attitude toward the entire health care system.

### Studying a Situation

It is not easy to serve all patients equally well. Sometimes there is a strong desire to escape—to carry out an assigned task and leave the patient as quickly as possible. If you find yourself trying to avoid a patient, consider the situation carefully. Why do you find this patient difficult to serve? Does this patient remind you of someone you dislike? Have you tried to understand this patient's personal and health needs? Have you tried to see the situation as the patient sees it (Figure 2-3)? If you make a habit of studying such situations, applying your knowledge about human behavior, you will grow in your ability to form effective relationships with your patients.

## PRACTICING A PHILOSOPHY OF INDIVIDUAL WORTH

It is easy to give lip service to the philosophy of individual worth. It is quite difficult to practice it day after day when there is a busy schedule and a wide variety of patients to take care of, unless you form certain ways of thinking about your patients. The following suggestions provide a starting point for developing and applying a philosophy of individual worth to your relationships with patients:

- Accept each patient as he is—an individual with a **unique** personality.
- Recognize that each person tries to meet his needs with patterns of behavior that have developed over a lifetime; these patterns cannot be changed easily.
- Make a conscious effort to understand each patient's behavior.
- Accept that many of your patients will not behave as you want them to behave.

**FIGURE 2-3** Try to understand the patient's point of view. *Delmar/Cengage Learning*

- Do not expect a sick person to adapt to you. As a health care provider and as a well person, you should adapt to the patient.
- Consider each patient with a cultural background different from yours as an opportunity for you to learn about the influence of customs, beliefs, values, religious practices, and socioeconomic level on human behavior.
- Make it a habit to treat all patients with respect, regardless of their backgrounds.

## REFERENCES AND SUGGESTED READINGS

Munoz, Cora, & Luckmann, Joan. (2004). *Transcultural communication in nursing* (2nd ed.). Clifton Park, NY: Delmar, Cengage Learning.

Runy, Lee Ann. (2008, Nov.). Building a culture of patient-centered care. *H & HN Hospitals & Health Networks, 82*(11), 44–45.

Tamparo, Carol, & Lindh, Wilburta Q. (2008). *Therapeutic communications for health professionals.* Clifton Park, NY: Delmar, Cengage Learning.

## REVIEW AND SELF-CHECK

1. Explain in writing your beliefs about individual worth.

2. State three reasons that cultural bias can affect the quality of patient care.

3. List five examples of differences that could lead to a misunderstanding between you, a health care provider, and a patient from a culture about which you know very little.

4. Explain "cultural bias" in your own words.

5. Explain "prejudice" in your own words.

## ASSIGNMENTS

1. Think about someone you know whose background is different from your own; list five ways in which this person's lifestyle is different from yours.

2. Think about each of the following situations, and then write a possible explanation for each patient's behavior.

    a. Mrs. M. has a private room. Her gowns appear very expensive and there are luxury cosmetics on her dresser. She is hospitalized for diagnostic studies. After the second day, she appears to lack interest in grooming; her hair is uncombed and she has not applied any makeup.

    b. Mrs. J. shows no interest in the food on her tray, has a messy unit, and shows no interest in other patients in the four-bed room. The doctor carefully explained the plan for Mrs. J.'s care, but she fails to follow the doctor's instructions.

c. Johnny has been admitted through the clinic for a tonsillectomy. When the laboratory technician tries to draw a blood sample, Johnny kicks and screams. When he is being prepared for the operating room, a string with a small bag attached is found around his neck. He tries to prevent this from being removed, saying he will die if it is taken off.

3. Participate in a class discussion about cultural influences of the following religious groups on food choices and lifestyle:

Catholicism

Judaism

Seventh-day Adventist Church

Church of Latter Day Saints (Mormonism)

Islam

> **Note:** Class members may add other examples for discussion.

4. Participate in a class discussion to list derogatory words that some people use to refer to members of a particular group (race, ethnic background, or nationality).

5. Write a brief description of a situation involving you and someone from a different culture. Was there any evidence of misunderstanding or distrust? If so, try to identify one or more cultural differences that may have contributed to the misunderstanding or distrust.

6. Consider each of the following situations in terms of your possible feelings about each patient:

    a. You are admitting a male patient from the emergency room; he has an unkempt beard, bad breath, and his clothes smell of stale perspiration.

    b. Your morning assignment includes an unconscious patient who was admitted during the night; the report states that this person is a known drug addict.

    c. Your patient is a 6-year-old boy who looks at you with obvious distrust; he responds to your "Good morning" by looking away from you and saying "Leave me alone." He then uses language you consider to be "gutter talk."

    d. Your patient is a Latino with a gunshot wound; he does not speak English.

    e. Your patient is 35 years old and weighs 300 pounds.

    f. You are admitting a patient who reeks of garlic.

7. You have learned that a person's socioeconomic level influences behavior patterns. List some possible differences in the behavior of people from three socioeconomic levels in each of the situations listed in the following chart.

| SITUATION | EXTREME POVERTY | LOWER SOCIOECONOMIC CLASS | MIDDLE CLASS |
|---|---|---|---|
| Example: A severe flu epidemic | Resignation to sickness and death as a part of life; little tendency to assume personal responsibility or take action to control the uncertainties of life | Some tendency toward resignation; perhaps seeking medical assistance from a clinic; possible reliance on home remedies, hearsay, or superstitions | Seeking flu shots from private physicians; medical help for victims from private physicians; perhaps criticism of medical profession for lack of precise methods for prevention and cure |
| Passage of a local ordinance requiring certain types of garbage containers, and a fine of $25.00 for not abiding by this regulation | | | |
| Serious illness in the provider of a family | | | |
| A public health campaign on the importance of obtaining a new type of immunization | | | |
| Hospitalization for the first time: adult patient; child patient | | | |

# Striving for Self-Understanding

## OBJECTIVES

Upon completion of this unit, you should be able to:

- List three responsibilities of the learner.
- Explain why learning is defined as "a change in behavior."
- Describe one technique for effective learning.
- List five essentials for developing one's potential.
- Identify one's life roles and appropriate behaviors for each role.
- Explain why role confusion is dangerous for a health care provider.
- List five time management strategies.
- List five guidelines for personal growth.

## KEY TERMS

| | | |
|---|---|---|
| Ethics | Potential | Role |
| Habits | Procrastinate | Similarities |
| Learning | Repertoire | Traits |

Today you are enrolled in a course of study that will lead to your becoming a health care provider. In the near future you will graduate and assume a position in an agency that provides health services to the community. What changes are needed before you, the student of today, can become you, the health care provider of tomorrow?

## YOU, THE STUDENT

Obviously, you must acquire knowledge, learn to apply it appropriately to a wide variety of situations, and develop skill in performing certain procedures. Your teachers have organized for you a meaningful sequence of learning experiences. They will guide your step-by-step progress toward a future **role** in the field. Your teachers, however, cannot do the whole job. The desire to learn, willingness to make the necessary effort, and determination to gain as much as possible from each learning experience must come from you.

## Learning versus Memorizing

**Learning** has been defined as a *change in behavior*. If you can answer the questions on a test, but do not apply that information in appropriate clinical situations, have you *really* learned? Do you approach assignments as though you are a tape recorder, storing information that can be played back on demand? Such an approach to study is not true learning.

## Developing Mental Skills

Do you constantly ask yourself how a new idea can be used? Does new information guide you in selecting appropriate behavior for situations where that information is relevant? If you can answer "Yes" to these questions, then you are truly learning. You are using mental processes such as thinking, reasoning, selecting, decision making, and evaluating for conscious control of your behavior.

## Developing Learning Skills

Unit 1 discussed guidelines for developing effective study habits. Learning new skills begins with studying but does not end when a test or an assignment is complete. Each time you begin a new topic of study in class, ask yourself the following questions: What do I already know about this topic? What do I want to find out about this topic? When you connect new information to ideas you have previously learned, the new information becomes more meaningful and easier to remember.

## Developing Your Potential

Think of yourself for a moment as a person who loves music, but does not have a musical instrument or teacher. Suddenly, your family obtains a piano, and a gifted piano teacher moves next door. After an appropriate period of study under the guidance of your teacher, you become an excellent pianist. Thus, through a combination of the right circumstances and effort, your **potential** for becoming a pianist has been fulfilled and you *are* a pianist.

This period as a student is your opportunity to develop your potential as a health care provider. The circumstances for learning are being provided in the form of many learning experiences, each designed to help you acquire new knowledge and develop skills. The effort necessary to develop your potential can only come from you.

Let us now explore some of the ways you can strive to develop your potential for learning. These same approaches, applied to your future career, will help you develop your potential for becoming a health care provider.

# TAKING A NEW LOOK AT YOURSELF

The immediate task is to undertake a study of yourself. "But," you say, "I already know myself." Do you really? If you do, you are a rare person indeed. True self-understanding is difficult to achieve. Even a beginning effort—just taking an honest look at yourself—may make you decide on some changes. The ability to be honest with yourself is absolutely necessary for achieving self-understanding.

## Will to Change

The first question to ask yourself is, "Am I willing to make changes in myself?" When someone criticizes you, do you nurse your hurt feelings or express anger toward your critic? Do you reject the criticism or make excuses for your behavior? Or do you see criticism as a possible indication that you need to change some aspect of your behavior? Willingness to change is necessary so that you can learn and grow as a person. Remember, learning was defined earlier as a change in behavior.

## Strengths and Weaknesses

Your next question might be, "What are my strengths and my weaknesses?" To develop your potential, you must know your weak points, for these will need your attention and greatest effort. For example, do you have a habit of putting off a task until the last minute? This habit can lead to many undesirable results: being late to class, not being prepared for a test, not practicing a skill until you have achieved a high level of proficiency. By correcting a tendency to **procrastinate,** you can spare yourself the emotional strain of doing things at the last minute. You may even escape the irritation others express when your last-minute efforts inconvenience them.

An honest appraisal of your personal **traits,** including your work **habits,** is the key to planning ways of developing your potential. If you eliminate those behaviors that interfere with good performance, you will improve your ability to perform well in a variety of situations.

## Adapting to New Conditions

A third question to ask yourself is, "How well do I adapt to change?" Are you still clinging to ineffective habits formed early in your school years? If so, these habits are probably not working very well in your present educational program. No longer can you depend on the teacher. No longer can you expect the teacher to go over the same material until you have passively absorbed it. Time is short, and there is much to be learned before you qualify as a health care provider. *You* must assume primary responsibility for learning.

Perhaps you once worked in the hospital as an aide. Now you are preparing for a different role. Will the habits you formed as an aide be acceptable in your new role? You will need to develop new habits appropriate to your new role and, possibly, to higher standards of performance.

In the future, you may be in a new situation and find yourself saying or thinking, "But I learned to do it such and such a way, not the way they do it here" (Figure 3-1). For most tasks, there is more than one acceptable procedure; adapting to the new setting requires that

**FIGURE 3-1** Old habits can hold you back. *Delmar/Cengage Learning*

you perform according to the procedures of the new setting. *Basic principles, however, do not vary.* For example, aseptic technique requires certain steps and certain precautions, regardless of the setting or the precise sequence of steps for the total procedure.

## Using Experience to Learn

A fourth question is, "Do I learn from my experiences?" Let us take a look at how two people reacted to an embarrassing experience. When Mary and Sue gave oral reports, they both showed signs of nervousness and performed poorly. For each of them, this was a very embarrassing experience.

Mary reviewed the situation, admitted to herself that she had put little effort into this assignment, and made plans to be well prepared for the next oral report. She decided to have her information better organized, to study the material until she understood it, to prepare good notes, and to rehearse her presentation until she could present the report with minimal use of notes. She also spoke with her instructor after class about ways to improve her performance.

Sue, on the other hand, used the same approach to prepare her next oral report, which proved to be another poor performance. She was no better prepared for the second report than she was for the first. In addition, she was developing a fear of oral reports that would have a negative effect on her future efforts to speak in front of others.

Mary used her experience constructively, making careful plans to prevent a recurrence of this particular embarrassment. With additional practice, Mary will give oral reports with confidence. Sue, on the other hand, allowed the experience to create self-doubt and fear of oral reports. Do you think she will develop either skill or confidence? Which of these students will grow as a person? Are you a Mary or a Sue, in relation to learning from experience? (Figure 3-2)

## Role Perception

A fifth question to ask yourself is, "What is my role?" The present program of study will help you understand your future role as a health care provider. For every role there are appropriate and inappropriate ways of behaving. Whether a particular manner of

**FIGURE 3-2** Education is an important objective for health care personnel.
*Delmar/Cengage Learning*

behavior is appropriate depends not only on the specific *type* of health care provider you are preparing to become, but also on the *level* of that role in relation to other health team members.

Certain behaviors that are appropriate for a specific health care role may not be appropriate for personnel in a different role. Also, there are differences in roles based on level. Nursing assistants, licensed practical nurses, registered nurses, head nurses, and supervisors all have specific roles within nursing. There are numerous roles within the hospital laboratory: pathologist, medical technologist, clinical laboratory assistant, laboratory aide, and others. These roles of laboratory personnel are distinct from those of nursing service personnel. The same is true of medical offices and other hospital departments: physical therapy, radiology, food service, and others. In the dental field, dentists, dental hygienists, dental assistants, and dental laboratory technologists are all concerned with oral health. Their roles have **similarities,** but vary according to the specific functions and educational preparation of each.

Knowing one's role is essential to effective functioning; it is also essential to self-understanding. Most roles within the health field require accepting instructions from someone at the next higher level. If you do not like "taking orders," then you may not be happy as a health care provider. If you feel anger or distrust toward persons in authority, you are likely to resent the **ethics** of the health field; the policies of your health agency; and relationships with those on the health team who have responsibility for giving instructions, making assignments, and evaluating performance. On the other hand, if you can accept a defined role, function within that role to the fullest extent of your educational preparation, and accept the limitations of the role without feeling "put down," then you are likely to find much satisfaction as a health care provider.

## YOU, A PERSON WITH SEVERAL LIFE ROLES

How many roles do you play? Probably several. You are a student now and hope to have a role as a health care provider in the future. You may be a husband, father, wife, or mother; or you may be living in your parents' home, still in a dependent role. Even if you are living on your own, you still have the role of child to your parents, if they are living, in addition to the other roles in your life.

### Role as an Influence on Relationships

There are similarities in the child-parent relationship and the teacher-student relationship during the school years. In a health occupations education program, the teacher-student relationship is between two adults, even though one adult is a student. What difficulties in role perception might occur if the student is a mature, 50-year-old person, and the teacher is a 25-year-old health professional? Or, if a doctor is 35 and the medical office assistant is 55, with 20 years of experience?

### Making a Distinction between Roles

The roles you play at home, in your church activities, as a health occupations student, and as a neighbor are all different. To some extent, each role requires different behavior patterns (Figure 3-3). Do not confuse the health care provider role with other roles in your personal

**FIGURE 3-3** Each life role requires certain behaviors. *Delmar/Cengage Learning*

life. Some friends may try to get "free medical advice"; but the role of friend and the role of health care provider are different. Medical practice acts, which are state laws, make it illegal for nonphysicians to diagnose and prescribe. Therefore, this type of role confusion is dangerous.

## GUIDELINES FOR GROWTH

Becoming an effective health care provider is a process that extends over a period of time. It requires continuous effort throughout one's career.

### Value of Self-Study

In undertaking a self-study, you will be making an investment in your own future. Hopefully, this study will start you on a lifetime process of striving for personal growth. You should continuously evaluate your habits and modify those that do not get the desired response from others. There will always be some people with whom you do not "hit it off," but you can learn to relate to most people in ways that promote understanding and minimize unfavorable feelings. As you become skillful in using a large **repertoire** of human relations skills, you will grow in self-understanding, in tolerance, and in your ability to accept others as they are.

## Value of Studying Human Behavior

Note that the sequence of growth is from understanding self to understanding others. Therefore, *the ability to understand others is limited until you have begun to understand yourself.*

Human behavior is very complex. In any situation, the behavior of a person is influenced by many different factors. The remainder of this course will introduce some of these influences. Striving to understand oneself and others must be based on knowledge about human behavior in general.

## Managing Your Time

An important aspect of understanding yourself is to recognize how you use your time. Have you ever asked yourself at the end of the day, "Where did the time go?" Have you ever wondered why some people seem to get everything done, whereas others are perpetually late or behind on their assignments? Learning to manage your time can make you more effective as a student and a professional.

To help you identify how you spend your time, try for a day or two to write down hourly what you are doing. You will gain a realistic estimate of how long household tasks or childcare actually take as well as how much time you spend on nonessential activities, such as watching television, talking on the phone, or surfing the Internet. Once you know how you are spending your time, you can decide what changes you would like to make in your daily routine.

The following strategies may be useful in using your time more effectively:

- Write down tasks or goals you hope to accomplish each day.
- Prioritize your goals so that you tackle the most important or most urgent first.
- As much as possible, focus on completing one task at a time.
- Throughout the day, stop periodically and ask yourself, "Am I working to meet my goals? Am I doing what I am supposed to be doing?
- If possible, review your list of goals each evening, mark off those that were completed, and plan the list for the next day.
- Start tasks well ahead of time to avoid the stress of having to rush.
- Break large tasks into small chunks and tackle one chunk at a time.

## Striving for Personal Growth

Now let us summarize some ways you can try to understand yourself and set goals for personal growth and achievement as a student and health care provider:

- Recognize that learning occurs only if you make the effort to learn, if you are willing to change, and if you recognize opportunities for learning.
- Study yourself in relation to specific traits, such as willingness to change, ability to be honest with yourself, and readiness to correct weaknesses and change habits.
- Identify your strengths and make full use of them to achieve your goals.

- Identify your weaknesses—the traits or habits you need to change in order to be more effective in each of your roles.
- Study your various roles in terms of desirable behavior. Identify differences, such as habits used at home that are not appropriate at school, interpersonal relations between a parent and child that are not appropriate between the health care provider and a pediatric patient, or relations between friends that are not appropriate between a hospital employee and a patient.
- Study your ability to make distinctions between different life roles and change behaviors accordingly.
- Study your tendency to use old habits in new situations. Do you allow habits to determine your behavior in any situation? Do you need to improve in adapting your behavior to each situation?
- Mentally review past experiences to understand how your own behavior contributed to the outcome. Consider the important question, "Would the outcome of that experience be improved if I had behaved differently?" This practice can serve as a "rehearsal" for future similar experiences.

## REFERENCES AND SUGGESTED READINGS

Jack, Kirsten, & Miller, Eula. (2008, Nov.). Exploring self-awareness in mental health practice. *Mental Health Practice, 12*(3), 31–35.

Leland, Karen, & Bailey, Keith. (2008). *Time management in an instant: 60 ways to make the most of your day.* Franklin Lakes, NJ: Career Press.

Siebert, Al, & Karr, Mary. (2008). *The adult student's guide to survival and success in college.* Portland, OR: Practical Psychology Press.

Tamparo, Carol, & Lindh, Wilburta Q. (2008). What is your style? Professional application. In *Therapeutic Communications for Health Professionals* (pp. 9–10). Clifton Park, NY: Delmar, Cengage Learning.

## REVIEW AND SELF-CHECK

1. List three responsibilities of a learner.

   _____

   _____

   _____

2. Explain why learning is defined as "a change in behavior."

   _____

3. Describe a technique that can help you become an effective learner.

   _____

4. List five guidelines for developing one's potential.

5. Explain why appropriate behavior for you as a health care provider differs from appropriate behaviors for your other roles in the family and community.

6. List five guidelines for developing your own potential.

7. Explain why role confusion can lead to problems for a health care provider.

8. List five time management strategies.

## ASSIGNMENTS

1. List some changes you have made in daily habits since you entered this health occupations program. Think of one additional change that may improve one of your life roles. Write out a description of the change and the steps necessary for making it part of your habitual behavior.

2. Which of the following roles do you play in your current life situation?

    Student in a health-related educational program

    Spouse or significant other

    Mother, father, or single parent

    Daughter or son

    Homemaker

    Worker/employee (part-time job)

    a. Beside each role that applies to you, enter the percentage of time per day that you devote to that role. The total of all roles should equal 100%.

    b. Indicate with an asterisk (*) the role that you value most.

    c. If other demands (job, school) limit the amount of time you devote to the role you value the most, list three ways to improve your approach to that role so that *quality* can compensate for lack of *quantity*. For example, "When in the role of ____, I will give it my full attention and not allow concerns about my other roles to distract me at that time."

3. Identify one habitual behavior in each of your roles that is not a desirable (or effective) behavior for your student role.

4. Identify one habitual behavior in your personal life that is not an acceptable behavior with patients or co-workers.

5. List five actions or behaviors that are appropriate in a friend/friend relationship, but are not appropriate in a health care provider/patient relationship.

6. Consider a situation in which you ran out of time to complete a task. Discuss how time management strategies might help you to handle a similar situation more effectively in the future.

7. Recall some unpleasant memory: an embarrassing experience, a failure, a situation in which a misunderstanding occurred, or one in which you behaved in a manner that you now recognize as inappropriate. Mentally review the situation and proceed with the following steps:

    a. Picture yourself in the actual setting.

    b. Who was there?

    c. What did other people say or do?

    d. What did you say or do?

    e. What happened after your behavior (whatever you said or did)?

    f. Was the consequence of your behavior a result of what you said or did? (Careful! Be honest with yourself in answering this question. Don't refuse to acknowledge that you brought about the consequences by inappropriate behavior. On the other hand, don't blame yourself for consequences over which you had no control.)

g. How did you feel about the undesirable consequences at the time? (Again, be completely honest with yourself.)

h. How do you now feel when you think about this experience?

i. Now, reconsider the situation to learn from it. What behavior on your part might have brought about a more desirable consequence? Is the experience something that might occur again in the future? What will you say (or do) if a similar situation occurs in the future?

> **Note:** The purpose of this exercise is to help you learn from a past experience. Everyone has unpleasant memories that recur at times, arousing the same negative feelings that were experienced at the time. When reflecting upon that experience, you can eliminate to a large extent (and perhaps completely) the emotional response associated with the memory of that situation. Trying to extract a lesson from the experience may prepare you to deal effectively with some future situation. The advantages of using the above exercise are twofold: (1) elimination of a recurring, unpleasant memory and (2) preparation, through mental rehearsal, for a future similar experience.
>
> We cannot change the past. So it is pointless to continue feeling angry, embarrassed, or guilty about something that cannot be changed. If you are "haunted" by past experiences that arouse negative feelings, you should talk with a professional counselor to learn how to resolve these feelings; otherwise, they can interfere with your present and future adjustment.

Section

# Striving to Understand Human Behavior

Health care providers deal with people whose lives have been complicated by illness. The reactions people exhibit toward illness and hospitalization must be understood and accepted by health care providers as behavioral responses to a stressful situation.

The interpersonal skills of health care providers are very important to the patient. The health care provider who can build rapport with patients increases confidence in the health team, promotes faith in the treatment plan, and is more likely to gain the patient's full cooperation. If a health care provider is unable to develop rapport, then the opposite may occur. The patient may have negative feelings toward members of the health team, may distrust them, and may not comply with the health care plan. The skillful health care provider can recognize behavior indicative of negative feelings and attitudes and make an effort to correct them. Section II explains some of the many factors that are basic influences on human behavior.

# UNIT 4

# Influences on Behavior

## OBJECTIVES

Upon completion of this unit, you should be able to:

- List five ways people are alike.
- Define heredity, chromosome, and gene.
- Define dominant, recessive, and sex-linked traits.
- List five possibilities that determine whether or not a particular trait will be inherited.
- Name four dimensions of the developmental process.
- Name two types of environment that influence a child's development.
- Name three important influences on development during childhood.
- Name three early childhood learnings that influence adult behavior.
- List four ways that one's interests influence behavior.
- Name the primary influence of one's value system on behavior.

## KEY TERMS

| | | |
|---|---|---|
| Addiction | Genes | Nurturing |
| Chromosomes | Genetics | Phenotype |
| Congenital | Genotype | Rapport |
| DNA | Hereditary | Teratogens |
| Ethnic | Human Genome Project | |

Human behavior is extremely complex. No one can understand behavior completely, but it is helpful to know about some of the many factors that influence behavior.

## HOW PEOPLE ARE ALIKE

All of us are alike in many ways. We have certain basic physical needs; we also have certain basic psychological needs. We have interests and value systems. We each have a unique hereditary endowment. We have all developed in a definite sequence that is characteristic of the human species. Behavior is influenced by factors that all people have in common and also by individual differences.

## HOW PEOPLE ARE DIFFERENT

Each person forms certain behavior patterns for meeting basic physical and psychological needs. Each person develops his own certain interests. Each of us has a value system that influences our life choices. In striving to understand behavior, then, it is necessary to be aware of ways people are alike, ways people are different, and factors that influence the learning of behavior patterns. Three major forces interact to create a specific individual: heredity, the developmental process, and the environment.

## HEREDITY

Each person is a unique individual. At the time of conception, **hereditary** traits are inherited from the mother and father to form a unique combination of traits. Since thousands of traits are involved, the possible combinations are limitless. That is why we say that no two people have exactly the same heredity, except in the case of identical twins. You are undoubtedly learning about heredity in other courses. Therefore, our concern here is to emphasize that *each person, from the time of conception, is endowed with a one-and-only combination of traits that will affect that individual throughout life.*

### The Physiology of Heredity

At the time of conception, 46 **chromosomes** are organized into 23 matched pairs (23 from each parent). There are two sex-linked chromosomes: X for females and Y for males. The combination of chromosomes from the two parents provides the individual's **genotype,** a unique set of inherited traits. The **phenotype** is the result of all genes that, in combination, provide traits that determine the individual's physical appearance.

**Genes** are locations, more than a thousand on each chromosome. Each gene is composed of molecules of a protein called deoxyribonucleic (de-oxy-ribo-nu-cle-ic) acid, or **DNA.** DNA is made up of four basic chemicals: adenine, thymine, guanine, and cytosine, arranged as strands that wrap around each other to form a spiral known as the double helix. DNA is present in every cell of the body in the form of genes. These chemicals are arranged on the gene in a particular sequence, and it is the sequence that establishes the trait or traits carried by that gene, just as the arrangement of letters makes up a specific word. The "words" are actually larger protein molecules, and each has a specific function—control of a specific cellular activity. The discovery of DNA and subsequent discovery of molecular sequences on strands of DNA were exciting scientific breakthroughs. This led to rapid development of human **genetics** as a scientific field of inquiry and the discovery of much new information on heredity.

### The Genetic Basis for Individuality

A particular characteristic of an individual may be due to:

- One specific gene,
- The sequential arrangement of molecules on each gene,
- A particular pair of genes,
- A group of genes interacting with each other, or
- The influence of environmental factors on a gene or genes.

Some traits are expressed, meaning that the individual will definitely manifest that trait. Other traits are unexpressed but predispose that individual to manifest the trait under certain conditions. For example, a person may have the gene for a specific hereditary disease but will develop the disease only if the life situation includes certain conditions. A person who has the gene for a disease but does not develop symptoms is a carrier; that gene can be passed on to the children, who may manifest the disease.

Like chromosomes, genes are paired so that a given trait is determined by the contribution of either or both parents. A dominant trait will be expressed, even if inherited from only one parent; a recessive trait will manifest only if matched with a recessive gene from each parent. Some traits are sex-linked, meaning they are inherited through the X chromosome of the mother or are linked to the Y chromosome of the father. For example, red/green color blindness is expressed only in males but is inherited from the mother because the gene for color blindness is carried on the mother's X chromosome.

## Health Implications

Genetics, the study of heredity, has expanded rapidly and is making significant contributions to medicine. Research to locate the genetic basis of diseases is ongoing, with new findings announced frequently.

A genetic disorder is one that results from an individual's genetic makeup. It may be apparent at birth, may appear as a developmental disorder, or may appear later in life as a disease or health problem. A single-gene disorder is due to the absence or alteration of one gene specific to that trait. Tests are available for many single-gene disorders, such as cystic fibrosis, hemophilia, and red/green color blindness. A multifactorial disorder is one involving variations in several genes. Obviously, identifying several defective genes is more complex than identifying a single gene. There are also chromosomal disorders; for example, persons with Down syndrome have three, rather than two, copies of chromosome 21.

Gene therapy is emerging as a specialty in medicine; therapy consists of modifying a defective gene in order to treat or prevent a specific disease. Genetic testing is already in use to identify certain single-gene disorders, confirm a diagnosis, identify carriers, and identify persons who are at risk for developing a disease but are currently free of symptoms.

From the moment of conception, then, an individual has a unique combination of hereditary traits, a blueprint that will guide growth, development, and numerous processes throughout that individual's life. Some genes are so specific that their traits cannot be modified by environmental influences or therapy. Other genes require pairing (one from each parent) in order for a trait or disorder to develop. Some genes are sex-linked—specific to the X or Y chromosome. Some genes provide a trait that will manifest only if environmental conditions foster its development.

## Genetic Testing

In 1990, the U.S. Congress funded the **Human Genome Project,** a 13-year project to map the sequencing of all of the genes on all of the chromosomes. The project was completed in 2003. This map, or pattern, of the chromosomal and gene arrangement is called the human genome, the basis for genetics in human beings. Identification of the genetic basis for certain disorders has resulted in the development of genetic testing that surpasses the development of improved therapies. During the 1990s, prenatal testing became routine; many pregnant women were given the maternal alphafetoprotein 3 (MSAFP3) screening test. Scientific advances in genetics have raised questions about privacy rights and the right of each patient to participate in health-related decisions.

DNA tests are proving valuable in areas other than health-related genetics. An individual's DNA can be used to determine paternity, to identify a body, to prove or disprove family relationships, and to investigate crimes. DNA samples have been used as proof to establish guilt or innocence of an accused person.

Genetic testing is expensive. It also involves certain risks that should be made known to anyone who is considering genetic testing. Insurance companies and employers (or potential employers) can demand the results of genetic testing. There are examples of people who were denied insurance or lost their jobs when genetic tests indicated the presence of a gene for some specific disease (e.g., breast cancer, Huntington's disease). Whereas a negative test can relieve one's anxieties, a positive test has profound psychological effects on the individual and his or her loved ones.

If your parent died at age 49 of Huntington's disease, you may or may not develop this incurable disease. Genetic testing could remove this terrible cloud over your life if you do not have the specific gene. On the other hand, if you do have the gene, you will be faced with the certainty of developing the disease, probably during your 40s. Would you choose to live with uncertainty? Or would you want to know, even if a positive test might cost you your job, insurance coverage, and relationships with those who cannot face the prospect of caring for you through a long illness? A positive approach to knowing that you have the gene would be to acknowledge your own mortality, accept that you will not have a long life, use your remaining years of health to live life to the fullest, and make end-of-life decisions while you are still in good physical and mental health.

### Behavioral Genetics

Genetics research has also given rise to the field of behavioral genetics, which seeks to understand human behavior in terms of hereditary or biological influences. Researchers note that some behaviors tend to run in families. Studies of twins and adoptees have been used for some time to explore the effects of heredity on behavior. More recently, researchers have worked to identify pieces of DNA that appear to be associated with particular behaviors.

## THE DEVELOPMENTAL PROCESS

Heredity establishes the basic physical/mental/emotional makeup and all the personality traits of each individual. But many other influences determine how these ingredients will be molded as the individual grows and develops from a helpless baby into an adult. One important difference is the built-in developmental rate, a hereditary factor. Thus, physical development proceeds at one rate for Johnny and at another rate for his brother, Joe. The study of a child must always consider the apparent rate of development.

### Prenatal Influences

The developmental process is subject to tremendous environmental influence, especially during the prenatal period. Ideally, the mother's body provides the embryo with a physical environment that is favorable to healthful development. This prenatal environment is affected by the mother's general health, her nutritional status, pathogenic organisms such as those causing syphilis or measles, and the presence in her blood of any substance that is toxic to the embryo.

The results of recent research indicate that the mother's daily habits have tremendous influence on the embryo. Even moderate use of tobacco, alcohol, and coffee can cause birth defects. Smoking during pregnancy increases the risk of complications of pregnancy, premature birth, low birth weight, stillbirth, and infant mortality. Consumption of alcoholic beverages by a pregnant woman places the infant at risk of various congenital defects. If the woman is a heavy drinker, the newborn infant may exhibit fetal alcohol syndrome (FAS), with various physical and mental abnormalities and behavioral problems that are not responsive to therapy.

Certain drugs, called **teratogens,** are known to cause **congenital** defects. Addictive substances used by a pregnant woman pass through the placenta to the baby. During the 1980s, cocaine **addiction** among women gave rise to a new type of patient—the "crack baby," a newborn baby addicted to cocaine. Because the pregnant woman's lifestyle has profound effects on the fetus, every expectant mother must avoid numerous substances if she is to have a healthy baby. Women who use alcohol or illegal drugs during pregnancy put their babies at risk for birth defects, learning disabilities, or other mental and physical impairments.

The role of nutrition during the prenatal period is critical to healthy prenatal development. For example, a serious congenital anomaly, spina bifida, is now known to be caused by a deficiency of folic acid. This developmental failure in the embryo occurs very early, so if a woman supplements her diet with folic acid *after* learning that she is pregnant, it is already too late to prevent this neural tube defect. The importance of this nutrient is indicated by the new government requirement that folic acid be added to certain commercial foods. Every woman who may become pregnant should be concerned about nutrition, especially adequate intake of vitamins and minerals. If a couple has decided to start a family, both should practice good nutrition and a healthy lifestyle.

The experiences and emotions of a pregnant woman have profound prenatal effects. Fear, anger, and grief—normal reactions to stressful and traumatic experiences—can affect the developing fetus. If the woman has an abusive spouse, the abuse is likely to accelerate during her pregnancy; the woman's emotional reactions to such abuse affect the fetus, even in the absence of physical trauma. On the other hand, positive experiences have a positive effect. Many expectant mothers listen to classical music daily; some read and talk to their unborn child. Studies of young children reveal that a child's personality and developmental rate are related to such prenatal influences.

## Aspects of Development

The developmental process involves physical, emotional, intellectual, and spiritual dimensions. There is an interrelationship among these various dimensions, but the development of one can proceed faster than another. The conditions of an individual's life may promote maximum physical development, yet fail to promote emotional or intellectual growth (Figure 4-1). The conditions that affect each aspect of development are different. An ideal environment promotes optimal physical, emotional, intellectual, and spiritual development. Most of us, however, have not been privileged to grow and develop in an ideal environment. The effects of environmental influences on the developmental process are discussed later in this unit in relation to specific periods of the life span.

FIGURE 4-1 Physically a man—emotionally a little boy. *Delmar/Cengage Learning*

## ENVIRONMENT

The environment is another major influence on development and the expression of certain hereditary potentials. Much has been written about the relative importance of heredity and environment. With increasing knowledge about heredity and with growing awareness of the power of the physical and social environment to affect the developmental process, it is now apparent that the interaction of many forces determines the traits of an individual. Heredity provides the basic ingredients and the blueprint, but environmental factors and events that affect the developmental process determine what aspects of the blueprint will be expressed as traits. The result is a unique person who reflects both how people are alike and how people are different.

### Physical Environment

Environment in its broadest sense means many things. The physical environment includes home conditions, climate, community conditions, means for meeting physical needs, and resources for developing one's potential. Children who live in a large city have a physical environment greatly different from children who live in a rural community. Many factors vary based on children's physical environments, from exposure to pollution to access to cultural resources. All aspects of the physical environment affect personality. Some personality traits tend to develop in one kind of environment, whereas a different environment fosters the development of other traits.

Those who care for a child create the child's immediate physical environment. It may be as safe as thoughtful adults can make it, or it may contain many hazards. Unless adults make a conscious effort to control risks in the home and child-care facility, the child may

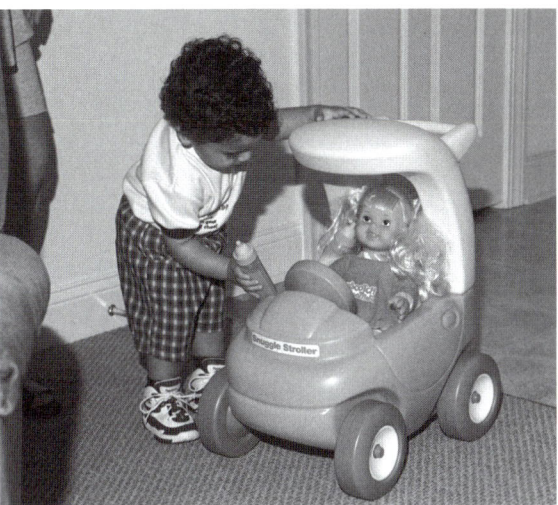

FIGURE 4-2 Attitudes, beliefs, and expectations learned as an infant and toddler influence behavior throughout life. *Delmar/Cengage Learning*

experience serious injuries from falls, burns, or poisoning. Although some such injuries are correctible, some are fatal and others leave lifelong scars. In addition to environmental hazards, some personal habits of adults also affect the child. Exposure to secondhand smoke increases the risk of sudden infant death syndrome (SIDS) in infants, and the chance of developing asthma is higher in babies and young children who are frequently exposed to secondhand smoke.

## Social Environment

The social environment involves people. A baby's experiences provide important first learnings about the world and people (Figure 4-2). The baby may learn that the world is a friendly place—that one can depend on others to correct such discomforts as hunger, cold, and a wet diaper. Or the baby may learn the world is a hostile place—that one cannot rely on others to relieve hunger and cold. These infant experiences lay the foundation for future relations with other people: distrust or trust, expectations of comfort and **nurturing** from others, or resignation to discomfort without help from others.

## Culture and Socioeconomic Level

Children are strongly influenced by the culture in which they grow up. Culture refers to the ideas, beliefs, values, and customs shared by a group of people. These shared ideas may be based on religion, ethnicity or nationality, geographic region, or a number of other factors. Put simply, children learn from the adults around them what is important and how they are expected to act in certain situations.

Socioeconomic level also influences children's early learning. According to the National Center for Children in Poverty (NCCP), 19% of children in the United States live in families whose income falls below the federal poverty level. These children are at increased risk for learning and behavioral problems (NCCP, 2009).

## INFLUENCES ON DEVELOPMENT DURING CHILDHOOD

The basic heredity of a child, plus environmental influences, exerts a powerful influence on development.

### The Preschool Years

Throughout the early years, a child continues to learn about people and the world. If these learnings are favorable, the child develops a sense of security and finds the world a place for exploring and satisfying curiosity. There are happy experiences and unhappy ones, but comfort is available when unhappy experiences occur. If the learnings of early childhood are unfavorable, the child learns to distrust other people and tends to fear new experiences or strange places.

Alex is a 15-month-old who is developing his walking, running, and climbing skills as he actively explores the environment. When Alex falls, his parents say "Uh-oh," and Alex gets up and resumes his activities. He now reacts to a fall by saying "Uh-oh" himself. The mother of Joey, a 20-month-old toddler, frequently calls out to her child, "Don't do that. You'll fall and hurt yourself." When Joey does fall, he starts to cry and his mother picks him up, often saying angrily, "You know you shouldn't do that!" These two children are being taught very different reactions to life experiences and will differ in their readiness to experience various activities. These early life experiences establish attitudes, beliefs, and expectations that may continue to influence behavior throughout life.

### The School Years

When the child enters school, the physical and social environments are greatly extended. If development has proceeded according to schedule, the child is ready for this expansion of experience (Figure 4-3). If the physical or social environment of early life inhibited some aspect of development, then the child may not be ready to benefit fully from school. Early school experiences may be so unsatisfying that they inhibit development of one or more dimensions.

First graders show marked differences in development and in behavior patterns. These differences reflect both hereditary and environmental influences. Some children readily adapt to being with a group of their own age; others hang back, afraid to join the group. Some see the teacher as absolute authority, to be obeyed without question; others show rebellion toward authority. Still others voice their opinions freely and may even expect to have a choice of whether or not to follow the teacher's instructions. Some first graders are quite self-reliant; others depend on the teacher for assistance with every task. Some are bubbling with ideas and participate fully in every activity; others sit quietly and participate only when urged. These differences are not accidental. They are the result of early influences on patterns of behavior.

### Social Influences on Development

The home environment is of great importance in the young child's development. How well does the family provide for the child's physical needs? What health practices are followed? Is the home atmosphere democratic or authoritarian? Do the parents "wait on" the child, or do

FIGURE 4-3 Early learnings influence readiness for new experiences. *Delmar/Cengage Learning*

they allow the child to develop self-reliance gradually? Is there an anxious parent who repeatedly warns the child about getting hurt?

The child's home may include an abusive parent. Child abuse is widespread; many abusive parents were themselves abused as children. The abuse may be physical, mental, or emotional. Mental and emotional abuse may be inflicted verbally (for example, with put-downs or guilt-arousing statements) or by specific actions (isolation, darkness). Physical abuse may be in the form of beatings or sexual activities. When a child is abused sexually, the abuser is most often a relative or family friend, someone the child trusts (or fears). All too often the abuser makes the child feel responsible for what happened; or the abuser convinces the child that the two of them have a secret that must not be shared with anyone. The abuser may even threaten to harm the child if this "secret" is revealed to anyone. The abused child has a heavy burden. In addition to physical trauma, the child has to deal with fear, anger, and guilt. And unless they get help, abused children may grow up to become abusive parents. This reflects the lifelong influence of adults on a child's future.

The child may belong to a minority group or be labeled "different" as a result of being the only individual of a particular culture in the peer group. If so, does the family maintain the lifestyle of the **ethnic** culture? How much rejection has the child experienced? Is the child's religion different from that of most classmates? What misunderstandings might this create?

What is the neighborhood environment? Is it safe or full of hazards for children? Are there opportunities for a wide variety of experiences? Are there relatives and neighbors who care about the child, or is the social climate of the neighborhood hostile? Are the parents from another country? If so, do they require the child to behave in ways appropriate for that country, but inappropriate in the present community?

Role models are powerful influences on children. Every adult in a child's world has the potential to serve as a role model, whether they be within the home (immediate or extended family), the neighborhood, the church, or at school. Role models influence children in many ways—value system, parenting style, career choice. The role model's influence may be positive or negative. It may last a lifetime or it may be temporary. A child may have only one role model or may adopt different role models at various life stages. An adult may even be unaware that he is serving as a role model for a specific child.

## CHANGING INFLUENCES DURING LIFE

Early learnings continue to influence behavior throughout life, often without the individual's awareness. On the other hand, one can learn to recognize certain early influences on behavior and, where desirable, modify the behavior patterns that have resulted. *Whereas a child is the helpless victim of developmental influences, an adult can become self-directing.* The adult can recognize an undesirable behavior pattern and choose to change it. An adult can seek to understand the basis for a particular behavior and, with such understanding, resist or eliminate that early influence. An adult can leave an unhealthy situation and seek a more favorable environment. These options are not available to a child, who is trapped in a specific living situation. It is now acknowledged that many runaway children are trying to escape abusive home situations.

### Modifying Early Learnings

Prejudice is one example of early learning that can influence a person's behavior throughout life unless the individual chooses to examine behavior patterns and their apparent origins. Prejudice is usually learned early in life from those people around us. In its most common form, prejudice consists of negative feelings toward people from a different race or subculture. If parents and their friends speak in unkind terms about members of another race, the child is influenced to develop negative feelings also. The child may exhibit hostility or disrespect toward members of another race. As adults, however, we do not have to cling to such early learnings. We can re-examine our attitudes in light of new knowledge and personal experience. Often, we find that our prejudice does not hold up against rational examination. *As adults, we can modify early learnings and take control of our own behavior, attitudes, and beliefs.*

An example of unexamined prejudice is the behavior of people who belong to one of the "hate groups." The leaders of such groups depend on "us versus them" thinking to arouse strong feelings and mobilize people to behave as the leaders wish them to behave. Televised reports of demonstrations show people who are controlled by their emotions, rather than by clear thinking. And those emotions probably have their roots in early learnings that have not been re-examined during adulthood. People who blindly accept the hate policies of a group, or even of a government, are allowing others to do their thinking, determine their beliefs, and control their behavior. *Throughout adult life, one should continuously evaluate and modify beliefs and value systems.*

**FIGURE 4-4** Having a variety of interests helps in forming effective relations with different people. *Delmar/Cengage Learning*

## Interests

Interests also influence behavior. They determine where we direct our attention. They even enter into the decisions we make, the activities we pursue, the occupations we choose, and the types of recreation we select for our leisure time. People who have many interests are well prepared for forming effective relationships with a variety of people (Figure 4-4). Those who have only their work and hours of television-watching do not have much to offer others in the way of interesting companionship. Developing a variety of interests is one way to become a more interesting person, find greater satisfaction in living, and form satisfying relationships.

## Value Systems

A value system is the degree of importance we attach (largely unconsciously) to various beliefs, ideas, or material things. Each person's value system has a strong influence on behavior. Each of us has a value system, even though we may not be conscious of it. Did you give up going to a movie in order to do an assignment for today? Then you placed a higher value on some aspect of being a student—responsibility, achievement, or perhaps duty—than you did on recreation, at least as far as this one sample of your behavior is concerned. Did you return the extra dime you received as change at the grocery store? Then you placed a higher value on honesty than on "getting the best of the other fellow." Did you cheat on that last test in order to improve your grade? Then you placed a higher value on a grade than on honesty or true learning.

The value system includes many things: character traits such as honesty and truthfulness, personal achievement, the symbols of achievement, love and friendship, material possessions, religion, recreation, work, and family living. Each person's value system begins to form early in life, influenced by the rewards or punishments that followed specific types of behavior. Throughout life, the value system exerts a powerful influence on behavior, particularly when there is a choice to be made. Your enrollment in this educational program indicates that you value education enough to attend classes and do your assignments.

## Standards of Behavior

Standards of behavior consist of our own personal rules and regulations, our own "dos" and "don'ts," that are part of our self-concept. There is a close relationship between one's value system and one's standards of behavior. They are both learned early in life and continually modified according to life experiences.

Standards of behavior should never be modified impulsively, especially if it involves lowering one's standards. Teenagers are often subjected to pressure from their friends to abandon home teachings and adopt the group's code of behavior. This can be a difficult decision for a young person, since peer acceptance is very important during adolescence. Sometimes, as an adult who is dealing with a difficult decision, one needs to examine *consciously* the standards of behavior, values, and beliefs that usually control one's behavior. Identification of these influences may facilitate making a decision. Or becoming clear about these influences may result in modifying a certain value or belief and the specific behavior that it supports.

There is a difference between current standards and those of the previous generation. Standards of behavior, therefore, are a frequent source of misunderstanding between parents and adolescents. There are also wide differences in standards of behavior from one subculture to another. Standards of behavior, including sexual behavior, vary between socioeconomic levels. Middle-class families tend to have the most rigid codes of behavior. Yet even within a particular socioeconomic level, there are wide variations from one family to another.

## Sleep and Nutrition

Our behavior is also influenced by whether we get sufficient sleep and appropriate nutrition. The need for sleep is discussed in greater detail in Unit 5. In short, insufficient sleep weakens the immune system, affects mood, and inhibits our ability to think clearly. You have likely noticed that you (or your family members) tend to be more short-tempered or accident-prone when you have not had enough sleep. Similarly, eating nutritious food without artificial colors or preservatives has been found to have a positive behavioral effect, particularly in children.

## ASSUMING RESPONSIBILITY FOR BEHAVIOR

You should now be aware that human personality is the result of many ingredients. It is continuously molded by the environment and by life experiences. It is always subject to further change as a result of future life situations.

As children, our early learnings were determined by circumstances beyond our control. As adults, we have a choice. We can continue to live without consciously directing our lives, or we can take control. We can foster certain aspects of our personalities and play down other aspects. We can learn to make sound decisions. We can learn to recognize ineffective behaviors that may prevent us from reaching our goals. Thus, we can become relatively self-directing instead of living by patterns of thought and behavior established during childhood. Even more important, as adults we can think through various issues, decide what our values are, set our own standards of behavior, and accept or reject the values and standards proposed to us by others.

## THE HEALTH CARE PROVIDER AND THE PATIENT

As a health care provider, you will find great satisfaction in your work if you make a conscious and continuous effort to study behavior—your own and that of other people. You will be meeting people from many different backgrounds. With some, it will be easy to establish a pleasant relationship, one in which the patient believes that *you understand* and that *you are sincerely concerned* (Figure 4-5). Such a relationship is called **rapport.**

There will be some patients with whom you find it difficult to communicate. Perhaps the patient's behavior arouses unfavorable feelings in you. Perhaps you just do not find the patient "interesting" as a person. Such a patient is likely to perceive you as "indifferent" or "cold." As long as this climate exists between you and the patient, rapport will not be established. It is easy to project blame or label the patient "difficult." The patient's behavior, however, may be a reaction to your unconscious rejection of the patient.

Any patient who has been labeled "difficult" needs special attention from the health team. The behaviors that cause the patient to be labeled "difficult" may actually be signs that the patient's needs are not being met. But, on the other hand, the pleasant, agreeable patient may be covering up true feelings and may have just as much need for understanding and

**FIGURE 4-5** Accept each patient in accordance with his stage of development. *Delmar/Cengage Learning*

concern. In other words, as a health care provider, you will need to apply interpersonal skills to *establish rapport with each patient* as an individual. Some patients will be more of a challenge than others, but all need your understanding and sincere interest if you are to make a positive contribution to their health care.

## REFERENCES AND SUGGESTED READINGS

Human Genome Program. (2008). *About the human genome project.* Retrieved from http://www.ornl.gov/sci/techresources/Human Genome/project/about.shtml

National Center for Children in Poverty. (2009). *Child poverty.* Retrieved from http://www.nccp.org/topics/childpoverty.html

National Institutes of Health. (2009). *Genetics home reference.* Retrieved from http://ghr.nlm.nih.gov/

U.S. Dept. of Health and Human Services. (2009). *Healthy pregnancy.* Retrieved from http://www.womenshealth.gov/pregnancy/

Van Hulle, Carol, et al. (2009, Nov.). Developmental structure of genetic influences on antisocial behavior across childhood and adolescence. *Journal of Abnormal Psychology, 118*(4), 711–722.

van Wormer, Katherine, et al. (2007). *Human behavior and the social environment, macro level: Groups, communities, and organizations.* New York: Oxford University Press.

Zallen, Doris T. (2008). *To test or not to test: A guide to genetic screening and risk.* Piscataway, NJ: Rutgers University Press.

## REVIEW AND SELF-CHECK

1. List five ways that people are alike.

    _____
    _____
    _____
    _____
    _____

2. Define the following in your own words:

    Chromosome _____

    Dominant _____

    Heredity _____

    Gene _____

    Recessive _____

    Sex-linked trait _____

3. List five factors related to genes that determine if a particular trait will be inherited.

4. Name the four dimensions of the developmental process.

5. What are the two types of environment that influence a child's development?

6. Name three important influences on development during childhood.

7. Name three learnings during early childhood that will later influence adult behavior.

8. Explain how one's interests influence behavior.

9. What is the primary influence of one's value system on behavior?

## ASSIGNMENTS

The following exercises are designed to give you an opportunity to apply some of the ideas discussed in Unit 4.

1. Using the following format, develop your family genetic chart as a guide to the possible contributions of heredity to your present and future health. Add additional lines as needed to list all members of your extended family. Add any cousins who have significant health problems, birthmarks, or congenital conditions.

| Relation | Current Age or Age at Death | Cause of Death | Health Problems |
|---|---|---|---|
| Father | | | |
| Grandfather | | | |
| Grandmother | | | |
| Uncles | | | |
| Aunts | | | |
| Mother | | | |
| Grandfather | | | |
| Grandmother | | | |
| Uncles | | | |
| Aunts | | | |
| Sisters | | | |
| Brothers | | | |

2. Mary grew up in a home where standards of behavior were quite rigid. Her requests for permission to do something were often met with the question, "What would people think?" As an adult, Mary often feels anxiety about the opinions of others.

   You, too, are affected in many ways by early learnings. List five learnings from your own childhood that still influence your behavior.

3. Refer to the list you made in Assignment 2. Which of these early learnings are no longer appropriate guides to your behavior? State why they are no longer appropriate.

4. List 10 things that are important to you. Number them from 1 to 10 in order of importance—*1* being most important and *10* least important. Describe a decision that may be influenced by this order of values. If you logged your daily activities in Unit 1, refer back to your log. Are you spending your time on the things you listed as most important?

5. Joan is hopeful that she will be admitted to a dental assistant educational program next month. Joan's mother wants her to take a secretarial course. How can Joan consciously use her interests and value system to make a choice that is in her own best interest?

6. List five of your interests. State how each interest will be helpful to you as a health care provider.

7. Review the list of interests you made for Assignment 6. Estimate the amount of time you have spent on each interest during the past seven days.

   a. Place a star by those interests to which you have devoted as much as five hours. (Reading assignments for your health occupations course do not count as evidence of reading as one of your interests!)

   b. Place an "X" by those interests about which you are sufficiently informed to carry on a conversation with someone who is knowledgeable on that subject.

   c. Evaluate your interests in terms of variety, keeping in mind that it is not really one of your interests *unless you devote time to it and are informed about it.*

   d. Select one activity for increasing the breadth of your interests. Plan how you will learn about this activity and develop the skills of that activity during the next six months.

8. Prepare a written plan for improving your ability to establish rapport with patients. The instructor will tell you how this plan is to be evaluated.

9. If one of your parents died at age 42 of a disorder that is known to be genetic, would you choose to have genetic testing to determine if you have the gene for that disorder? Yes or no?

   a. Write a brief explanation for your answer.

   b. If the test result is positive, what is the likely effect of that information on your life?

# UNIT 5

# Physical Needs

## OBJECTIVES

Upon completion of this unit, you should be able to:

- List the five levels of human needs as proposed by Maslow.
- Explain why Maslow stated these needs as a hierarchy.
- List and explain four influences on the formation of behavior patterns.
- List five physical needs that are essential to survival.
- Explain the effect of need-satisfaction on behavior.
- State two reasons that responsible behavior includes practicing safe sex.

## KEY TERMS

| | | |
|---|---|---|
| Biorhythms | Dehydration | Necrosis |
| Circadian rhythms | Dependency | REM sleep |
| Compensation | Hierarchy | Sleep debt |
| Consequences | Melatonin | Suffocation |

All of us have certain basic needs. In having such needs and inner forces that drive us to satisfy these needs, we are all alike. In the ways we attempt to satisfy these needs, we are all different. We are also different in the goals we set. What satisfies one person does not satisfy another. The tremendous variability in human behavior patterns makes the study of human behavior a continuing challenge.

Psychologists and sociologists engaged in the study of human behavior have described these needs in various ways. The most useful approach for our purpose is the model provided by psychologist Abraham Maslow. This model is known as Maslow's Hierarchy of Needs (Figure 5-1). The term **hierarchy** means arranged in a specific order or rank.

## MASLOW'S HIERARCHY OF NEEDS

In Maslow's hierarchy, human needs for survival are primary; the need for safety is secondary. Following in sequence are needs related to love and belonging, the need for esteem, and the need for self-actualization. These five levels of human needs are shown in hierarchical arrangement in Figure 5-1.

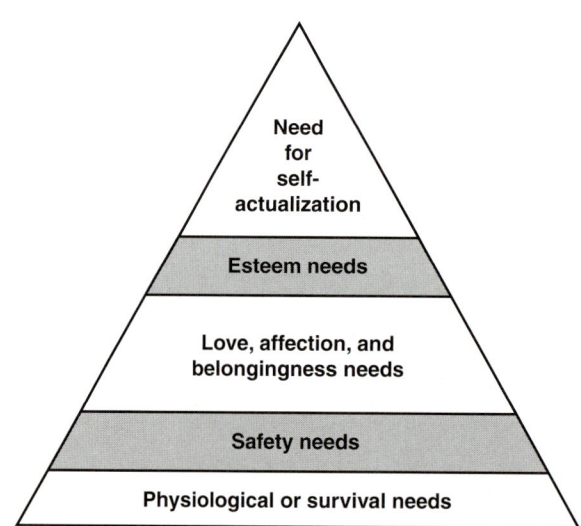

**FIGURE 5-1** Maslow's hierarchy of needs. *Delmar/Cengage Learning*

Each level of need must be satisfied before an individual is ready to strive for satisfaction of the next higher level of need. The highest level refers to full development of one's human potential. The remainder of Section II will focus on needs relevant to the first four levels. Unit 5 is devoted to the physical needs, which are related to levels 1 and 2.

## ESSENTIAL PHYSICAL NEEDS

Some physical needs are essential to life; others contribute to comfort and satisfaction. The physical needs that are essential to life are oxygen, water, food, protection, and sleep. These needs are not only essential to the life of the total organism, but also to the survival of individual cells. For example, a body part that does not receive a continuous supply of oxygen and nourishment will die. If this body part is a vital organ, then the individual will also die. If, however, the body part is a finger, the affected finger can be surgically removed and the individual will survive, minus the finger. Death of tissues in a limited area is called **necrosis.** It is usually due to lack of an adequate blood supply that deprives the cells of oxygen and nourishment. As you work in the health field, you may see patients with necrosis of some body part or area.

### Importance of Oxygen

The physical need for oxygen pertains to every cell in the body. Submersion of the face in water for more than a few minutes can result in death due to drowning. Although some people have been resuscitated after about 20 minutes under water, in such cases there is serious risk of permanent brain damage, because the brain needs a continuous supply of oxygen. If deprivation of oxygen is due to the face being covered, as in a cave-in, the death is called a **suffocation.** Accidental drowning or suffocation may be the result of carelessness, failure to use appropriate precautions (e.g., not wearing a life jacket when going out in a boat), or inappropriate sleeping arrangements (in the case of a baby). Because of so many instances of crib death, it is now considered safer to place babies on their backs to protect against suffocation. Remember the motto, "Back to sleep."

## Importance of Water

The body must have adequate water for various functions, preferably at least eight glasses of water each day. Water provides liquid and is the carrier for various nutrients that cannot be digested and absorbed without a liquid medium. Drinks such as tea and coffee, and especially soft drinks, do not contribute to this basic need for water.

When the body does not receive adequate water each day, chronic **dehydration** develops and certain body functions are affected. When the body loses water, as through diarrhea, persistent vomiting, or high fever, dehydration develops. Severe dehydration leads to an imbalance in body chemistry, a life-threatening condition. In hospitals, intravenous fluids are used for patients who cannot drink enough fluids to prevent dehydration. Persons who are stranded where there is no water available, as in a desert, can survive only about six or seven days. For this reason, survival training includes learning how to extract water from plants and use liquids from other sources to maintain life until rescued. Sometimes it is hunger rather than thirst that signals the body's need for water.

## Importance of Food

Because of its ability to store food in various tissues and organs, the body can survive lack of food for longer periods of time than it can survive lack of oxygen or water. Prolonged lack of food results in stored nutrients being used for basic metabolic processes and for the energy needed for physical activities. Even thinking requires energy! Muscle movement requires a lot of energy. If lack of food continues, tissues shrink and body wasting occurs. When body reserves have been exhausted, death occurs due to starvation.

Regular intake of food, then, is essential for providing the body with the nutrients needed to carry out metabolic processes, build and repair tissues, and produce energy for various activities. The nutrients needed include proteins, fats, carbohydrates, vitamins, minerals, amino acids, and essential fatty acids. Optimal health requires that *all* of these nutrients be included in one's daily diet, since even a slight deficiency of certain nutrients results in less efficient body functions.

Even more significant, a slight deficiency in certain nutrients, especially vitamins, minerals, and amino acids, can lead to symptoms. For example, a prolonged clotting time or a tendency to bruise easily may indicate a serious health problem or may simply indicate that the individual needs additional vitamin C or vitamin K. A deficiency of magnesium can result in a cardiac arrhythmia that may be misdiagnosed as a heart disorder. There is currently a trend in health care to acknowledge the relationship of certain nutrients to specific body functions. (This will be discussed further in Section VII.) Health care providers should become informed about nutrients in order to protect their own personal health and that of their families. Sometimes it may be appropriate to suggest dietary changes to a friend or patient or recommend a consultation with a nutritionist.

## Importance of Protection

In its broadest sense, protection includes the safety and security of having a home that protects one from the elements, using safety precautions to avoid accidents, having a lifestyle that includes healthful eating and drinking clean water, avoiding exposure to extremes of heat and cold, and avoiding substances that can harm the body.

Commonsense measures, such as avoiding times and places where one might be attacked and practicing safe driving, can decrease the likelihood of a serious accident or traumatic experience. Small children, especially, need protection against a variety of hazards in the community and in the home. It is a responsibility of adults to "child-proof" the home, so that children do not have access to household cleaners, medicines, and other harmful substances. Adults have a responsibility to provide safe and healthful lifestyles for themselves and their children.

## Importance of Sleep

Sleep is essential to life and health, but people are more inclined to deprive themselves of sleep than of water, food, and air. The body's demand for sleep can be resisted, or even ignored, more easily than hunger, thirst, and the need for air. Of the various aspects of lifestyle that are *essential* to health, recent research indicates that sleep ranks third, behind diet and exercise.

Although individual needs for sleep vary, the average person needs one hour of sleep for every two hours of wakefulness. Sleep needs are biologically determined; a person who needs 10 hours of sleep is not "lazy" and will be healthier if that need is respected. On the other hand, persons who claim to need only a few hours of sleep per night place their health at risk. Some researchers believe that loss of sleep contributes to at least one-third of all accidents, decreases efficiency, and increases a person's tendency to anger and violence.

## THE SLEEP CYCLE

Numerous body functions involve specific rhythms or cycles, known collectively as **biorhythms.** The frequency of these rhythms ranges from fractions of a second to months or years; **circadian rhythms** are based on the 24-hour period that makes up one day. The need for sleep is regulated by the brain's circadian pacemaker, influenced by the earth's electromagnetic fields. As the sun sinks in the sky, daylight shifts to dusk and then to darkness. This shift in light signals the pineal gland in the brain to secrete **melatonin,** the hormone that causes us to yawn and our eyelids to become heavy. As the level of melatonin increases, one finds it more and more difficult to stay awake. Eventually, the individual falls asleep, even if trying hard to stay awake. This is a natural rhythm that represents the body's response to decreasing light and the body's inherent need for sleep to round out the 24-hour period.

Sleep consists of two phases that alternate throughout the sleep period: **REM** (rapid eye movement) **sleep** and non-REM sleep. The latter phase is a period when most body processes slow down, the muscles are relaxed, and the eyes are relatively still. This phase includes four stages of progressively deeper sleep. Following a complete cycle of the four stages, the REM phase begins. In this phase, there is an increase in mental activity, dreaming occurs concurrently with bursts of rapid eye movement, breathing is irregular, and pulse and blood pressure rise and fall. In normal young adults, the first non-REM phase lasts about 90 minutes and is followed by about 15 minutes of REM sleep. The frequency and duration of REM sleep periods increase during the final hours of sleep, especially between the sixth and eighth hours.

The dreaming that occurs during REM sleep is thought to be a major factor in stress management. The entire sleep period is a time when the brain cleanses itself of the day's accumulated sensory input and prepares for the next day's mental activity; it is also the time when the brain replenishes its stock of neurotransmitters. Although people vary in the amount of sleep they need to awaken rested and refreshed, less than eight hours of sleep deprives the body of some periods of REM sleep. Research conducted in sleep laboratories has revealed that deprivation of REM sleep has the same effects as sleep deprivation.

### Effects of Sleep Deprivation

After the loss of one night of sleep, a person has poor concentration and coordination; usually irritability is increased. Anyone who is deprived of sleep for several days will experience hallucinations and exhibit psychotic behavior.

Sleep deprivation is an increasing problem in American society. The temptations of late-night television and the lure of the Internet are causing large numbers of people to get as little as two or three hours of sleep per night. Eventually, continued sleep deprivation will exact a price.

### Sleep Debt

Chronic loss of sleep, called **sleep debt,** may affect as many as two-thirds of the adults in the United States, but that estimate does not include the adolescents who are watching late-night television or surfing the Internet instead of going to bed. Supervisors know that workers who are sleep-deprived do not perform well and are more likely to commit errors. Traffic engineers know that many automobile accidents result from a driver falling asleep. Now medical researchers are finding evidence that sleep deprivation weakens the immune system, increasing one's susceptibility to infections. Some researchers suspect that chronic lack of sleep contributes to the current epidemic of obesity and diabetes, and may even be a factor in the increasing rates of cancer. As a health care provider, you need to understand that the sleep cycle is an essential part of one's 24-hour day.

Some health care providers work a double shift; those who regularly work the night shift may experience 24- to 30-hour periods without sleep before or after their days off. These people should make a special effort to ensure adequate sleep and rest, for both personal health and avoidance of errors due to fatigue and lack of sleep.

## SATISFACTION OF PHYSICAL NEEDS

The physical needs have an important characteristic that sets them apart from psychological needs—*they can be satisfied in only one way.* An abundant supply of oxygen cannot make up for a lack of food. Abundant food stored within body tissues cannot provide survival for the worker who has just been buried in a cave-in and has no supply of oxygen. The need for sleep can be satisfied only by sleeping; though eating may enable one to delay going to sleep, food cannot satisfy the body's need for sleep. *Each essential physical need can be met only by a specific substance or condition.* Neither substitution nor **compensation** is possible. This will become more meaningful as we explore comfort needs in the next section and the social and emotional needs of people in the following topics.

## COMFORT AND SAFETY NEEDS

There are also physical needs that are highly desirable but not essential to life. These needs are related to comfort and a sense of well-being. Labor-saving devices, soundly built homes, running water, comfortable clothing, and automatic heat seem like essential needs to those who are accustomed to them. Though some of these comforts are not essential for survival, they do meet safety needs and contribute to health and well-being.

The satisfaction of sexual needs falls into two categories: emotional needs and physical needs. Intimacy can contribute to a sense of belonging—an especially important need of adolescents. Sexual activity was formerly considered an adult activity, but currently many young people—adolescents and children—are sexually active. This is an issue for families and individuals to address in terms of beliefs and standards of behavior. The issue of *responsibility*, however, extends beyond the family to the larger community because of health issues and the risk of pregnancies that produce children who are unwanted or whose parents cannot or will not provide for them.

Anyone who is sexually active, regardless of age, should practice safe sex. For young people who are not prepared to assume adult responsibilities of parenting (which includes financial support), prevention of pregnancy requires the use of protection. For everyone who is sexually active but is not in a stable, one-partner relationship, responsibility means protecting oneself against sexually transmitted diseases. Safe sex, then, has two very important purposes: (1) avoidance of an unwanted pregnancy and (2) prevention of a sexually transmitted disease. Although both sexes are affected, it is the female whose life is most likely to be disrupted by the results of unprotected sex.

## PHYSICAL NEEDS AND BEHAVIOR

Each person has specific ways for trying to meet needs. The baby cries when hungry but is dependent on others to provide nourishment. Throughout childhood each of us learned which behaviors were successful or unsuccessful in meeting our needs within the home and in the subculture. *The child tends to repeat any behavior that results in satisfaction of a need and to abandon behaviors that do not get results.* Behavior patterns are established on the basis of **consequences**—what happens following a specific behavior.

### Cultural Influences

A city person purchases food at the grocery store but is dependent upon a complex system of marketing and distribution to keep a supply available. A rural person may purchase only staples and depend on a garden and livestock to provide most of the family's food. A rural family living at a subsistence level may depend upon hunting or fishing for food. A family living in poverty in a large city may depend upon the welfare department for food. The pattern of striving that is learned from childhood on is influenced by the customs and practices of the family, neighborhood, and community. The pattern of striving is also influenced by individual factors, such as the desire to obtain the comforts of life and the value placed on conforming to group standards.

### Self-Reliance versus Dependency

Some people are largely self-reliant in obtaining food, clothing, and shelter. Some people depend on others to provide their basic needs. **Dependency** may involve so much of the person's life that any change is extremely upsetting. The farm wife whose husband is hospitalized with a serious illness may seem to you to be unnecessarily upset. Actually she is realizing that unless her husband recovers in time to plant or harvest the crops, their family will be without

FIGURE 5-2 Our life situation influences behavioral patterns for meeting basic needs. *Delmar/Cengage Learning*

income for a year. Patient and family reactions to illness are closely tied to the role of each member and their life situation.

## UNDERSTANDING BEHAVIOR IN TERMS OF PHYSICAL NEEDS

There are certain physical needs that people must meet in order to survive. There are other needs that make people more comfortable or free them from routine tasks so they may do other things that are more satisfying. In having these needs, people are alike. In the specific ways they strive to meet these needs, people are different. But each person strives in ways that have been learned by imitating members of one's subculture and from personal experiences (Figure 5-2). Each person tends to repeat the behavior that has been successful in satisfying a particular need. This repetition becomes established as a behavior pattern.

Most people meet their needs in ways acceptable within the laws, customs, and religious beliefs of their group. Some people choose or are forced by circumstances to violate the laws or customs of the group in order to satisfy their needs. These people too may be striving in their own way—the only way they know. Here, too, the health care provider's philosophy of individual worth can be applied to understanding, rather than judging, a patient.

## REFERENCES AND SUGGESTED READINGS

Babson, Kimberly, et al. (2009, Sept.). An experimental investigation of the effects of acute sleep deprivation on panic-relevant biological challenge responding. *Behavior Therapy, 40*(3), 239–251.

Lara-Carrasco, Jessica, et al. (2009, June). Overnight emotional adaptation to negative stimuli is altered by REM sleep deprivation and is correlated with intervening dream emotions. *Journal of Sleep Research, 18*(2), 178–187.

Schmutte, Denise. (2006). Maslow's hierarchy of needs. In Kristine Krapp (Ed.), *The Gale encyclopedia of nursing and allied health* (Vol. 3, pp. 1500–1503). Farmington Hills, MI: Gale, Cengage Learning.

Tamparo, Carol D., & Lindh, Wilburta Q. (2008). Overview of Abraham Maslow's humanistic psychology. In *Therapeutic communications for health professionals* (3rd ed., p. 233). Clifton Park, NY: Delmar, Cengage Learning.

## SOURCE OF ADDITIONAL INFORMATION

National Sleep Foundation 1522 K Street, NW, Suite 500, Washington, DC, 20005, http://www.sleepfoundation.org

## REVIEW AND SELF-CHECK

1. List the five levels of human needs in Maslow's hierarchy.

2. Explain why Maslow arranged these various needs as a hierarchy.

3. List four major influences on the formation of behavior patterns.

4. List five physical needs that are essential to survival.

5. Explain the effect of need-satisfaction on behavior.

6. State two reasons why responsible behavior includes the practice of safe sex.

## ASSIGNMENTS

1. In your mind, review some early influences in your life that shaped the patterns of behavior you now use to meet your physical needs. Do your patterns reflect dependence on others? Or self-reliance? How would these patterns be affected if you should become disabled? Visualize yourself in such a situation. How might your reaction to this forced change be reflected in your behavior?

2. If you have ever experienced any of the following, describe how it affected you physically, mentally, and emotionally:

    a. Difficulty in getting air for several minutes

    b. No water (or any other beverage) for eight hours

    c. No way to obtain food for two days

    d. Exposure to severe weather, without any way to get to shelter for several hours

    e. Deprivation of sleep for 36 hours

3. Think of a situation in your community where someone drowned. Using all the information available to your class, discuss the circumstances and identify actions someone (including the victim) could have taken in advance to prevent this drowning.

4. You know that there is a cave in some woods near your home and several children play in the cave. How could you, as a health care provider, assume the leadership in determining if there is danger of these children getting trapped in a cave-in?

5. Think about your usual sleep pattern. How many hours do you sleep on weeknights? On Saturday nights? On Sunday nights? If you are sleeping less than eight hours each night:

    a. List reasons that you stay up too late to get a full night's sleep.

    b. List reasons you get up before you have had eight hours of sleep.

6. Describe how you feel when the alarm clock goes off and you have to get up, even though you are still sleepy.

7. If you average less than eight hours of sleep each night, list changes in your habits or lifestyle that would enable you to get more sleep.

8. Participate in a class discussion about the importance of safe sex from the standpoint of:

    a. Adolescent boys

    b. Adolescent girls

    c. Parents of a girl between the ages of 10 and 18

    d. Parents of a boy between the ages of 10 and 18

9. Consider the implications of safe sex for you personally.

10. Consider the implications of safe sex for you as a health care provider.

UNIT

# The Need for Self-Approval

## OBJECTIVES

Upon completion of this unit, you should be able to:

- Explain social needs.
- Describe three important influences on one's self-concept.
- Compare self-concept and self-esteem.
- Explain the influence of success and failure experiences on self-concept and self-esteem.
- Describe the relationship between "success expectation" and "performance."
- List two essential steps for modifying a habit.
- List six steps of the problem-solving process.

## KEY TERMS

| | | |
|---|---|---|
| Appraisal | Autonomy | Derogatory |
| Aptitudes | Compensation | Hindrance |

In the previous unit, you learned about influences on the ways people strive to meet their physical needs. There are other human needs that are just as important to comfort and happiness as physical needs. These other needs are also powerful influences on behavior, but they are less obvious than the physical needs. This unit will help you learn about social and psychological needs.

## SOCIAL NEEDS OF PEOPLE

For the most part, physical needs can be met either alone or in the company of others. However, sharing with others is more satisfying than meeting these needs alone (Figure 6-1). You enjoy your dinner more if you have pleasant companionship than if you eat alone or in the company of someone you dislike. When physical needs and social needs are met simultaneously, enjoyment is greater and there is more likely to be a sense of well-being.

A social need involves relationships with other people. As used here, "social" does not mean "socializing." Socializing is participating in recreational activities with other people.

FIGURE 6-1 Basic physical needs can be met by the self alone. Basic social needs require satisfying relationships. *Delmar/Cengage Learning*

## Types of Social Needs

There are many different kinds of social needs: psychological, emotional, intellectual, spiritual, diversional, and recreational. These terms overlap, because each term refers to groups of needs that are closely related.

Some social needs can be partially met alone, but relationships with other people are necessary for full satisfaction. For example, the person who enjoys studying a subject can partially meet intellectual needs alone. Greater satisfaction might be experienced, however, if there are opportunities to discuss the subject with others who share the same interest. *Satisfying relationships with other people lead to full satisfaction of the social needs.*

Some social needs are related to the self; other needs are related to contact with other people. Each of us needs to feel important as a person, to have a sense of achievement, and to feel worthy. We also need to feel that we are important to others, that other people approve of us, and that we are accepted as a member of the group. These two sets of needs are closely tied together, for feelings and beliefs about oneself affect acceptance by others.

## Compensation

You have learned that each of the physical needs can be met only in a specific way. With the social needs, a type of substitution known as **compensation** is possible. *Compensation does not satisfy a basic need.* It is a device that provides temporary relief from the discomfort felt when a basic social need is not being met (Figure 6-2).

Do you know a person who habitually talks loudly, tends to brag, is a showoff, or dresses in loud clothes? Is this person popular? Is this person accepted by the group? Probably not, for these are attention-seeking behaviors. For some people it is better to be noticed, even disapprovingly, than to be ignored. Behavior that gets attention can relieve the inner discomfort of being ignored. Attention-seeking behavior is an example of compensation. This behavior temporarily relieves inner discomfort and gains attention from the group. Obtaining approval meets a basic need; getting attention compensates for not gaining approval. People who compensate are usually unaware that they are getting temporary relief from inner discomfort

**FIGURE 6-2** Compensation provides temporary relief when a basic social need is not being met. *Delmar/Cengage Learning*

instead of the full satisfaction that comes only from meeting basic social needs. Now that you have a general understanding of social needs and their importance, let us consider self-approval and its relationship to social needs.

## THE SELF-CONCEPT

Each of us has an image of "self." We think of ourselves as a certain kind of person, possessing specific characteristics. Self-concept may be thought of as all the things a person thinks are true about the self. It is a mental image of "me."

A particular person's self-concept may be realistic or unrealistic. Suppose Joe thinks of himself as an honest person, yet he takes advantage of any situation in which he can gain something, regardless of whether it is honest or dishonest. Joe's concept of "Honest Joe" is not in agreement with his behavior when he is acting like "Joe the Cheat." Jim, on the other hand, thinks of himself as just an average guy, whereas his teachers see him as a person with exceptional ability. Neither man has a realistic self-concept.

### Behavior as an Indicator of the Self-Concept

The person with a realistic self-concept thinks of the self in terms that are consistent with behavior. Usually, behavior is an accurate indicator of a person's self-concept. Joe's behavior indicates that he is not honest, but if Joe's self-concept includes honesty as an attribute, then his behavior and his self-concept are not consistent. Which reflects the real Joe?

Behavior is not always an accurate indicator of a person's true characteristics. Behavior may not be consistent with a person's beliefs and values. Suppose a person in the health field talks about the philosophy of individual worth and treats all patients courteously and with impartial efficiency, yet actually has strong prejudice against members of certain groups. This prejudice may not be revealed in day-to-day behavior but would be reflected in an important decision. Such a person's public self—the self revealed to others—is inconsistent with the private self, the self known only to the individual.

## A Realistic Self-Concept

The person who has a realistic self-concept is able to be honest about the real self. Such a person's behavior accurately reflects the person's own beliefs, values, and standards.

The person whose self-concept is unrealistic is not ready to set goals for personal growth until the self-concept has been revised. "What is" must be acknowledged before considering "what can be." An unrealistic self-concept may be either idealized or self-derogatory.

For example, Crystal has great difficulty with high school subjects, but thinks of herself as a person who can do anything she attempts. Her ambition is to be a scientist. Crystal's *idealized self-concept* may trap her into setting goals that she cannot achieve. In contrast, Crystal's friend, Erica, is an excellent student but lacks self-confidence. Erica has an older sister who is a good student, is very pretty, and sings extremely well. Erica does not seem to have any artistic talent. She is average in appearance. Because she has always compared herself unfavorably with her sister, Erica thinks of herself as a second-rate person, yet she has tremendous potential and can probably succeed in any field of study she undertakes. Erica has a **derogatory** *self-concept,* meaning that she is overly critical of herself and does not fully recognize her abilities and talents. Unless Erica revises her self-perception, she may settle for goals less challenging than those she could achieve.

## Formation of the Self-Concept

The self-concept begins to form at a very early age and is well established by about age 6. It can be modified later in life, but only with conscious effort over a period of time. The self-concept is greatly affected by all life experiences, but it is most susceptible to the influence of other people *during the early formative years and during adolescence.* The young child's relationships with other people establish the early pattern. Is the child considered a person with rights and feelings? Many adults demand expressions of courtesy from a child, yet fail to use courteous behavior toward the child. The old saying "Children are to be seen and not heard" reflects an attitude that children are not really worthy as persons, that what a child thinks and says is not important enough for an adult to hear.

A positive self-concept develops if the young child has positive experiences and positive verbal interactions with the important adults of his or her social environment:

> *"You are sweet."*
> *"I love you."*
> *"You are so strong."*
> *"You are special."*
> *"It's fun being with you."*
> *"I like for you to ask questions."*

A busy adult may forget to tell a child that he is loved and is important. A child needs to hear such positive statements in order to think of "me" as one who is loved and is important to other people. Children also need positive nonverbal messages: hugs and kisses, a squeeze of the hand, a pat on the shoulder, and other appropriate forms of touch. The most important message is conveyed through time spent with the child, time in which the child is the primary focus of a parent's attention. Working parents should plan for quality time with the child each day—reading, playing, walking, and talking. The amount of time is less important than the quality.

The form of discipline used with a child also has an extensive influence on the child's self-concept. If Greg is repeatedly told that he is a bad boy, he will begin to think of himself as being bad. Why should Greg try to be good if he has learned to think of himself as "bad" and believes that "everyone expects me to be bad"?

During adolescence, the peer group exerts a powerful influence on self-concept. Teens experience pressure to conform to the group's standards and values. Adolescents may label those who do not conform. A teenager must have a strong self-concept to resist those pressures, to stand up for personal beliefs and values, and at the same time gain acceptance from the peer group.

In these and many other ways, the people around a young child mold the developing child's self-concept. In the following sections, we will explore two aspects of personality development: self-reliance (a strong, capable person) or dependence (a weak, incompetent person who relies on others). Obviously, the tendency to remain dependent on others, versus the tendency to become progressively more self-reliant, influences a person's self-concept.

## Learning Independence

One of the most important aspects of development during childhood and adolescence is a gradual increase in independence, with less and less dependence on others. The need for self-reliance is an inborn force. Many infant behaviors reflect the need for this type of development: efforts at self-feeding, attempts to help with dressing and undressing, and attempts to "do it myself!" A child's angry reaction when an adult interferes in something the child is trying to do reflects this need for independence.

## Autonomy versus Dependence

The struggle between self-reliance and dependence on others continues throughout life. Each of us has a need for **autonomy,** the ability to function independently without outside control. No one ever achieves complete autonomy. We are social beings, and in many ways our welfare depends upon our being able to function as a member of the group. The mature person has learned to live harmoniously with his fellow man, functioning autonomously in many ways and accepting that dependence on others for some things is a matter of necessity.

Autonomy must be achieved over a period of time, by gradually learning to be self-reliant in the simple tasks of daily living (e.g., dressing and eating) and then progressing to self-reliance in more complex situations. It is impossible to be dependent on others throughout childhood and adolescence and then suddenly, at age 18 or 21, become a self-directing, autonomous adult. Effective parenting provides for the gradual development of independence throughout childhood by encouraging the child to do simple tasks. It also requires being available when help is requested or frustration becomes more than the child can handle.

This struggle for a compromise between autonomy and dependence reaches its peak during adolescence. The young person struggling for autonomy rebels against dependence on others. The parents may resent the young person's insistence on greater independence than they believe the child can handle. Young people who do not successfully resolve this conflict may carry the struggle for autonomy into adulthood, usually as rebellion toward any form of authority, such as the teacher or the "boss." You may find it interesting to study examples of rebellious behavior in terms of the struggle for autonomy.

The self-concept can be modified in adulthood, either by experiences that change one's perception of self or by a conscious approach to self-study. A realistic self-concept is based on thinking of oneself as a worthy person with a high level of capability for some activities, but not for others. You need to *accept yourself as a worthy person* before you will be able to make a constructive appraisal of your strengths and weaknesses.

## SELF-ESTEEM

Self-esteem refers to one's *feelings about self at a given moment* or period of time. Self-esteem is closely related to self-concept, but is not the same. Whereas self-concept is established during the early years and is relatively permanent, self-esteem is quite changeable and is affected by life experiences. A person's self-esteem may be high in the morning; then, some negative experience may plunge that person's self-esteem to a very low point. For most people, a period of low self-esteem is short-lived. If a negative experience, such as being unemployed, extends over a period of weeks, then self-esteem may remain low throughout that period. Effectively dealing with a life problem usually restores self-esteem to a high level. Good life experiences tend to maintain self-esteem at a high level, whereas negative experiences can lower a person's self-esteem (Figure 6-3).

**FIGURE 6-3** Illness and dependency are serious threats to an adult patient's self-esteem. *Delmar/Cengage Learning*

## INFLUENCE OF OTHERS ON ONE'S SENSE OF SELF

Other people have a strong influence on one's sense of self, beginning with the interactions of adults and the newborn baby. A sense of self-and-others begins to develop during infancy. The struggle for autonomy, "self" as separate from others, begins during the toddler stage, continues throughout childhood, and becomes intense during adolescence. During the infant and toddler periods, family members and caretakers influence the early sense of self. The child's exposure to the world widens with entry into preschool programs and school itself; from that time on, teachers and others make significant contributions to the formative sense of self. These early interactions help to establish the child's self-concept, which then acts as a sort of filter for the effects of later experiences and relationships.

The struggle for self-identity, a clarification of the "Who am I?" question, intensifies during adolescence and early adulthood. Dating and marriage introduce another influence, so powerful that it may lead to modification of some aspect of the self-concept. Any intimate relationship can have a powerful effect on one's self-concept, as well as day-by-day effects on self-esteem.

New social contacts and relationships influence one's feelings about self, and one's feelings about self affect relationships and social interactions. Communication style, a major component of one's behavior patterns, is so important that Section V consists of two units devoted to practicing effective communication, both verbal and nonverbal.

You should now become more aware of the role other persons play in determining how you feel about yourself at any given time. Your interactions with some people almost always make you feel good. Some people say and do things that make you feel good about yourself. Other people tend to have the opposite effect: they make put-down statements, are often critical, play the one-upmanship game, or otherwise have a diminishing effect on your sense of self. If there are many such people in your daily life, you are probably struggling to maintain a positive level of self-esteem. In order to correct the situation, you have certain choices:

1. Avoid such people.
2. Be assertive about not accepting negative statements.
3. Refuse to participate in their games.
4. Learn ways to respond to communications that have a negative effect on you.

Obviously, the first choice is not available to you if members of your family or your co-workers have a negative effect on you. In that case, you can begin to learn how to deal with such people through various activities, such as reading about effective relationships and participating in assertiveness training and communication skills workshops.

During the 1980s, some psychologists began to focus on differences in the way men and women communicate, the different values and expectations of the two sexes, and different emotional needs of men and women. As a result, many workshops and seminars on human relationships and family dynamics emphasize the need for men to understand the emotional needs and communication styles of women, and for women to understand that the emotional needs and communication styles of men differ from their own. By learning to relate to the other sex effectively, a person can not only be more effective in meeting the other's needs, but also achieve greater satisfaction of one's own needs.

Patricia Evans (2006), who works with abused women, describes the destructive effects derogatory statements can have on self-concept, gradually undermining self-confidence and fostering a growing belief in one's incompetence. In most cases, derogatory statements are made only in private; the abuser does not reveal to others the use of put-downs and criticism. When the woman begins to realize that she is being abused verbally, she cannot find understanding from friends or relatives because the abuser has not revealed this tendency to them. Not finding emotional support, and hearing from others that she should be thankful for such a wonderful relationship, simply increases her self-doubt and further erodes her self-concept.

Evans emphasizes that most verbally abused women *believe what the abuser says,* without considering that there is no real basis for the criticism, accusations, and put-downs. Any woman who suspects that she is being verbally abused should consult a professional counselor, rather than seek understanding from friends and relatives. A counselor can help restore her belief in herself and also help her learn ways to cope with the verbal abuse. Verbal abuse usually accelerates and eventually includes physical abuse, which the abuser always explains as being the woman's fault. Abusers are not likely to agree to marital counseling. Most abusers derive satisfaction from *having power over another person* and are not willing to work toward establishing a mutually fulfilling relationship.

In summary, positive relationships can help one to develop a strong self-concept and maintain high self-esteem most of the time. Negative relationships can have a destructive effect on self-concept and may result in a chronic state of low self-esteem.

## EFFECTS OF SUCCESS AND FAILURE

Have you ever had a task so difficult that you did not believe you could complete it? Perhaps it was a reading assignment that just did not make sense when you read it. Perhaps it was a written assignment, and you did not know how to proceed.

What was your approach to this task that appeared so hopeless? Did you pitch in, try your best, and find that you could do it, after all? How did you feel about your accomplishment? You should have felt good, for you overcame obstacles and successfully completed a difficult task. Each successful experience should be consciously recognized as a success. Each success should help you believe in *yourself as a person who can overcome obstacles.*

On the other hand, you may have found a particular task just as hard as you expected and were unable to complete it. No doubt you still have some negative feelings about this experience. Perhaps you were angry at yourself for not finishing it. Perhaps you were angry with the person who assigned the task to you. In either case, your self-confidence was threatened. You were discouraged and probably approached the next difficult task with greater self-doubt.

### Meaning of Failure Expectation

Discouragement and a sense of failure can be quite damaging to self-confidence, especially if experienced frequently. But this is only part of the problem. When failure occurs too frequently, there is a tendency to develop "failure expectation" (Figure 6-4). Each failure adds to self-doubt; self-doubt creates failure expectation; failure expectation interferes with performance (Figure 6-5). Thus, there is increased probability that the next task will result in another failure. If this cycle becomes well established, the individual may need professional help to break the pattern and believe in the possibility of future successful performances.

Unit 6: The Need for Self-Approval  81

**FIGURE 6-4** The failure-expectation cycle: Expectations can affect results. *Delmar/Cengage Learning*

**FIGURE 6-5** What if I strike out? *Delmar/Cengage Learning*

### Success Expectation

For most people, however, the problem is lack of self-confidence rather than an established failure expectation. Self-confidence might be thought of as "success expectation." The key to building self-confidence is conscious recognition of each successful experience, with awareness that life includes both successful experiences and disappointing experiences.

Success expectation is an attitude that affects the way you attack a task. Your approach, to a great extent, will determine the outcome. Two personal traits that are helpful in the performance of any task are persistence and determination. Successful performance may be dependent upon time—some tasks require a slow, careful performance, whereas others should be performed quickly. A skill that is helpful in many situations is the problem-solving method. Successful performance as a health care provider requires that you choose the appropriate method of performance in a wide variety of situations.

Confidence comes from having a reasonable balance of successes and failures. Perhaps you have such a balance, but give undue attention to failure experiences and do not consciously acknowledge your successes.

Everyone has some failures and some disappointments in spite of a conscientious effort to do well. It is possible to use such experiences as opportunities to identify factors that may have contributed to a poor outcome:

- Did I begin the task without proper preparation?
- Did I attempt to do the task too rapidly? Did I give enough attention to details (or technique)?
- Did I allow too little time for the task?
- Did I use efficient work habits? If not, what work habits might have been more effective?
- Did I use the appropriate method for this task? If not, what method would have been better?
- Did I give up too soon?
- Did I have control over the outcome, or was the outcome controlled by someone else? If the outcome was controlled by someone else, then the failure is not yours. Habitually blaming others, however, can prevent you from taking responsibility for your actions, and therefore inhibit learning from experience.
- If you used the problem-solving approach, which alternative solution might have resulted in a better outcome?

Successful experiences in life make it easier to accept the occasional failures that all of us have. If you can maintain a reasonable balance between successes and failures and experience satisfaction after each success, then your self-esteem will likely be high most of the time, and any periods of low self-esteem will be brief.

## SUCCESS

Do you think of "success" as making a lot of money, gaining power, having a late-model car, or perhaps even becoming a movie star? Only a few people get to the top, and some of those who do get to the top in their field find that their "success" does not provide happiness.

### Influence of Success

Each of us has many opportunities for success if we recognize daily accomplishments and grant ourselves the right to feel good about them. Each time a job is done well, you should feel inner satisfaction. If others notice and express approval, this should add to your enjoyment. But even when you do not gain approval from others, you should feel good when you know, deep inside, that you did a job well.

If you recognize and acknowledge daily successes, each one will build your self-confidence and prepare you for succeeding in the next task you undertake. Each success diminishes the probability that self-doubt will interfere with success in future undertakings.

### As a Student

As a student, you will have many opportunities to experience success. New information, new insights, new understandings, and new skills can give you a sense of accomplishment. Take pride in each achievement, seeing it as another step toward becoming a health care provider. Remember, however, that none of us can experience success in every task. There are times when we do not do as well as we would like. From the disappointments, however, we can learn what to avoid in the next similar situation. Thus "failures" can be used constructively as learning experiences, instead of being allowed to create destructive self-doubt.

### As a Health Care Provider

When you have become a full-fledged health care provider, recognize your successes each day and gain satisfaction from them. Regard your "nonsuccesses" as learning experiences that will help you perform more effectively in the future. Set goals for developing those traits that are fundamental to self-confidence: persistence, determination, and adaptability. Learn to use a systematic, problem-solving approach. Develop efficient work habits. As successes increase, disappointments will be less damaging to your self-esteem. Thus, you can build belief in yourself as a competent person.

## STRIVING FOR SELF-APPROVAL

### Modifying Habits

In striving to build self-confidence, you must be realistic. You have many, many personal traits. Some are so highly developed that they characterize you as a person; in trying to describe you, someone would mention those traits. Other traits are not so prominent, but can be developed if you give your attention to them. Some traits are favorable; others are unfavorable. Try to identify the traits that will help you as a person and as a health care provider and strive to develop those traits to a high degree. Also, identify those traits that are a **hindrance** to you; strive to minimize or eliminate those traits from your behavior patterns.

You cannot overhaul yourself on a moment's notice. In fact, revising habits is a somewhat slow process. It takes effort and persistence to replace an undesirable habit with a more desirable one. You must practice the new habit at every opportunity. Do not let an exception occur; each time you lapse into the old habit, it becomes harder to establish the new habit. For example, if you tend to procrastinate, it will take much effort to overcome this one habit.

Resist the temptation to put things off. Gradually, the habit of "do it now" will replace the habit of thinking, "I'll do that later."

### Developing Problem-Solving Skills

You can deal with problems more effectively by using a systematic method. The following steps to choosing successful behavior can be applied to a variety of situations:

1. Identify the problem. Think it through. Discuss it with someone who might help you to understand it or to see the problem in a new light. Write out a statement of the problem.
2. Collect information and/or ideas that might help you to understand the problem better.
3. Consider all available information, then look at your statement of the problem. Reconsider what the problem is and rewrite the statement, if necessary.

> **Note:** At this point, your perception of the problem may have changed completely. You may eventually see the problem as being entirely different from what you initially thought.

4. Write down every imaginable solution. In a second column beside each possible solution, write out the possible consequences of trying that solution.
5. Select the solution that seems most likely to lead to the desired outcome and carry out the actions required.
6. Evaluate the outcome. If the result was not satisfactory, try another solution that appears likely to succeed.

It requires practice to become skillful in using a problem-solving approach, but if you apply it to daily problems, you will soon become skillful in thinking through these steps. In other words, thinking through a problem may become a work habit. Skill in problem solving enables a person to choose a specific behavior for a desired result.

### Building a Realistic Self-Concept

A realistic self-concept requires conscious and thoughtful consideration of "what is." By honestly appraising your strengths and weaknesses, identifying your interests, and clarifying your values, you will get in touch with the "real you." This is the starting point for planning ways to develop your potential and gaining greater satisfaction from living (Figure 6-6).

### Setting Goals

Your true interests and **aptitudes** influence the success you are likely to experience and the satisfaction you are likely to gain from certain types of activities. Each of us tends to do best those things that we enjoy doing. Also, we learn more easily and perform best those activities for which we have an aptitude. A realistic **appraisal** of "what is" provides the foundation for setting goals, "what may be."

**FIGURE 6-6** Strive to develop a realistic self-concept—neither derogatory nor idealized. *Delmar/Cengage Learning*

Goals that are in accordance with your true interests and aptitudes are more likely to be achieved than goals set for you by someone else. If your goals offer a challenge, then reaching them will provide much satisfaction—the feeling of having overcome obstacles and of being a person who can achieve goals. This is self-approval. When goals are too high for your aptitudes or readiness, then you may experience disappointment, failure, and self-doubt. Goals that are too low are easily reached, do not challenge you to develop your potential, and provide only limited satisfaction.

It is desirable to have both short-range and long-range goals. Short-range goals are the stepping-stones that lead to long-range goals. If JoAnn wants to study medicine and is qualified to do so, her high school curriculum and college courses will be a series of short-range goals leading to the long-range goal of becoming a physician. If there are financial problems, JoAnn may use a health occupations course as a short-term goal, obtaining job skills that enable her to work part-time while attending college. Thus, JoAnn may eventually reach her long-range goal through a series of intermediate goals. Intermediate goals provide inner satisfaction and a sense of achievement that help one persist in striving for the long-range goal.

## REFERENCES AND SUGGESTED READINGS

Amini, Mitra, et al. (2008, Oct.). A qualitative study of factors associated with medical students' academic success. *Journal of Social Sciences, 4*(4), 347–352.

Evans, Patricia. (2006). *The verbally abusive man, can he change?* Avon, MA: Adams Media.

Lerner, Harriet. (2005). *The dance of anger: A woman's guide to changing the patterns of intimate relationships.* New York: HarperCollins.

McKay, Matthew, et al. (2005). *The self-esteem companion: Simple exercises to help you challenge your inner critic and celebrate your personal strengths.* Oakland, CA: New Harbinger.

van Wormer, Katherine. (2007). *Human behavior and the social environment: Micro level: Individuals and families.* New York: Oxford University Press.

## REVIEW AND SELF-CHECK

1. Explain the meaning of "social needs" and list five kinds of social needs.

2. List three influences on one's self-concept and explain the importance of each.

3. Compare self-esteem and self-concept.

4. Explain the influence of a success experience on a person's self-esteem and self-concept.

5. Explain the effects of a failure experience on a person's self-esteem and self-concept.

6. Explain the relationship between expectations of success and performance of a task.

7. What are the two essential steps for modifying a habit?

8. List six steps of the problem-solving process.

---

## ASSIGNMENTS

1. Briefly describe one experience you have had in regard to each of the following:
   a. You attempted a task but gave up without completing it.
   b. You attempted a difficult task and finished it.
   c. You expected someone to praise your performance, but no one commented.
   d. Someone complimented you on how well you did something. It was a routine job that you do regularly without giving it much thought.

2. Review each of the above situations. Describe how each experience made you feel about yourself.

3. Consider how you feel when you complete a task satisfactorily, in your opinion, but your boss (or your teacher) criticizes the result. What does your reaction indicate in terms of your need for self-approval? What does it mean in terms of your need for approval from authority figures?

4. Select a problem you have had recently in your role as a student. The problem may involve a disagreement with a classmate, daily adjustments necessary in becoming a full-time student, a task you found difficult, or a patient situation in which there was a misunderstanding. Briefly describe the situation. Now use the problem-solving method to study the situation, including your own behavior and the outcome. Identify an action that probably would have had a better result.

5. Select a problem you now have and apply the problem-solving method. Write out several possible solutions; beside each, list the probable results. Select the solution you think will have the most desirable outcome. Try this solution. After one week, review the problem, your action, and the outcome. Evaluate your use of the problem-solving method. Did you select the best action? Do you now think another action would have had a better result?

# UNIT 7

# The Need for Acceptance

## OBJECTIVES

Upon completion of this unit, you should be able to:

- Explain the relationship of social needs to one's sense of worth.
- List two specific needs that are related to the need for acceptance.
- List three behaviors required for effective use of approval.
- State two components of caring.
- Differentiate between sympathy and empathy.
- Recognize behaviors that may represent an effort to meet the need for approval, acceptance, or appreciation.
- Express approval, caring, or appreciation appropriately.

## KEY TERMS

Conformity  Martyr complex
Empathy  Sympathy

You have learned that social needs can be met fully only through satisfying relationships with other people. Satisfaction of social needs requires both self-approval and approval and acceptance by others. The person who has achieved self-approval finds it easier to gain approval and acceptance by others. On the other hand, acceptance by others makes us feel more comfortable with ourselves. So these two needs are closely tied together; the person who can grow in self-approval can become increasingly acceptable to others and vice versa.

The need to belong can be satisfied through (1) frequent, positive interactions with the same people and (2) a life situation (framework) that provides a long-term, stable climate of caring and concern. A person who has established a relationship that fulfills some of these belonging needs is reluctant to end the relationship, even when it includes destructive elements such as abuse.

## THE IMPORTANCE OF ACCEPTANCE

Each of us needs to believe that others accept us as a worthwhile person. To satisfy this need, we must see and hear expressions of approval from time to time, in order to remain convinced of this acceptance. We also need to believe that others understand our viewpoint, our feelings, and our problems. Obviously, satisfying the need for acceptance requires receiving indications of approval and caring from other people.

Friendships develop and are maintained on the basis of whether or not two people meet each other's needs. You may find it difficult to understand why your friend, Melanie, seeks Helen's companionship in preference to your company. Perhaps you do not care for Helen at all. In reality, the Melanie/Helen relationship continues because it provides mutual satisfaction of needs. Perhaps Helen is very ready to express approval or admiration of Melanie, whereas you assume that Melanie knows you approve of her. Friendships grow stronger or they weaken on the basis of the extent to which the relationship satisfies the social needs of those involved (Figure 7-1).

Ideally, a relationship between two people involves a balance of give-and-take. This ideal can be met only if the behavior of each person helps the other to satisfy basic social needs. In some relationships, the balance of give-and-take appears to be one-sided. One person exerts much effort to please the other and seems to get little in return. If the relationship continues over a long period without change in this balance, both parties are satisfying certain needs. Self-sacrificing behavior is sometimes referred to as the "**martyr complex,**" meaning that the individual actually derives satisfaction from being taken advantage of by another person (Figure 7-2).

To a great extent, we can understand our behavior and that of others in terms of basic needs—behaviors that satisfy a basic need, and behaviors that compensate for not being able to satisfy a basic need. Usually, a person puts up with certain circumstances or with the behavior of others because some need is being met. Perhaps compensation is taking place. Perhaps the need is a "sick" one, as illustrated by the martyr type of behavior. If no need is being met, the individual will usually engage in behavior that changes the situation or provides escape. Now let us consider some specific needs that are related to the overall need for acceptance.

**FIGURE 7-1** A relationship deteriorates when it no longer satisfies the social needs of one or both parties. *Delmar/Cengage Learning*

**FIGURE 7-2** A continuing relationship satisfies some need of each person in the relationship. *Delmar/Cengage Learning*

## THE IMPORTANCE OF APPROVAL FROM OTHERS

Have you ever expected to be praised for something you did, but instead you were criticized? How did it make you feel? How did you behave? How did you feel about the person who was critical instead of approving? This person, in failing to give approval, deprived you of a basic need. Each of us has had such experiences. The one who failed to give us our earned approval may have been a parent, friend, classmate, teacher, or boss. The hurt associated with such experiences is proportional to the importance we attach to the other person.

Now consider the other side of the coin. Have you ever had a friend show you something new, yet you failed to express approval? Has a friend ever won an honor, but for some reason you could not bring yourself to offer congratulations? If so, you were depriving this person of approval. Why did you withhold your approval?

### Hunger for Approval

Being deprived of approval early in life can create a hunger for approval that never seems satisfied. Do you know someone who "looks for compliments"? How do you feel about this person? Seeking compliments usually indicates a strong need for expressions of approval. The next time you observe such behavior, will you recognize the need for approval? Assuming it is deserved, will you express your approval freely and sincerely? If so, you will be helping that person meet an important need. You will be contributing to that person's inner comfort, but the cost to you is only the effort it takes to state your sincere approval.

### Failure to Offer Approval

Some people fail to notice others. Some are indifferent to a job well done, but very ready to react to a job or a person not meeting their approval. Some people may notice that a job has been well done, but make no comment. Some, for reasons of their own, deliberately avoid saying nice things to others. The habit of not expressing approval can be easily overcome, once you are aware that approval is a need we all have. Deliberately withholding approval is another matter, however. To understand this trait may be more difficult, because it indicates negative feelings toward others and, probably, toward oneself.

### Appropriate Use of Approval

Approval should be given freely for everyday tasks—not just for the big tasks that come only occasionally. The child who voluntarily does a task at home deserves expressions of approval. The student who does an assignment well deserves approval. The person who serves a tasty meal deserves approval. Each of us has opportunities throughout the day to express sincere approval to others. It only requires that we form the habit of noticing others and expressing approval when it has been earned.

When will you have your next opportunity to express approval to someone? Perhaps your young son washes his hands for dinner without being told. Perhaps a patient shows the first interest in grooming since an operation. Perhaps the teacher presents an especially interesting class. All of these people need approval, too!

This is not a recommendation that you rush around paying compliments freely. Insincerity is worse than silence. The desirable behavior is *noticing others and unselfishly expressing approval when it has been earned.* This is an easy way to meet your own needs while also helping someone else satisfy a basic need. Giving approval to others can be quite enjoyable.

## CONFORMITY

**Conformity** means acting in accordance with the behaviors, beliefs, and values of a specific group. Conformity expectations of group members may extend to lifestyle choices, including manner of dress, foods, sexual behavior, and relationships with the group's authority figures. In groups that emphasize conformity, individuality is not valued and may be perceived as rebellion against the group's beliefs. The person who "dares to be different" may be excluded from the group; if allowed to remain within the group, that person may be viewed with suspicion and watched closely for evidence of unacceptable behavior.

Being overly concerned about conformity places one at risk of allowing others to make decisions that mature people make for themselves. A person who readily accepts the opinions of others, without becoming informed and giving thought to the situation, depends upon conformity as a means of gaining acceptance. Many people accept without question the word of any authority figure and may even be fearful of expressing a different point of view.

### Importance of Acceptance during Adolescence

Have you ever arrived at a party and found you were dressed differently from most of those present? Perhaps you dressed casually and the others "dressed up." If among friends, you were probably not overly uncomfortable. But if you were trying to gain acceptance by the members of this group, discovering that you dressed inappropriately may have made you very uncomfortable.

During adolescence the need for acceptance by the peer group is very strong, and conformity is almost necessary to gain acceptance. Parents are often distressed to find that their teenager is more concerned about the opinions of friends than about their parents' beliefs. Some people never outgrow depending on conformity to win the acceptance of the group to which they wish to belong.

Lauren has just entered high school. She and her classmates notice that many girls in the sophomore class have various body piercings: eyebrows, nose, tongue, "belly button," and two or more in the ears. Lauren wears stud earrings, but now she and many of her classmates see additional piercings as the means for acceptance into the high school culture. When Lauren asks her parents for permission (and money) for additional piercings, they refuse. Lauren uses the argument, "Everybody is doing it." Her parents respond, "That doesn't make it sensible." Over the next several weeks, Lauren is uncomfortable as many of her friends acquire additional piercings; she even feels "left out" as she witnesses the attention and admiration generated from members of the peer group as each new piercing is displayed. Lauren has not yet learned that acceptance does not require conformity to each new fad.

### Group Standards and Conformity

Some of the policies of your health care preparatory program may seem unreasonable to you, but they are probably based on sound reasons. The ethics of the health professions are based on high principles and establish what is "appropriate" behavior for health care providers. As a health care provider, you will be expected to conform to the standards and practices of the health care field. There will be some minor differences in policies and procedures from one clinical facility to another, but emphasis on appropriate dress, ethical behavior, and high standards of performance extends throughout the entire field of health care.

There are many situations where conformity is desirable, perhaps necessary. Military service, for example, requires conformity to rules, regulations, procedures, dress codes, and almost all aspects of daily life. Many other situations require conformity to a particular group's expectations in order to gain acceptance. This need for conformity in certain situations is reflected in the familiar expression, "When in Rome, do as the Romans do." In all situations, however, it is important to maintain your integrity and your own high principles.

If you find yourself in a group whose standards are not acceptable to you, you must either change your beliefs, convince the group that their standards should change, or find another group whose standards reflect your own. In other words, use good judgment in deciding when to conform to a group's standards and when to go by your own standards, even at the risk of disapproval.

## THE NEED TO BELIEVE THAT OTHERS CARE

Another social need that requires appropriate responses from other people is the need to believe that other people care. The extent to which we believe that a particular person does care about us has an influence on how we feel about that person. To put it another way, the more important a particular person is to us, the more strongly we need to believe that person cares about our feelings. Expressions of caring promote strong ties between people.

## Sympathy

As a health care provider, you will be hearing the terms **sympathy** and **empathy.** Perhaps you think of sympathy as "feeling sorry for someone." Actually, few people want or expect pity from others, and some would react to expressions of pity with anger. But most people, when sick or experiencing some type of difficulty, need to believe that their loved ones and friends care, share their feelings, and regret that they are having a bad experience. Sympathy, then, implies sharing and feeling with another, while retaining one's own point of view.

## Empathy

Empathy is similar to *some* of the meanings of sympathy, but it is not the same. Empathy means identifying with another person in such a way that we see another person's situation from her point of view, rather than from our own perspective. Do you remember the previously mentioned farm wife who was extremely upset about her husband's accident? Another farm wife would have no difficulty in feeling empathy; she would understand this threat to the family's livelihood. On the other hand, a person who has never lived on a farm and has no understanding of the complexities of farm life may think, "Instead of being so upset, that woman ought to be thankful her husband didn't die."

As a health care provider you will be exposed to many situations in which an effort to feel empathy for the patient and the family—*to see the situation as they see it*—will help you to understand their behavior. Most patients do not want others to feel sorry for them. They *do* want others to care about them, to understand what they are experiencing, and to care about their feelings and beliefs (Figure 7-3).

**FIGURE 7-3** Patients want to believe that others care about them and understand what they are experiencing. *Delmar/Cengage Learning*

## THE NEED FOR APPRECIATION

Each of us needs to believe that someone appreciates us. We especially need to feel appreciated by those who are important to us. Appreciation may mean "to be grateful," by saying "thank you," or "to have respect," as shown by the statement, "She has great appreciation for modern art."

Expressing appreciation might indicate either of these meanings and might even imply approval or caring as well. For example, a child's first attempt to help with a household task will be unsuccessful by adult standards, yet the child may be proud of the effort. The adult reaction will affect future efforts. For a positive effect, the parent could show gratitude for the attempt to be helpful, could show respect for the child's effort, or could show caring and pleasure with the child's intent to help. All of these should be shown sincerely, even though the result of the child's performance may not meet adult standards.

Expressions of approval, appreciation, and caring provide a sense of satisfaction. The absence of any such expressions can have as negative an effect as open criticism or disapproval. If a task has been attempted but not performed well, sincere *approval* cannot be given; yet it is quite likely that an expression of *appreciation* would be appropriate. If suggestions for improvement are needed, these suggestions are less likely to appear as criticism if they are preceded by an expression of appreciation, caring, and understanding. Thus, there are some situations where approval should be expressed, but indications of appreciation or caring are not necessary. At other times, approval is not needed or has not been earned, but appreciation could be shown. Sometimes neither approval nor appreciation can be expressed, yet an expression of caring would be appropriate.

Our social needs are interrelated. The person who is aware of social needs and their importance in interpersonal relations will recognize opportunities to contribute to the satisfaction of another's needs. The person who is unaware may blunder through life, contributing little to the needs of others and lacking personal satisfaction from meeting social needs.

## SOCIAL NEEDS AND BEHAVIOR

Perhaps you are now more aware of the complexity of human behavior. One person seeks approval by strict conformity to a group's standards of behavior, another by getting good grades, another by acquiring symbols of success, another by doing favors for people, still another by being the life of the party. Some people find effective patterns of behavior that lead to self-approval and acceptance by others. Some people compensate with behavior that temporarily relieves their inner discomfort but fails to satisfy basic social needs.

All behavior is caused; it does not just happen. However, it is seldom possible to pinpoint one particular cause of a specific action. The causes of behavior are numerous and complex. Some of these causes lie in the situation in which the behavior occurs; other causes are within the individual, as a result of past learnings and their continuing influence on behavior. Many behaviors are goal-oriented; that is, they represent an individual's efforts to achieve some goal, such as satisfying the need for acceptance. We can increase our understanding and tolerance for behavior of others by being more aware of possible contributing causes, some apparent and others hidden. It is also helpful to study behavior in terms of its effectiveness—the degree to which it satisfies some basic need.

## BEHAVIOR AND THE HEALTH CARE PROVIDER

For health care providers, being aware of the social needs of others can mean the difference between effective and ineffective relations with patients and their families. People under the physical and psychological stress of illness are more likely to cope with their illness successfully if caregivers help them meet social and emotional needs, as well as physical needs.

As a health care provider, you can be more effective if you are also a student of human behavior. You know that there is no ready answer to the "why" of any one person's behavior. You know that basic needs, both physical and social, continue during illness. However, the need for relieving distress and releasing emotions such as fear may temporarily push the need for approval or acceptance into the background. On the other hand, some patients try to cover up their own emotional distress to win acceptance from health care providers by being pleasant and cooperative.

As you observe people in apparently similar situations reacting in very different ways, you are seeing evidence of individual differences. Patients differ in their behavior used to cope with stress, in the strength of different needs, in relative importance given to specific needs, and in the capacity to find behavior patterns to meet their needs in a particular situation.

The human scene provides a never-ending variety of situations for thoughtful study. You will become less critical of others, more accepting of behavior that you do not understand, and more tolerant of human weakness as you apply your learnings about human behavior to people around you.

## REFERENCES AND SUGGESTED READINGS

Breggin, Peter R. (2006). *The heart of being helpful: Empathy and the creation of a healing presence.* New York: Springer Publishing Company.

Chamberlin, Christine, & Zhang, Naijian. (2009, Spring). Workaholism, health, and self-acceptance. *Journal of Counseling and Development, 87*(2), 159–170.

## REVIEW AND SELF-CHECK

1. Explain the relationship between social needs and a person's sense of worth.

   _____

2. List two specific needs that must be met in order for a person to feel accepted.

   _____

   _____

3. List three ways to express approval effectively.

   _____

   _____

   _____

4. What are two essential components of caring?

5. Compare empathy and sympathy: How are they alike, and how are they different?

6. List one or more behaviors that could indicate a person is seeking:

    a. Approval_____

    b. Acceptance_____

    c. Appreciation_____

7. List two or more guidelines for expressing each of the following appropriately:

    a. Approval_____

    b. Caring _____

    c. Appreciation_____

## ASSIGNMENTS

1. Consult a dictionary and list all meanings given for "sympathy" and "empathy."

2. Describe how you could use sympathy and empathy in the following:

    a. Your relations with patients and their families

    b. Your relations with coworkers

    c. Your personal life

3. Consult a dictionary for all meanings of "appreciation." Select those that relate to social needs and explain briefly how you could use each meaning as a basis for improving your relations with others.

4. Observe yourself and others for one week. Describe, in writing, examples of behaviors that illustrate the following:

    a. Need for acceptance by others

    b. Need for conformity

    c. Need for believing that others care

    d. Need for appreciation

5. In your work as a health care provider, you have seen several patients who have infections that resulted from body piercings and one who developed hepatitis C after getting a tattoo. Today, your 15-year-old son announces that he wants to have his girlfriend's

name tattooed on his forearm, "where everyone will see it." You know that many of his classmates already have a tattoo. Using your awareness of the importance of conformity and peer approval during adolescence, how will you handle this request?

6. Refer to the examples you collected for activity 4. List ways you could have helped each individual meet a social need.

7. Engage in a small-group discussion to identify various ways to satisfy one's social needs.

8. Develop a plan for meeting your own social needs more effectively.

# UNIT 8

# Emotions and Behavior

## OBJECTIVES

Upon completion of this unit, you should be able to:

- List five effects of emotions on the quality of life.
- Describe the physiological effects of emotional arousal.
- Define stress, distress, and stressor.
- List two positive emotions and three negative emotions.
- Describe five influences on the formation of emotional patterns.
- State five guidelines for using emotions constructively.
- State five ways a health care provider can use knowledge about emotions to foster effective relationships with patients.
- Modify communication habits to include "I talk" and eliminate accusative statements.

## KEY TERMS

| | | |
|---|---|---|
| Adrenalin | Hostility | Resentment |
| Altruism | Mind-talk | Stress |
| Compassion | Noradrenalin | Stressors |
| Cynicism | Physiological | Suppression |
| Emotions | Psychosomatic | TLC |
| Homeostasis | Repressed | |

## MEANING OF EMOTIONS

**Emotions** are the inner feelings that all of us have. They are responses to life situations, varying in type and intensity according to the experience of the moment. Many different terms are used to describe emotions. Some of these terms describe the *type* of feeling; other terms imply the *intensity* of the feeling.

*Emotions are neither good nor bad.* We all experience these inner feelings according to what is happening to us and how we perceive the experience. To think of any emotion as good or bad, in a moral sense, is as pointless as considering hunger to be morally good or bad. Both positive and negative emotions are natural reactions to life experiences.

## IMPORTANCE OF EMOTIONS

Emotions have physical and mental effects. Indirectly, emotions determine the amount of satisfaction one gets from life, the degree of success in solving life problems, the satisfaction found in relations with other people, and, ultimately, one's *physical* and *mental* well-being throughout life.

The relationship between negative emotions and physical health is now well established, both by research and clinical findings. Anger, when experienced frequently, tends to evolve into **resentment** (chronic, low-level anger), **hostility** (an angry attitude toward a specific person or group), or **cynicism** (an attitude of contempt or distrust of others). Thus, anger can become incorporated into the personality.

Since our emotions have powerful mental and physical effects, it is important that we learn to use emotions effectively, rather than allow emotions to control our behavior (Figure 8-1). The person who has learned to express feelings in socially acceptable ways is competent in dealing with life situations—both good and bad. A person who has not learned to use emotions constructively is likely to lose control when feelings become strong. The sudden eruption of powerful feelings may result in behavior that is ineffective in dealing with a situation (Figure 8-2). Appropriate expression of emotions in any job situation influences relations with coworkers, supervisors, and patients/clients.

**FIGURE 8-1** To use emotions constructively, one must be in control.

*Delmar/Cengage Learning*

**FIGURE 8-2** Suppressed emotions can erupt suddenly and propel an individual into undesirable behavior. *Delmar/Cengage Learning*

## PHYSIOLOGICAL EFFECTS OF EMOTIONS

Emotions influence physical functioning, with particular effect on the autonomic nervous system, which influences the functioning of internal organs. Through this indirect influence, the emotional state can stimulate certain organs and inhibit the activity of others. If the emotion is strong, the effect is of short duration. If it is a long-term emotion, as in chronic anxiety, internal processes are kept in a state of "semi-emergency alert." Over a period of time, this long-term **physiological** situation can lead to actual physical changes.

The human body is an organized system that carries out numerous life-sustaining processes. The body makes certain adaptations in response to a variety of life situations so that **homeostasis** is maintained. Homeostasis is the balance of chemicals and hormones necessary for ideal physiological functioning. When the body is unable to make this adaptation (i.e., homeostasis does not exist), there is serious threat to physical health until homeostasis is reestablished.

Studies of body reactions to situations that arouse fear or anger show that the adrenal glands discharge large amounts of **adrenalin** and the sympathetic nervous system produces **noradrenalin.** These two hormones speed up the circulation of blood, accelerate blood clotting, dilate the blood vessels that serve the skeletal muscles, and increase the respiratory rate. The purpose of these changes is to prepare the body for unusual activity, that is, a "fight or flight" state to deal with the emergency situation. While the body's resources are being mobilized to strengthen the musculoskeletal system, other areas of the body have a diminished supply of blood. These physiological changes are adaptive, meaning that they enable the individual to deal physically with a threatening situation.

## STRESS

Dr. Hans Selye studied the physiological effects of unusual life situations for over 30 years. Dr. Selye noted that there is a *generalized* body reaction in addition to the alarm ("fight or flight") reaction. He labeled the latter response **stress** and the generalized reaction *general adaptation syndrome*, the sum total of physiological changes that occur in a state of stress. The stress response is essential to survival; it occurs in response to either a positive or a negative emotional state. Thus, a happy event such as marriage or the birth of a baby, as well as an unhappy experience, can trigger the generalized stress reaction.

Extreme emotional states are generally of short duration; they can be measured in terms of minutes or hours. The "fight or flight" arousal generally subsides as soon as the emergency has passed, although the after-effects, such as sweaty palms and trembling, may continue for several hours, until the amount of adrenalin and noradrenalin in the bloodstream has returned to normal. On the other hand, stress (the generalized response) does not subside quickly; when this aroused state exists for a long period, the body is in a state of distress. The physiological arousal interferes with normal body functions. Stress over a period of years can lead to depletion of the adrenal glands. The term *stress* refers to the adaptive response itself. The outside influences that create a state of arousal are **stressors.**

Dr. Selye's research led to the discovery that the stress reaction includes increased body resistance to outside agents such as infectious organisms. This is the basis for immunity to specific diseases (i.e., production of antibodies). During a period of increased resistance to a specific stressor, resistance to other stressors is decreased. For example, working long hours, eating improperly, and not getting sufficient sleep and recreation add up to stress. A person with such a lifestyle is likely to have lowered resistance and therefore be more susceptible to infection.

The person whose stress reaction is due to invasion by a specific infectious agent, such as the measles virus, has the physiological response specific to that infectious agent (e.g., in case of measles, fever, rash, runny nose). At that time, the measles victim has lowered resistance to other organisms, such as the bacteria or viruses that cause pneumonia. While the body mobilizes its resources to deal with the measles virus, only limited resources are available to deal with other threats to health.

Unfortunately, resistance to psychological stressors does not automatically develop, as is the case with immunity to some infectious organisms. Nor does the stress reaction subside as quickly or as completely after a psychological threat is no longer a part of the immediate life situation. Because of mental/emotional/physiological interactions, we can experience stress by remembering a past event, by anticipating some undesirable future event, or even by imagining that something has happened or is happening. When one's thoughts are directed to an undesirable event (e.g., failing a course, being fired, being overworked), the emotional reaction to this *mental activity* triggers the adaptive response (Figure 8-3).

Another major source of stress for many people is "**mind-talk.**" This almost continuous stream of thoughts and memories is most likely to occur when an individual is performing routine tasks (i.e., ironing, raking leaves) that do not require concentrated thought or during quiet times when trying to relax. Mind-talk contributes to insomnia, since the physiological reaction to thoughts can lead to increasing wakefulness. Mind-talk, as used in this discussion, is ongoing, not fully under conscious control, and not purposeful. It is different from conscious use of mental processes for thinking, planning, evaluating, analyzing, and remembering.

**FIGURE 8-3** "I'll never finish on time." A heavy workload can be a major source of stress. *Delmar/Cengage Learning*

Mind-talk that deals with past events may include an embarrassing situation, a failure or an unsatisfactory performance, a disappointment, a lost opportunity for a smart response, or an extensive review of a conversation. But past events cannot be changed; only the present and the future can be altered. This habit of frequently recalling past events that aroused a negative emotion results in a state of chronic stress that can lead to permanent physiological changes—the basis for **psychosomatic** (psycho—mind; soma—body) illness.

Mind-talk can also focus on future possible events, rather than memories of past events. These thoughts may involve rehearsal of an expected conversation, something "bad" that could happen to oneself or to a loved one, a loss, or the possibility of abandonment. If worrying about possible future events is habitual, the individual maintains a state of anxiety, and a state of stress exists.

Mind-talk can also include remembering good things that happened or anticipating some type of good experience. Mind-talk concerned with "good" things is satisfying, rather than stress-inducing. Everyone experiences mind-talk, but people vary in the extent to which they react emotionally. Stress management requires learning to control mind-talk so that it does not arouse negative emotions or interfere with sleep.

## POSITIVE EMOTIONS

The positive emotions, primarily joy and love, contribute to our feeling good. Words such as *elation* and *ecstasy* describe extremely high states of joy, whereas *pleasure* and *satisfaction* imply a less intense state of joy. Love is a complex emotion; there are various types of love and the intensity varies according to type, the object of the love, and circumstances of the moment.

These two emotions are essential to the state we call "happiness." Some degree of joy is experienced whenever good things happen, when life is relatively free of difficulties, and when we are aware of loving others and being loved. Yet happiness is possible even when our life situations include problems, some degree of stress, and times of negative feelings. The experience of happiness is dependent upon one's ability to focus on positive aspects of life and minimize negative feelings by dealing competently with the challenges of daily living.

## Love

Love is an important positive emotion. Strong feelings of warmth for another person might be thought of as *love,* with milder feelings of the same type being termed *friendliness. Affection* implies a feeling less intense than love, but stronger than friendliness. Love implies caring about someone else, being concerned enough to help, understand, and respect the person loved. The capacity for feeling love influences one's outlook on life and attitudes toward people and has a powerful effect on physical and mental health.

### Kinds of Love

There are many kinds of love: the love of a mother for her child; the child's love, at first self-centered and then extended to others; love for one's playmates; love for material things associated with pleasant memories; love for friends with whom life experiences have been shared; love for unfortunate ones wherever they might be; and love for a patient and his family who are all struggling with their stressful situation. Spiritual love is different still and varies according to one's concept of the Divine. Each kind of love is expressed in specific ways. Newspaper accounts of some family's misfortune often result in a flood of contributions from strangers, illustrating the capacity of many people to express love for strangers who are less fortunate than themselves. This type of love is an example of **compassion.**

### Learning to Love

Love is essential to an infant's normal development. Babies who must remain in an institution tend to waste away and die, unless the staff makes certain that the babies are frequently touched or held. The importance of tender loving care (**TLC**) for institutionalized infants has only been recognized in the past few decades. If you ever work in a nursery or neonatal unit, you may see "TLC" orders for certain infants. The infant who receives the love of parents and other caretakers also learns trust and develops a sense of security.

Throughout childhood, one gradually learns to extend love to others: parents, siblings, other family members, caretakers, and eventually a widening circle of friends and associates. This learning is basic to the development of such traits as generosity, **altruism,** respect, and courtesy toward others. During adolescence, romantic love becomes a primary concern, which may extend throughout adulthood. Mature love is a special type of love that evolves through a long-term adult relationship. Each of these types of love can flourish only if the individual's early experiences fostered the development of self-love.

### Self-Love

Self-love is basic to the experience of love. Without self-love, a person is not able to truly love others. Self-love is not selfish, nor is it egotistic. It is an awareness of "self" as a worthwhile, lovable being who deserves to be cared for. A religious person may experience self-love through the belief, "I am a child of God." Loving oneself and believing oneself to be lovable are fundamental to a positive self-concept, the best protection one can have against threats to self-esteem as various difficulties of life are experienced.

Self-love enables a person to experience joy and happiness. It also contributes to health and well-being, in part because those who have self-love care enough about themselves to practice habits of safety and health maintenance. They do not abuse their bodies with toxic substances, such as alcohol, nicotine, or other addictive drugs. They eat right, exercise appropriately, get enough sleep, wear seat belts in the car, and do not drive recklessly or otherwise place themselves at needless risk. In other words, a person who has self-love takes responsibility for "self" in all aspects of living.

### Unconditional Love

Love should be *unconditional,* which means that it is not subject to being withheld whenever one is displeased. Conditional love has an "if/then" basis: *if* you do (or do not do) such and so, *then* I will love you. All too often, conditional love is used as a manipulative tool to control another person. This is destructive to a relationship, but is especially damaging when used by parents to control a child. Conditional love teaches, "You're only lovable when you do as I say." This style of parenting can lead to a negative self-concept, the belief that one is only lovable when meeting the demands of another.

Unconditional love, then, not only provides a growing child with a strong, positive self-concept, it also prepares the individual for a more healthful future life. Unconditional love does not mean that one must put up with undesirable behavior from others. It is important to differentiate between the person and that person's behavior. It is also important to realize that you can *love* someone even when you do not *like* them. Unconditional love is available at all times; it survives the ups and downs of a relationship.

Insofar as behavior is concerned, love for a child includes teaching appropriate behaviors at each stage of development; boundaries must be set in terms of what is acceptable behavior and what is not. Setting boundaries—making it clear that one will not tolerate a specific behavior—is a way of clarifying a relationship; it is not a matter of withholding love.

## NEGATIVE EMOTIONS

Negative emotions are uncomfortable. The intensity of each emotion can range from mild to very strong, causing one to feel a vague restlessness, a feeling of dissatisfaction, or a state of intense agitation. Negative emotions such as anger, fear, guilt, or sadness may occur as a response to the behavior of another person, a specific event or piece of information, or mind-talk. These emotions result in stress and physiological changes.

### Anger

Anger is aroused by obstacles, threats, or otherwise offensive situations. It is usually short-term and directed at a specific object or person, but can be generalized as anger at the world or society. *Hate* may be thought of as intense anger felt toward a specific person or group. *Annoyance* is used to describe a mild form of anger. *Rage* describes intense anger and implies that the anger is expressed through violent physical activity. *Hostility* is a mild form of anger/hate directed to a specific person or group. *Resentment* is chronic anger, which can be a powerful influence on one's behavior.

Anger is the emotional response to one's perception of a situation. The perception usually involves feeling wronged, neglected, cheated, deprived, ignored, or exploited. If the anger is not resolved, it becomes resentment. Many resentments have their origins in childhood, with a parent or sibling as the object of the resentment. Both anger and resentment can arise from feeling powerless to change a situation or to fight back. Anger may be aroused by an unsuccessful effort to control another person, or by awareness of being controlled or manipulated by another person. When anger is shared by a large number of people and control is held by a faceless group ("administration" or "the owners" or "government"), the anger of powerlessness can erupt as rebellion.

As individuals, we may generate our own anger. Dr. Thomas Gordon, a psychologist who works with parents to help them improve family relationships, believes that anger is often secondary to some other emotion. A parent feels fear when a child cannot be found; once the child's safety is assured, anger is directed at the child for having "caused" the situation. Anger may be secondary to other primary feelings, such as embarrassment or disappointment. When one experiences anger toward a friend or family member, it is advisable to consider whether or not the anger is due to some need of our own not being met. If the anger is due to some type of problem/situation, it is better to state that one is experiencing anger, and then suggest that an effort to solve the problem or situation be undertaken by all parties involved. If the anger is not used constructively, it may develop into smoldering resentment, hostility, or even hatred. **Suppression** of these feelings is likely to result eventually in an explosive verbal outpouring or even destructive physical actions.

One unfortunate example of destructive anger is domestic violence, now recognized as a growing problem in American society. (Perhaps it is a long-standing problem that is only now being acknowledged.) Violence against another person is an inappropriate expression of anger. Domestic violence involves directing anger toward one's spouse or child, usually through physical assault; it also includes verbal assault and any menacing actions that arouse fear in the victim.

The problem of child abuse has received increasing attention over the past two decades. Studies of child abusers reveal that many were themselves abused as children. This is a tragic example of how inappropriate adult behavior influences the child's future patterns for emotional expression. The child who grows up in a home where violent behavior occurs perceives this pattern of family interaction as "normal." Unless that perception is changed through education and counseling, the pattern of violent behavior within the family will continue through succeeding generations. Unit 11 provides a more extensive discussion of this subject.

## Fear

Fear is aroused by the threat of physical harm or danger to one's sense of security. Fear of physical harm is usually short-lived; the danger passes or the person copes with the dangerous situation. *Terror* and *panic* are terms for describing intense fear; the person who is in a state of terror or panic may flee the situation or may be immobilized by the intensity of the emotional reaction.

Fear is a natural reaction to threat or danger. It mobilizes the body for action—for fighting or fleeing a threatening situation. The body releases adrenalin, which increases the flow of blood, raises the rate of respiration, and stimulates muscle tone. If physical activity does not occur, this readiness for action may be released through "the shakes." Perhaps you have been involved in a dangerous situation, remaining calm until the danger was over and then finding yourself shaking all over or "weak in the knees." Many examples of heroic action involve physical exertion that the individual could not repeat after the excitement had subsided. The outpouring of adrenalin resulted in physical strength far beyond the person's usual abilities.

Fear can also be a reaction to mind-talk. *Worry* is fear based on thoughts about a *possible* event, such as losing one's job, losing a loved one, losing some type of property, or displeasing someone. *Anxiety* involves a higher intensity of fear than worry; it is likely to be a chronic pattern of emotional response to mind-talk. *Apprehension* and *dread* describe fear based on thoughts about some pending event that one perceives as threatening.

Fear is healthful when it is a reaction to a threatening event or situation. When self-generated through mind-talk, fear is pointless and destructive, unless it is used to plan ways to deal effectively with an expected situation. If one is apprehensive about a speech to be delivered on Monday, the best way to deal with the fear is to prepare well, practice the speech until completely comfortable with it, mentally picture oneself delivering the speech effectively, then remember to take several deep breaths before starting to deliver the speech. In the process of preparing for an effective delivery, self-confidence will replace apprehension.

## Grief

Grief is the emotional response to loss. It can range in intensity from momentary disappointment to deep sorrow that completely absorbs the individual. *Grief* describes intense feelings; *sorrow* implies grief without indicating intensity; *sadness* implies grieving of moderate intensity; *disappointment* implies a mild form of grief. Whereas fear and anger tend to arouse one physically, grief has the opposite effect. A person who is grieving may find it difficult to perform simple tasks. The body seems to reserve energy at this time for the individual to work through the grief. It is highly desirable, even healthful, to consciously grant oneself time to grieve when loss has been experienced.

## Guilt

Guilt as discussed here refers to self-blaming, rather than to any legal/criminal aspects. A clinical psychology professor once referred to guilt as the "most useless emotion there is." We can feel guilty about many things: something we did or said in the past, something we now wish we had done but did not do at the proper time, words we could have spoken but didn't.

*It is impossible to change the past, so it is pointless to wallow in guilt about what cannot be changed.* Some things can be remedied by doing now what could have been done in the past. Another remedy is forgiveness—of self and others. But forgiveness is not easy; self-forgiveness is especially difficult for people who have been controlled by guilt. Those who try to control others, especially family members or lovers, may use guilt as a manipulative tool.

Striving for self-understanding and learning effective interpersonal skills are one's best protection against the damaging effects of guilt. Anyone who realizes his or her behavior is strongly influenced by guilt feelings, or that someone is controlling him or her through guilt, will find professional counseling helpful.

## FORMATION OF EMOTIONAL PATTERNS

Emotional patterns are learned through the satisfaction or distress that accompanies various life experiences. Each person's capacity to feel specific emotions may be hereditary, as indicated by the fact that newborn infants show marked differences in their responses to distress. In spite of this hereditary factor, the great differences in adult emotional patterns are primarily the result of learning.

The people of a baby's world—the social environment—determine to a great degree whether the baby's experiences are pleasing or distressing. Throughout infancy, childhood, and adolescence the formation of emotional patterns is influenced by the emotional expressions and behaviors of others, especially primary caregivers and family members. Later in life, the balance of successes and failures in daily living has great influence on emotional expression. Also, the reactions of other people influence the tendency to show one's feelings or attempt to hide them. Patterns for expressing feelings develop within a framework of various influences on behavior: heredity, environment, basic needs, the consequences of behavior that follow specific life experiences, and interactions with other people.

Family patterns of emotional expression influence the formation of a child's emotional patterns. Ideally, the child receives loving care from both parents and other family members, thereby learning love and trust. In these days of single-parent and two-wage-earner homes, the primary caregivers may be the staff of a childcare facility, rather than a parent. The demands of a full-time job plus homemaking responsibilities limit the amount of time and energy a parent has for parenting. And so, the child may be exposed to a hectic schedule, rushed to the childcare center in the morning and picked up later in the day by an exhausted parent. At times, the balance of emotional expression may be more negative than positive. The behaviors of the adults are the behaviors the child will learn. In addition, the behaviors of childcare personnel and their beliefs about the expression of feelings are important influences on the child's developing emotional patterns.

Although these patterns are learned early in life, they are influenced later through exposure to widening circles of relatives, friends, schoolmates, coworkers, and various peer groups. As you study the remainder of this unit, be aware of your own patterns for expressing each emotion. As you remember specific behaviors you saw in your home as a child, speculate about the emotions that were being expressed. Also, consider (1) whether or not you, as a child, adopted that pattern of behavior and (2) what modifications you have made in expressing feelings during adolescence and adulthood.

## INDIVIDUAL DIFFERENCES IN EMOTIONAL PATTERNS

Everyone experiences negative and positive feelings. The tendency to respond to a certain type of situation with a specific emotion, the intensity of our emotional responses, the ways in which we express our feelings, the balance between positive and negative feelings, and the duration of a particular emotion are all characteristic of each person as an individual. People differ, then, in regard to the inner experience (feeling) and in the outward expression (behavior) of emotions.

Sometimes we suppress, or choose not to express, an emotion while in the situation that arouses it, then express it later; this is especially common with anger. If an emotion is extremely intense, and/or the situation that aroused the feeling is painful or unacceptable, then the emotion may be **repressed.** The memory of a traumatic event and the feelings associated with that event may both be repressed, meaning that they are not available to conscious memory. Therapy can help a person access repressed memories/feelings.

### Intensity and Frequency

Some people have the capacity for very strong feelings, whereas others seem to feel less intensely. Some people react frequently with strong emotion, even to daily annoyances such as traffic slowdowns. Other people react with strong emotion only to situations in which an intense emotional reaction is justified. Some people hide their feelings, which can result in a chronic state of stress.

### Temperament

The type of emotion (positive or negative) that a person feels most of the time is known as *temperament*. An optimistic person is one whose feelings are primarily positive; a pessimistic person is one whose feelings are primarily negative. Temperament is indicated by the way emotions are expressed: words and tone of voice, facial expression and other nonverbal behavior, and actions.

Most of us prefer the company of people who usually reflect positive emotions. Sometimes people with a pessimistic outlook find mutual satisfaction in each other, which brings to mind the saying, "Misery loves company." Some people do not show their feelings readily; their appearance is somewhat the same whether they are feeling good or bad inside. This lack of expressiveness may indicate suppression of emotion, rather than lack of feeling. It is difficult to know how such people feel, and therefore difficult to adapt your own behavior appropriately.

### Mood Swings

Another difference in individual emotional reactions is the tendency to have mood swings. Each of us has times when we are "blue"; each of us has times when we feel especially good for no apparent reason. This swing from up to down is normal. Some people, however, swing from one extreme to another or remain "down" for long periods and "up" for long periods. Extreme mood swings and/or a prolonged mood at one extreme or the other may indicate a need for professional counsel. Those whose mood swings are within normal range can learn to make full use of the times when they feel good and develop techniques for coping with periods when they feel "low."

The tendency to have long "down" periods can indicate that a person is clinically depressed, a condition now referred to as "unipolar." Extreme mood swings, down periods alternating with periods of high energy and productivity, may indicate that a person has bipolar disorder (formerly known as manic depressive illness). The line between "normal" mood swings and those indicative of a mood disorder is not clear-cut. Many unipolar and bipolar people function relatively well at jobs and within the family, especially if they are under psychiatric care. In fact, bipolars tend to be highly productive when they are in the "hypomanic" state; this is especially true of creative people, such as writers, poets, composers, musicians, and others in the performing arts. If the mood swings are serious enough to interfere with work, study, or family relations, then the individual should seek medical evaluation. If destructive or threatening behavior accompanies the "up" cycle, the individual should have a psychiatric evaluation as soon as possible.

## GENDER DIFFERENCES IN EMOTIONS

In the past, it was generally believed that women tended to be more "emotional" than men. At one time, women may have felt that society frowned upon their showing negative emotions such as anger. Recent research suggests that these stereotypes do not hold true today. In a 2004 study, researchers found that men and women surveyed reported similar numbers of emotional experiences, including the experience of anger. However, men reported a higher number of positive emotional experiences, while women reported more negative ones. Though men and women reported similar rates of experiencing anger, women's anger tended to last longer, and women were more likely to feel that their anger was appropriate to the situation (Simon & Nath, 2004).

While cultural stereotypes about men and women's emotions may be unfounded, researchers continue to identify differences in the way emotions affect brain chemistry and health in men and women. For example, in a study of patients over age 65, researchers found that symptoms of depression measurably affected the cardiac function of the male patients. The same symptoms did not have a measurable cardiac effect among female patients (Chen et al., 2010). Another study found differences in the way men's and women's brain chemistry changes as they age (Kovacs et al., 2010). New information about gender differences continues to develop. As a health care provider, you should be aware of which gender differences are based on evidence and which are based upon opinions or stereotypes.

## USING EMOTIONS CONSTRUCTIVELY

### Accentuating the Positive

Happiness is determined by how we react to both pleasant and unpleasant experiences in life (Figure 8-4). Some people use their unhappy experiences for endless conversational material. Others give only short notice to unhappy experiences, rapidly turning their attention to activities that give them satisfaction.

Each of us is free to choose between a negative and a positive outlook. We cannot eliminate all of life's disappointments, but we can refuse to let negative emotions dominate our lives. It is important, however, to consider each negative experience in terms of any lesson that can be learned. By learning from negative experiences, we become more competent for coping with life events.

### Open and Honest Communication

Dr. Gordon recommends a number of techniques for handling situations effectively. Owning your feelings involves stating how a situation is affecting you. Suppose you have a supervisor who frequently changes the schedule for no apparent reason. Some of your coworkers rearrange their personal plans in order to work the changed hours, but criticize the supervisor to other coworkers and the family. One person confronts the supervisor in anger and refuses to accept the changed hours. Still another worker says nothing about the change, but takes sick leave on the day for which the hours were changed. Each of these three approaches has disadvantages. None is likely to alter the supervisor's habit of changing hours on short notice. A cooperative approach is preferable; but first, the supervisor must become aware that there is a problem.

**FIGURE 8-4** Everyone has "ups" and "downs." *Delmar/Cengage Learning*

Suppose you approach the supervisor at an appropriate time and calmly state, "I have a problem when my hours are changed. I have to make different arrangements for care of my children." You have made statements of fact, using "I" to describe the effect of the schedule changes. This is "open and honest" communication. No accusation has been made; no blame has been laid on the supervisor. The climate is right for a discussion of the problem and a cooperative approach to finding a solution.

Perhaps there is a good reason for the change in hours. It is easier to accept an undesirable situation if you know that it exists because of unavoidable circumstances, rather than because of someone's poor planning. Perhaps the supervisor was not aware of your childcare needs and therefore was unaware of the inconvenience created by a change in schedule. Regardless of how the supervisor responds, you would have diffused any anger that was felt; it will not erupt later in an uncontrolled outburst of feeling. Even more important, the anger will not be displaced onto patients, coworkers, or members of the family who did nothing to cause the anger.

This approach is called "I talk," meaning that *feelings* are expressed in a statement beginning with "I" rather than a "you" statement that accuses or blames the other person. Compare the suggested "I" statement with an accusative statement: "You are always changing the hours! You are forcing me to change my babysitting arrangement! Why can't you make up a schedule and stick to it?" These statements would result in an angry supervisor. Certainly being on the defensive would not put the supervisor in a problem-solving frame of mind.

"I talk" is valuable as a means of expressing both positive and negative feelings. This technique can lead to improved interpersonal relations. Dr. Gordon warns, however, that when an "I" statement is used to express anger, it may be perceived as an accusation ("you made me angry"). Consider the possible effect of the following statements:

- "You always keep me waiting."
- "I really get angry when I have to wait."
- "I was disappointed when I arrived and you were not here yet."
- "You are fifteen minutes late."

Obviously, the "you" statements put the other person on the defensive, may create angry feelings toward you, or may arouse feelings of guilt. On the other hand, the "I" statements simply state how you feel. The other person cannot deny you your feelings. There is no basis for argument. And you have expressed the feeling verbally and are no longer burdened with anger.

Open and honest communication of positive feelings will greatly improve relations with others. All of us like to hear good things. Open and honest communication is especially important as a means of dealing with negative emotions. The following sections deal with approaches to handling specific negative emotional states.

## Dealing with Anger

Negative emotions must be dealt with constructively, or they will have destructive effects. When inner tension builds up from anger, this tension needs release. If a patient makes you angry, you cannot throw a bedpan or physically attack the patient. It is not desirable to "blow up" at your supervisor; not is it fair for you to bottle up your anger until you get home, and then let it loose on your family. (This is called "displaced anger.") Perhaps the tension built up from your anger can help you mow the grass, repair that broken gate, or whip up a cake. In other words, use energy generated by anger in some type of constructive physical activity. While you are in the situation, use "I" statements as appropriate or ask questions that will help you understand the other person's views or the circumstances. As you gain understanding, your anger may subside.

Once you are out of the situation in which you became angry, try to understand the reason for your anger. Is the reaction related to old resentments? Do you have a "response set" for becoming angry with this person or in this type of situation? Were you frustrated in your efforts to meet some need? Did you have expectations that the other person failed to meet? Were you treated unfairly (in your opinion)?

If you still feel anger, there are several techniques for safely diffusing the feelings. Talk with someone who knows how to listen. Just talking about the situation—the facts and also your feelings—can provide effective release. If you cannot talk to someone about it, set up a tape recorder, visualize it as the person at whom you are angry, and tell it exactly how you feel. Then, listen to a playback of the tape. Continue until your anger has been released. (Don't forget to erase the tape!) Another technique for working off feelings is to "punch out" a pillow, preferably a large, firm one. The physical activity provides for release of energy generated by the anger.

Many therapists consider that the most effective technique for dealing with anger is forgiveness. It is difficult to forgive someone who has hurt you or cheated you. Yet the anger you carry with you is actually harming *you*—your health and well-being—rather than the one who is the object of your anger. Learning to forgive may be one of life's most difficult lessons.

But the power of another person to harm you psychologically is diminished when you are able to forgive. Forgiveness of those who are deceased is just as important as forgiveness of those who are still living.

Self-forgiveness is especially important. It is only human to make mistakes. We all have regrets about things we did or didn't do, about what we said or didn't say. Some matters can be corrected by taking action, sometimes referred to as "mending fences." If the other person is deceased, then the only recourse is self-forgiveness. It is desirable that we learn from the past, however, so that new regrets do not accumulate.

## Dealing with Fear

To deal with fear effectively, we must first acknowledge the fear. We all encounter situations that arouse mild fear: a test, an oral report, returning to care for the patient who was critical of you yesterday, reporting to the supervisor that you broke a piece of equipment. In some situations the fear is justified, and the only recourse is to deal with the situation as effectively as possible. Sometimes mentally rehearsing the event in advance as a successful experience prepares you to deal with the situation with less fear.

Sometimes a person's fear is out of proportion to the expected event; fear tends to magnify the dreaded aspects of the situation. Fear can interfere with realistic thinking about a problem, but the problem-solving approach often reveals that there is an acceptable solution. Once a solution is apparent, fear tends to decrease.

**Phobias** Some people have an intense fear, known as a phobia, regarding something that most people do not find fearful (i.e., heights, being closed up in a small space such as an elevator, flying in an airplane). These fears are "abnormal" when they interfere with daily activities or cause the individual to take extreme measures to avoid the feared experience. Psychotherapy often results in the identification of some past traumatic event that the person had repressed, so that it was not available to conscious memory. In severe cases, the phobia requires a process of systematic desensitization, which may be done by various licensed mental health practitioners.

**Post-Traumatic Stress Disorder** A more serious example of fear-related memory is known as post-traumatic stress disorder (PTSD). This is manifested by panic attacks, in which the individual relives a traumatic experience through sudden flashbacks or nightmares. This disorder came to the attention of the public after many Vietnam veterans had difficulty adapting to civilian life following discharge from military service. PTSD can have a severe disabling effect if left untreated.

PTSD is experienced by many people who have been involved in a serious accident or experience a frightening event such as a flood, hurricane, or tornado. For several weeks or months after such an experience, the individual may relive the experience when trying to go to sleep, or wake up suddenly in a cold sweat with rapid heartbeat, clammy skin, and uncontrollable shaking—a panic attack. Usually this tendency passes after several weeks, as physical healing occurs. If not, the individual should have professional counseling; it requires skilled professional intervention to desensitize survivors of traumatic events and free them from recurrent panic attacks.

### Dealing with Grief

Grief is an emotion that lasts over a period of time. It may take weeks or months to work through the intense feelings and readjust one's life pattern. Whenever a loss occurs, permit yourself to grieve. When feelings of guilt are associated with grief, professional counseling may be needed to work through both emotions; such a combination is difficult to handle alone.

## EMOTIONS AND BEHAVIOR

### Self

In striving to understand yourself and your behavior, you must give attention to your emotional patterns. Do you usually react to unpleasant situations with fear or anger? If you tend to overreact, you may need help in understanding reasons for your strong feelings.

Do you give too much attention to negative feelings, perhaps even "enjoying" them? Enjoyment of misfortune is manifested through conversation, pessimism, self-pity, and other attention-getting behavior. You have only to think of one person who manifests such behavior to recognize the unfavorable effect on others. Obviously, such behavior is not appropriate for health care providers.

Emotions do exist, and they do affect us physically, psychologically, and mentally. To deny these feelings is a form of suppression. Suppressed emotions will have their effects sooner or later, through "blowing up" in an uncontrolled display of emotion, illness, poor coping mechanisms, or poor interpersonal relations (Figure 8-5).

Self-control is a constructive way of using emotions, rather than not showing emotions. Self-control is a learned behavioral pattern for expressing feelings in socially acceptable ways while dealing with a situation intelligently. The following guidelines can be used to increase self-control:

- Express your feelings at the time they are experienced; if for some reason that is not appropriate, express the feelings as soon as possible in a "safe" setting.
- Own your feelings; use "I" statements rather than accusative "you" statements in your interactions with other people.
- Acknowledge (do not deny to yourself or others) that you experienced a particular emotion in a specific situation.
- Ask yourself, "Is this situation important enough to me to justify these feelings?" If the answer is "No," turn your attention to other matters. If "Yes," then deal with the situation effectively, perhaps using some of the guidelines that follow.
- Work with others to clarify a problem and find a solution acceptable to all—a "win-win" situation.
- If you begin to experience anger, ask questions about the situation, then *listen* to the answers; better understanding of the other person's point of view may dissipate your anger.
- When you become aware of fear or apprehension, ask yourself whether or not you are in *real* danger. If the answer is "Yes," take appropriate action; if "No," analyze the basis for your feelings and take preventive action if needed.
- Use problem solving to deal with a situation, present or future, so that you feel competent to find a solution and no longer need to feel apprehensive.

**FIGURE 8-5** Suppressed emotions eventually lead to a blow-up. *Delmar/Cengage Learning*

- Take responsibility for your feelings and your behavior; avoid blaming others for "causing" your feelings.
- Avoid negative mind-talk. If your thoughts involve future possible events and you become anxious, realize that mind-talk, not a real event, is the source of your anxiety.
- If you have a particular phobia, seek professional help so you can free yourself from this unrealistic fear. Once you have exposed the basis for your phobia, it no longer has the power to control your behavior.
- Use and enjoy humor; be willing to laugh at yourself for getting upset over something trivial. Defuse a tense situation, as appropriate, with a humorous comment or anecdote.
- If you are still "worked up" after a situation that aroused strong emotions, use the energy for some type of constructive physical activity, such as mowing the grass, working out, running, or walking.
- Allow yourself to grieve for any loss you have experienced.
- Become aware of the events of your daily life that give you pleasure and allow time at the end of the day to enjoy thoughts of these good experiences.
- Love yourself. Take credit for your strengths, your competence, your willingness to grow; forgive yourself for being less than perfect.

The foregoing suggestions are intended to help you understand yourself and your emotions better. As you become more open and honest with yourself and others about your feelings, you will have a favorable effect on others. As you learn to replace impulsive emotional behavior with actions based on reasoning, you will be free to control situations more effectively. As you develop greater sensitivity to the feelings of others, you are more likely to react appropriately to their behavior.

## Others

Emotions are somewhat like a chain reaction. Hostile behavior by one person tends to bring out hostility in others. Aggressive behavior by one person brings about defensive behavior in others. When someone else expresses a negative emotion, do not allow that behavior to arouse a negative emotion in you. Instead, maintain a positive feeling and show your concern with such statements as, "I sense that you are angry" or "I sense that you are really feeling down today." This approach is called "reflecting," meaning that you act as a mirror for the person's feelings. Reflecting indicates that you are "tuned in" to what that person is experiencing, that you care, and that you are giving that person your full attention.

Although you can choose how to express your feelings most of the time, you cannot *control* the feelings or behavior of another person. However, your behavior can *influence* another person's behavior. It requires practice to develop sensitivity to the feelings of others. We can best adapt our own behavior and respond effectively to another person only if we are aware of the other person's emotional state.

As you work with patients and their families, strive to understand their feelings. Notice behavior that may indicate fear, anger, or grief. Avoid adding to such feelings by your own behavior. Take a little more time with the fearful patient, giving effective reassurances as best you can. Acknowledge the grieving person's right to sorrow, recognizing that this emotion needs expression and cannot be worked through quickly. Grant your patient the right to be angry in certain situations; instead of becoming defensive, listen. Then try to resolve the problem that aroused the patient's anger.

Through continuing effort, you can become a health care provider who practices the *art of human relations* along with the technical skills of your field.

## REFERENCES AND SUGGESTED READINGS

*Indicates a "classic" reference that introduced new ideas.

Chen, Hsi-Chung et al. (2010, March). Gender differences in the relationship between depression and cardiac autonomic function among community elderly. *International Journal of Geriatric Psychiatry, 25*(3), 314–322.

*Gordon, Thomas. (1975). *Parent effectiveness training*. New York: New American Library.

Kovács, Zsolt et al. (2010, April). Gender- and age-dependent changes in nucleoside levels in the cerebral cortex and white matter of the human brain. *Brain Research Bulletin, 81*(6), 579–584.

McKay, Matthew et al. (2007). *Thoughts and feelings: Taking control of your moods and your life*. Oakland, CA: New Harbinger.

Positive emotions increase resilience and life satisfaction. (2009, December). *IDEA Fitness Journal, 6*(10), p. 76(1).

*Selye, Hans. (1987). Stress without distress. *Psychological Bulletin, 131*(6), 925–972.

Simon, Robin, & Nath, Leda. (2004, March). Gender and emotion in the United States: Do men and women differ in self-reports of feelings and expressive behavior? *American Journal of Sociology, 109*(5), 1137–1176.

*Simonton, O. Carl, Matthews-Simonton, Stephanie, & Creighton, James. (1974). *Getting well again*. New York: St Martin's Press.

## REVIEW AND SELF-CHECK

1. List five effects of emotions on a person's quality of life.

2. Describe the physiological effects of experiencing a strong emotion.

3. Explain each of the following in your own words:
    a. Stress
    b. Distress
    c. Stressor

4. Name two different positive emotions; for each, list several words that describe various degrees of that particular emotion.

5. Name three different negative emotions; for each, list several words that describe various degrees of that particular emotion.

6. What is the essential characteristic of unconditional love?

7. Name five influences that affect the formation of emotional patterns.

8. Write out five guidelines that could help you to use emotions constructively.

9. Describe five ways that you, as a health care provider, can use knowledge about emotions to build effective relationships with patients.

10. Explain the value of using "I talk."

## ASSIGNMENTS

1. Consider how you are affected by anger and how you usually express it:
   a. Can you think clearly when you are angry?
   b. Do you usually express your anger *verbally* by:
      saying something you later regret?
      calling the other person a "dirty name"?
      raising your voice? shouting or screaming?
      threatening to do something the other person would not like?

c. Do you usually express your anger *physically* by:

   throwing things or kicking something?

   slamming a door?

   attacking the other person with your fists?

   slapping the other person?

d. Do you try to express your anger, but burst into tears?

e. Do you usually leave a situation when you become angry?

f. Do you manage to appear completely calm even though you are seething with anger inside?

g. Do you express your anger later, "taking it out" on someone other than the person at whom you are angry?

h. Do you believe that other people or events *cause* your anger?

2. Consider how you are affected by sadness and how you usually express it:

   a. Can you think clearly when you are unhappy?

   b. Can you concentrate when you are unhappy?

   c. Is it difficult to do things you know you should do?

   d. Is it difficult to make decisions?

   e. Have you ever made a decision while feeling sad, then later realized you did not use good judgment?

   f. Do you believe another person or some situation is the cause of your unhappiness?

3. Do you tend to feel anger toward those you believe caused your unhappiness? What are some alternatives to holding this anger?

4. Your husband has just come home and states that he and a colleague "really got into it today." You sense his anger and want him to talk about what happened. Instead, he changes clothes and goes out for a five-mile jog. What do you think of this behavior?

5. Mary Ann is 17 years old. Her mother died the day before her seventeenth birthday. Mary Ann occasionally states, somewhat proudly, "I didn't even cry." You know that she and her mother were very close. What do you think of Mary Ann's behavior?

6. You are assigned to Mr. J. today. You enter his room and say "Good morning" in your most cheerful voice. Mr. J. answers in an angry tone, "What's good about it?" What would be an effective response? What are some possible reasons for Mr. J. responding in such a way? How would you feel about Mr. J.?

7. Mrs. K. is scheduled for heart surgery. She is cheerful, never has a complaint, and tries to be helpful to the other patients. Your coworker says, "Mrs. K. is certainly unusual. She is not at all worried about her surgery." Do you agree with your coworker? Explain your answer.

8. Your supervisor calls you to the office and angrily says, "I'm changing the hours. You will have to work Saturday and Sunday." You have no plans, but it is your turn to have a weekend off. You become angry and say you will not work, even if it means being fired. Later that day you learn that two members of the staff are sick and one has been called out of town because of family problems. Describe the supervisor's probable emotional state when she called you into the office. List five ways you could have responded that might have prevented the unpleasant scene.

9. Consider each of the following statements. Be prepared to discuss each in terms of possible effects on the listener's emotional patterns:

   a. "You must not cry. You're a big boy now!"

   b. "If you do that again, I'll shut you in the closet."

   c. "You're a bad boy!"

   d. "It's wicked to hate someone. You must love everyone."

   e. "My friend had that same operation you're going to have. She had a terrible time and hasn't been the same since the operation."

   f. "Oh, you don't have a thing to worry about" (to a patient scheduled for surgery).

   g. "Shame on you! I expect you to get all As."

   h. "How dare you stomp your foot! You're a little girl; you must be sweet."

10. During the remainder of this course, collect examples of the following:

    a. "Innocent" statements that could arouse fear or anger in the listener, especially a child

    b. Ineffective reassurance offered to a patient or member of the family

    c. Effective reassurance, either verbal or nonverbal

    d. "You" statements in which the speaker projects blame instead of using open and honest communication

    e. Failure to express anger in a situation where anger is justified

    f. Denial of grief when there has been a great loss from one's life

    g. Statements that discourage the honest expression of feelings

    h. Statements that imply *conditional* love

11. Your child usually goes to his room whenever his older brother teases him. What does this mean, in terms of his pattern for expressing feelings? Now that you've noted his behavior, what should you do?

# UNIT 9

# Adjustment and Patterns of Behavior

## OBJECTIVES

Upon completion of this unit, you should be able to:

- List five characteristics of a person who is well adjusted.
- List three characteristics of a person who is poorly adjusted.
- Explain why poor adjustment can be a vicious cycle.
- State one reason change may affect adjustment.
- State five guidelines for improving adjustment.
- State four steps for adapting to a new situation.
- State two requirements for adapting to the role of health care provider.
- Name four ways one's emotional patterns influence adjustment.
- List five examples of daily hassles that can affect adjustment.
- List five examples of satisfying daily experiences that affect adjustment.

## KEY TERMS

| | |
|---|---|
| Adjustment | Hassle |
| Burnout | Vicious cycle |

**Adjustment** refers to how well an individual has learned to deal with life situations. Each person's adjustment is variable, depending upon circumstances. A person may be well adjusted most of the time, but poorly adjusted during a period when there is a serious problem. Some people are poorly adjusted most of the time. They have not learned to deal with ordinary life situations effectively.

## GOOD ADJUSTMENT

A person who is "well adjusted" deals effectively with problems and finds much satisfaction in living. Such a person has developed the habits and skills needed to solve common problems and has developed patterns of behavior that satisfy basic needs. Such a person is well prepared to weather a crisis and re-establish good adjustment within a reasonable period of time.

## POOR ADJUSTMENT

A person who is poorly adjusted is not living a full life. Such a person feels dissatisfied much of the time. Actually, the poorly adjusted person may not have any more problems than a well-adjusted person. *The difference is that the poorly adjusted person has not learned to cope with obstacles or effectively deal with everyday problems of living.*

The biggest obstacle for the poorly adjusted person is the poor adjustment itself. The habits, attitudes, emotional reactions, and behavior patterns that are a part of poor adjustment create additional problems for the individual. Poor adjustment is a **vicious cycle.** Ineffective behavior often creates additional problems that the individual handles with more ineffective behavior. For that reason, poor adjustment can be modified only if the individual learns to deal with life situations more effectively.

## EFFECTIVE BEHAVIOR VERSUS INEFFECTIVE BEHAVIOR

The key to adjustment is learning to recognize ineffective behavior and replacing it with another behavior that gets better results. The person who is willing to change can improve adjustment. The person who is unwilling or unable to change behavior patterns will not improve adjustment.

### *Transitions*

*Life is transitions*
  *professional and personal.*
*Transitions help us to grow*
  *and force us to change.*
*It is our choice—*
  *to make these transitions or not.*
*Listen for cues,*
  *follow the signs.*
*Life is transitions!*

Courtesy of Larry Hudson
University of Central Florida

Change is a test of one's ability to adjust. If familiar habits are used in new situations, the results may be quite different from results in the old situation. Change is an opportunity for growth that calls for conscious evaluation of habitual behavior. Ineffective habits should be discarded and new, more effective ones established. To acquire new friends, to fit into a new community, to succeed in a new job, and to do well in a course of study all require that some old habits be discarded and that some new ones be developed.

Change is always a threat to adjustment. It is easy to continue using familiar habits; it requires effort to form new habits. It is distressing to find that established patterns of behavior do not bring the familiar result. Such inner discomfort may lead to criticizing the new situation, telling new companions about the old situation, or even trying to change the new situation to make it more like the old one. These types of behavior indicate poor adjustment.

Larissa and Kay are two high school juniors enrolled in the health occupations course. Both are new in the school, faced with a new and unfamiliar setting. Kay wants desperately to be popular; when her new classmates ignore her, she feels resentment. She becomes critical of the class leaders, looking for opportunities to make uncomplimentary remarks about them. Her classmates soon tire of her negativity. They do not understand that Kay gets some relief from inner discomfort by criticizing those she envies. Kay is using ineffective behavior. Criticizing others makes her feel better momentarily, but it interferes with her forming new friendships. Unless Kay gains insight into her own behavior, she is likely to continue to use a behavior that provides only temporary satisfaction.

In the meantime, Larissa decides to broaden her interests. She becomes more active in school affairs, helping with the newspaper and joining several clubs. Each new activity leads to new friends for Larissa. She is also learning new skills and acquiring new outlooks through these various activities. Larissa is using effective behavior to improve her adjustment. She took action to adapt to her new situation and that action proved to be effective. Larissa's goal was to become comfortable in the new situation and broaden her range of interests; gaining many new friends was only one of several benefits.

Julia is a student in the surgical technician program. She knows the procedures must be performed correctly, but her performance often includes errors. The instructor has talked with Julia about her performance. Every error and every problem, according to Julia, was the fault of someone else: the circulating nurse, another student, whoever set up the tray or pack, some member of the surgical team. Julia does not learn from her mistakes or from the instructor/student conference, because she is unable or unwilling to admit that she can make a mistake. She has not learned to take responsibility for her actions, and she denies the consequences of her errors by claiming "It wasn't my fault." Unless Julia changes this pattern of behavior, she will have problems throughout life (Figure 9-1). She will not be acceptable as a health care provider, because she would not be a safe practitioner.

**FIGURE 9-1** Improving your adjustment requires giving up ineffective habits.
*Delmar/Cengage Learning*

## EMOTIONS AND ADJUSTMENT

Emotions are a major influence on one's adjustment. A person who experiences positive emotions several times a day is likely to have better adjustment than one who frequently experiences negative emotions. Sometimes the emotion one experiences is a matter of choice. For example, you drop your keys as you try to unlock the car door. You feel annoyed as you pick them up and try again to fit the key into the lock. Somehow the keys slip out of your fingers and fall to the ground a second time. At this point, you can utter a string of four-letter words to express your anger and exasperation. Or, you could pick the keys up again, laughingly comment that you seem to have butterfingers today, then pay close attention to getting the key into the lock successfully.

Everyone has daily experiences that represent some type of difficulty. Everyone has daily experiences that proceed smoothly, without any problems. At the end of the day, one person remembers a number of these "good experiences" and gives little thought to the things that did not go well. Another person may finish the day feeling angry about several problem situations that occurred, and have little or no conscious awareness of any good experiences. Each of us may *choose* the type of experience to which we give most of our attention. In most situations, we may either choose to be angry or to deal with a situation unemotionally, working toward a resolution of the difficulty. Dr. Norman Shealy, whose work is discussed in Unit 23, stated in a workshop that he regards anger to be a destructive emotion that serves no useful purpose; by this, he means that it is better to deal *effectively* with an anger-arousing situation than to indulge in angry feelings and ineffective behavior. Another workshop leader commented that when he begins to feel angry, he goes for a walk and thinks about *why* he is angry; often, the answer involves a way to resolve the situation and his anger simply dissipates.

Fear is also a powerful influence on adjustment. A person who lives in fear of what "might happen" is expecting bad things to happen. Such expectations influence behavior and also affect how that person perceives events. It is normal to experience fear when faced with a real threat; the well-adjusted person reacts appropriately to such threat. A person who is chronically anxious, however, is living with fear that arises from negative thinking, rather than any real threat. Habitual negative thinking represents a state of poor adjustment.

Sadness also may be experienced appropriately or inappropriately. Each of us has life experiences that arouse sad feelings. Each of us is exposed to world news revealing the terrible things that are happening, events that we are powerless to change. Someone who is truly grieved by conditions in a third-world country might join the Peace Corps and devote two or more years to try to improve those conditions. Many people address their prayers to such situations; persons who meditate may focus a daily meditation on peaceful resolution of a specific problem, wherever it exists. Others might feel real empathy for the victims of some distant tragedy and send a contribution to an organization that is providing help. Others may feel a brief period of sadness and then shift their attention to their own affairs. These reactions indicate healthful use of sadness.

A person who chooses to focus on tragic events may remain in a sad state, indulge in "Ain't it awful" talk, yet take no action to correct the situation. This focus of attention on tragic events allows sadness to interfere with adjustment. As with anger and fear, a person can *choose* the extent to which sadness is allowed to affect one's overall feeling (Figure 9-2).

**FIGURE 9-2** When you look in the mirror, do you see a person who finds much satisfaction in life, or one who focuses on negative experiences? *Delmar/Cengage Learning*

## DAILY HASSLES

**Hassle** denotes "any event that causes you to feel irritated, annoyed, frustrated, fearful, or angry." How one copes with "daily hassles" is a reflection of one's adjustment. However, one's usual state of adjustment is also a factor in how well one copes with "daily hassles."

Box 9-1 is designed to help you identify hassles in your life. Box 9-2 permits you to identify the "good" things that occur. You choose which type of events receive most of your attention, and therefore which type of emotions dominate your daily life.

## IMPROVING ADJUSTMENT

How does one improve adjustment? It is easier to make the effort while in a familiar situation. The following guidelines can be useful in directing your efforts to improve adjustment. First, focus on one or two of the guidelines until you have made significant progress, then select one or two others. If you attempt to focus on all of the guidelines at the same time, you are likely to become discouraged.

- Find patterns of behavior that satisfy basic needs.
- Assume conscious control of your behavior.
- Use problem solving to find the best possible solution for a problem situation instead of acting impulsively.
- Use emotions constructively. When appropriate, express feelings at the time they are experienced.
- Evaluate your behavior in a specific situation. Was the outcome favorable for you? What other possible behavior on your part would have been appropriate? Is it likely that another behavior would have been more effective?
- Self-evaluate in a constructive sense. Look for ways to improve but avoid feelings of guilt or inadequacy.
- Select appropriate goals in terms of "all that I can be" and plan how you will reach these goals.

## BOX 9-1

### Hassles in My Life

**Instructions:** In the following list circle (1) for each event you experienced yesterday and (2) for each event you experienced during the past week or month. Substitute appropriate words (e.g., "my glasses" for "keys") to adapt a statement to your situation. If a statement just does not apply to you, leave it blank.

| | | |
|---|---|---|
| 1. I couldn't find my keys. | 1 | 2 |
| 2. My neighbor's dog barked all night. | 1 | 2 |
| 3. My sister called to talk about her problems. | 1 | 2 |
| 4. There's no way I can pay all my bills this month. | 1 | 2 |
| 5. My spouse is thrilled with our new sound system; I'm not, because our charge card is now "maxed out." | 1 | 2 |
| 6. I had to make a difficult decision. | 1 | 2 |
| 7. My coworkers take extended breaks and I end up doing more than my share of the work. | 1 | 2 |
| 8. One of my clients was especially unpleasant, even though I had given him extra time. | 1 | 2 |
| 9. I am having a plumbing problem (again!). | 1 | 2 |
| 10. I'm having a really bad hair day. | 1 | 2 |
| 11. I tossed and turned all night. (I went to bed really sleepy, then couldn't go to sleep; or, I woke up at 2 a.m. and couldn't get back to sleep.) | 1 | 2 |
| 12. My car wouldn't start. | 1 | 2 |
| 13. I locked my keys in the car. | 1 | 2 |
| 14. Traffic was terrible this morning. | 1 | 2 |
| 15. The news is full of crime reports; I just don't feel safe anymore. | 1 | 2 |
| 16. There's a rumor that administration plans to "downsize" the patient care staff. | 1 | 2 |
| 17. Even on my day off, I just couldn't relax. | 1 | 2 |
| 18. Someone (insert name or title) took advantage of me; I'm afraid to confront him or her. | 1 | 2 |
| 19. Someone (insert name) smokes too much; I'm afraid he or she will develop lung cancer. | 1 | 2 |
| 20. It's harder and harder to please my spouse; he or she complained all through breakfast this morning. | 1 | 2 |

Total your score for each column. Note that items 1–14 deal primarily with anger and frustration; items 15–20 are more closely related to fear and anxiety. Now follow the same procedure with Box 9-2 to identify some "good" experiences in your life.

## BOX 9-2

### Satisfactions in My Life

**Instructions:** In the following list circle (1) for each event you experienced yesterday and (2) for those you experienced during the past week or month. Substitute appropriate words to adapt statements to your situation. If a statement does not apply to you, leave it blank.

| | | | |
|---|---|---|---|
| 1. | I had a good night's sleep. | 1 | 2 |
| 2. | My supervisor complimented me on my work. | 1 | 2 |
| 3. | I am scheduled to be off on my birthday. | 1 | 2 |
| 4. | I found a good buy on my family's favorite food. | 1 | 2 |
| 5. | I enjoyed talking with a new coworker during break. | 1 | 2 |
| 6. | One of my patients said, "You are the best!" | 1 | 2 |
| 7. | When I reconciled my checkbook with my bank statement, I found a $50 deposit I had failed to enter. | 1 | 2 |
| 8. | My energy level has been up lately. | 1 | 2 |
| 9. | I stopped smoking. | 1 | 2 |
| 10. | I ate less fat (sugar, snacks, caffeine). | 1 | 2 |
| 11. | I exercised for 20 minutes. | 1 | 2 |
| 12. | I managed my time so that I had free time in the evening. | 1 | 2 |
| 13. | I included some recreation in my schedule. | 1 | 2 |
| 14. | I spent time with friends and really enjoyed it. | 1 | 2 |
| 15. | I confronted (insert name) about (insert issue) and, to my surprise, we had a very satisfying discussion. | 1 | 2 |
| 16. | I weighed myself this morning; I have lost 3 pounds. | 1 | 2 |
| 17. | I was able to relax and enjoy my day off. | 1 | 2 |
| 18. | My neighbor got rid of his barking dog. | 1 | 2 |
| 19. | My sister liked the birthday present I gave her. | 1 | |
| 20. | My child's grades have improved and he or she likes the new teacher. | 1 | 2 |
| 21. | I didn't think I could handle an assignment, but I did and was complimented on my work. | 1 | 2 |
| 22. | I received a favorable work review (grade). | 1 | 2 |

Total the two columns. Now, compare your "hassles" scores with your "satisfaction" scores. Which score is higher? Was it easier to recognize hassles than satisfactions? Or were the satisfactions more recognizable? Do you tend to focus more on your satisfactions or hassles?

If you can achieve reasonably good adjustment in your usual life situation, then you will be prepared for the challenge of adapting to new situations and dealing with the occasional crisis situations that are an unavoidable part of life.

### Maintaining a Healthful Lifestyle

The suggestions just listed for improving your state of adjustment are somewhat broad and require conscious effort over a period of time. Steps for improving your daily habits can be taken immediately, and these daily habits definitely contribute to one's state of adjustment. A diet that consists largely of junk food, the use of addictive substances, lack of balance in work and play, lack of exercise, and inadequate sleep can all interfere with good adjustment. Your diet should include generous amounts of fresh vegetables and fruit, some eaten raw. Drink at least eight glasses of pure water each day. Exercise regularly. Avoid harmful and addictive substances. Participate regularly in recreational activities that help you release stress and regenerate your energies. Allow adequate time for sleep. Most of these habits are discussed elsewhere, and some you are probably learning about in other courses.

One daily habit that is essential to good adjustment, yet is seldom included in a course of study, is sleep. You learned about the physical need for sleep in Unit 5. The purpose here is to re-emphasize that seven to eight hours of sleep are necessary in order to get the full benefit of REM sleep, which tends to occur most often during hours six to eight. So be aware that an important first-line defense against stress overload is getting your full quota of sleep. When you start your day well rested, it is easier to work toward other aspects of achieving good adjustment.

### The Role of Joy and Laughter

The therapeutic effects of laughter came to the attention of the public and the health community with the publication in 1979 of Norman Cousins's book, *Anatomy of an Illness as Perceived by the Patient*. Cousins described how laughter had helped him recover from a debilitating illness for which there was no known cure. Since Cousins was an internationally famous journalist, his story had such a high level of credibility that it had an impact on health care delivery. Within a year or two, conferences were being held to teach health care providers about the value of humor and laughter.

Research since that time has revealed that there are physical, mental, and emotional benefits of laughter and joyous experiences. The physical benefits include improved circulation, higher oxygen levels, enhanced immune functions, and increased levels of hormones that influence how one copes with stress. With so much to be gained from experiences that make us laugh, why is laughter not more commonplace in our daily lives?

Dr. Lee Berk, of the College of Medicine at the University of California–Irvine, proposes that sometime between childhood and adulthood people tend to lose the joyful aspects of living. He notes that the average child smiles or laughs 400 times a day, but the average adult smiles or laughs only 15 times a day.

Laughter, then, is now acknowledged as a factor in health, whether for the purpose of maintaining health, managing stress, or coping with illness. Some simple techniques for purposely putting more laughter into your day include:

- Look in the mirror at least once a day and tell the image you see there to laugh with you; even that moment of forced laughter will be beneficial.

- At least once a day, remember some funny incident or joyful experience; take a few minutes to laugh or experience joyful feelings.
- Place a keepsake from some fun or joyful experience where you can see it and enjoy a laugh or feelings of joy, even if only for a moment.
- Share funny experiences with other people; when you make them laugh, you also laugh and everyone benefits.
- Choose friends who like to laugh; it is hard to be "down" when you are around people who laugh often.
- Seek out humor that you can share with others.

## Avoiding Burnout

Every health care provider is at risk for developing burnout syndrome. **Burnout** is a state of deterioration that affects an individual physically, mentally, and emotionally. It develops gradually over a period of weeks, months, or years of living or working in a high-stress situation, during which the individual may not eat properly, gets minimal rest, has few opportunities for recreation and self-renewal, experiences much frustration, receives little emotional support from others, and/or ignores signs of illness in order to keep going. Anyone with a tendency to be a "workaholic" is risking burnout.

A conscientious worker who begins to make errors, take longer to perform tasks, or fail to complete assigned work may be in the early stages of burnout. Other early signs include increasing frustration and loss of interest. The worker may believe that his or her efforts are unappreciated and develop a negative attitude about the job. As the condition worsens, it becomes increasingly difficult to fulfill job responsibilities. Coworkers may notice increased irritability or complaints. Physical symptoms include fatigue, frequent minor illnesses, gastrointestinal disorders, headaches, or various aches and pains. There may be increased consumption of caffeine, tobacco, or alcohol or a tendency to seek relief through drugs, either legal or illegal.

The causes of burnout may lie within the individual—unhealthful life habits, failure to take responsibility for one's own well-being, a dedication to the job that results in too much work and not enough self-care, and failure to use effective stress management strategies. Often the causes of burnout are within the work environment—stressors such as uncomfortable physical conditions, unpleasant working relations, supervisor or management behavior, lack of encouragement and emotional support, and lack of recognition or reward for work done well.

In any individual case, the contributing causes of burnout syndrome may be a combination of personal habits and working conditions. The period of service in a high-stress area (i.e., air traffic controllers, intensive care personnel) should be limited, with periodic rotations to less stressful work assignments. Supervisors in high-stress occupations should be alert for early signs of burnout. Early intervention can prevent errors and accidents by a worker whose functional capacity is diminished. In the final analysis, it is the individual worker who has responsibility for avoiding burnout.

The best protection is a lifestyle that includes all of the above suggestions for improving adjustment plus the regular use of effective stress management techniques (discussed further in Unit 27). If the stressors of the work setting affect numerous workers, management should eliminate as many stressful conditions as possible. If work conditions cannot be improved and the worker is not able to deal effectively with the resulting stress, then it is time to seek employment elsewhere!

## Adapting to New Situations

When a change occurs in your life situation—for better or worse—modify some of your patterns of behavior in order to achieve a state of good adjustment in the new situation. If the change is rather minor, you may adapt with little awareness of stress. If the change is great, however, you may go through a stressful period before you achieve adjustment. You may even be very unhappy at first, wishing that you could return to the old situation (Figure 9-3). As you successfully adapt, you will gradually begin to feel comfortable in the new situation.

The degree of disruption a change causes in one's usual pattern of living is dependent upon the type of change. Some changes you are likely to encounter include job changes, moving to a new neighborhood, a change of supervisors, a new administration in your place of employment, and changes in operational procedures and policies. A major change all of us have to face at some time is the loss of relatives and friends.

In general, adapting to change requires acceptance of the new situation and a conscious effort to adapt. If the change involves new tasks and new people:

1. Study the situation carefully.
2. Observe the behavior of others.
3. Learn the policies and regulations of the new situation.
4. Consciously adopt behaviors that are appropriate for that situation.

If you find that the new situation requires you to follow procedures that are unsafe (for you or your patients) or are unethical, you have a conflict: you can lower your standards and

**FIGURE 9-3** Clinging to old situations indicates poor adjustment to the present situation. *Delmar/Cengage Learning*

console yourself with the thought, "I'm just doing what everybody else is doing"; you can use appropriate procedures to try to change practices, a risky approach for a new employee; or you can leave the situation. Conflicts are discussed in detail in Unit 13.

There is also the possibility that the new situation has more rigorous standards than your previous position. In that case, you have a challenge: to improve your performance in order to be acceptable to your new coworkers and supervisors. Willingness to learn and to improve performance will earn favorable evaluations for you; rebelling against the higher standards will mark you as an unsatisfactory employee.

A type of behavior that interferes with adapting to a new situation is clinging to the old situation. Comparing the old situation to the new, especially in terms that indicate your preference for the old, reveals that you do not yet accept the present situation. One sure way to antagonize new coworkers is to tell them repeatedly how you did things on your previous job. This behavior indicates poor adjustment to one's present job situation.

### Adapting to the Role of Health Care Provider

You are already aware that becoming a health care provider requires certain modifications in behavior. Perhaps your previous job permitted smoking at any time while you worked; this is not appropriate in your new role. Perhaps you have had a job in which you were allowed to do many different tasks and accept as much responsibility as you were able to handle. As a health care provider you will have a well-defined role. You may find it annoying to have limitations placed on your role, especially if others perform tasks you believe you can do. Performance within one's defined role is necessary within the health field; to exceed that role may endanger a patient and also may have legal implications. You are already aware of the change you must make in giving health care suggestions to your friends. Refrain from any advice or actions that appear to be efforts to diagnose or prescribe. Essentially, adjustment to being a health care provider requires knowing one's role and performing within it, while also accepting and abiding by the code of ethics appropriate to that role.

## REFERENCES AND SUGGESTED READINGS

*Indicates a classic reference that introduced new ideas.

*Cousins, Norman. (1979). *Anatomy of an illness as perceived by the patient.* New York: W. W. Norton.

Hallowell, Edward M. (2007). *Crazy busy: Overstretched, overbooked, and about to snap! Strategies for handling your fast-paced life.* New York: Ballantine.

McCreaddie, May. (2008, April 23). You must be joking: Using humor to benefit patients' health could be a risk worth taking. *Nursing Standard, 22*(33), 22–23.

Tamparo, Carol T., & Lindh, Wilburta Q. (2008). *Therapeutic communications for health professionals* (3rd ed.). Clifton Park, NY: Delmar, Cengage Learning.

Winter, George. (2006, Dec. 13). Laughter therapy: Don't be surprised when people laugh in the face of illness or disaster. *Nursing Standard, 21*(14), 14–16, 28–29.

## SOURCES OF ADDITONAL INFORMATION

Humor Matters, http://www.humormatters.com
American Association for Therapeutic Humor, http://www.aath.org
The Humor Project, Inc., http://www.humorproject.com

## REVIEW AND SELF-CHECK

1. List five characteristic behaviors that indicate a person is well adjusted.

2. List three characteristic behaviors that could indicate a person is not well adjusted.

3. Explain why poor adjustment can be a vicious cycle.

4. Explain why any change in a person's life situation can affect adjustment.

5. List five guidelines that you could use to improve adjustment.

6. State four steps a person could follow to adapt to a new situation.

7. What are two requirements for adapting to the role of health care provider?

8. How do one's emotional patterns influence adjustment?

9. List five examples of daily hassles that can affect one's adjustment.

10. Name five examples of daily experiences that can provide satisfaction and thereby contribute to good adjustment.

## ASSIGNMENTS

1. List 10 observable behaviors that may indicate poor adjustment.

2. List 10 observable behaviors that indicate a person is relatively well adjusted.

3. Using the above lists, place an X beside each behavior that is characteristic of you. Count the number of Xs beside "poor adjustment" behavior; count the Xs beside "good adjustment" behavior. Subtract the "poor" score from the "good" score. If the remainder is less than 5, begin *now* to plan ways to improve your adjustment.

4. Select one behavior listed under "poor adjustment" in your previous list and plan how you will modify or eliminate that behavior. Set a time limit (for example, three months) at which time you will evaluate your success in modifying, or eliminating, this behavior.

5. Your classmate says, "I think all this study about understanding yourself is a waste of time." Write a brief response to this statement. Use the following as a basis for your reasoning: (a) the importance of adjustment to living a full life and (b) the importance of self-understanding for health care providers.

6. Refer to your scores for Boxes 9-1 and 9-2 and review the items that you marked. Tonight before going to bed, list the hassles you experienced today; select one particularly annoying event and consider ways you could prevent that particular hassle from recurring.

Now, list the satisfying events of the day and consciously experience "good feelings." As you drift off to sleep, feel a sense of gratitude for the good experiences you had today.

7. List five behaviors you will modify in order to adjust to the role of health care provider.

8. List four behaviors that could help you adapt to a new situation.

9. Participate in a class discussion about the following events, each of which has the potential to change one's life significantly; consider ways a person could experience personal growth through dealing with each situation.

    a. Divorce

    b. Diagnosis of a health problem requiring lifestyle changes

    c. Moving 1,000 miles away from your hometown

    d. Loss of your job

    e. Extensive changes in your job responsibilities

Section

# Behavior and Problems in Living

Life does not always flow smoothly. There are many problems in daily living. The goals we set for ourselves can be reached only through continual striving, and progress is often blocked by some type of difficulty. Behavior in the face of threat, blocking, failure, and other unsatisfying experiences can resolve the difficulty or create additional problems. This is especially true if a defensive reaction or aggression occurs.

Anyone with a health deviation has new problems in addition to those of the usual life situation. Health care providers must be aware that many patients are reacting to threat and, possibly, overwhelming problems. The patient needs acceptance, understanding, and caring from those who provide health care.

Section III is designed to help you understand some types of behavior likely to result from threat. By learning to cope effectively with personal threat and its effects, the health care provider prepares to understand and accept the behavior of others who are reacting in their own way to threats in their life situations.

# UNIT 10

# Common Threats to Adjustment

## OBJECTIVES

Upon completion of this unit, you should be able to:

- List six stages of life that present new challenges to a person's adjustment.
- Name one significant change that occurs in each of the six life stages.
- Name three experiences that represent a major life change.
- Explain the significance of peer pressure on an adolescent.
- List three examples of sexism.
- Describe three learning problems that can make school difficult for a student.
- Explain the difference between healthy and unhealthy family relationships.
- List two cultural stressors that can occur in each of these life stages: childhood, adolescence, adulthood.
- List three strategies parents can use to improve a child's behavior.

## KEY TERMS

Attention deficit disorder (ADD)
Attention deficit hyperactivity disorder (ADHD)
Autism spectrum disorders
Coping skills
Developmental disorders
Discrimination
Dyslexia
Family dynamics
Resilience
Separation anxiety
Sexism

The adjustment of any one person can be very poor, very good, or anywhere in between. Each person has a relative state of adjustment that characterizes that person most of the time. Adjustment, however, is always subject to change. Life experiences require changes in behavior to adapt to new situations and cope with new problems. Our state of adjustment can always be threatened by difficult situations.

A state of good adjustment *most of the time* is the best protection a person can have against the difficulties of life. By developing skills that help us deal effectively with our daily life problems, we prepare ourselves for dealing with big problems.

## CHANGE AS A THREAT TO ADJUSTMENT

Most people are reasonably well adjusted to their usual life situation. They are able to deal with routine problems, and they get along fairly well with family and friends. Then a change occurs. Perhaps the change appears rather ordinary—a move to a new neighborhood, a change of schools, even a change of jobs. We adapt to "ordinary" changes with slight modifications in our behavior. Perhaps the change is major, such as going away to college or leaving a protective home to enter military service. When major changes occur, we may have to learn new patterns of behavior.

Any type of change is a threat to one's adjustment. Since change is inevitable, learning to adapt our behaviors to new situations will help us maintain a state of good adjustment.

## LIFE STAGES AND CHANGE

As human beings, we are designed to grow, change, and develop throughout our lives. Each stage of life brings new opportunities but also presents new challenges (Figure 10-1). Sometimes these normal changes threaten our adjustment and require us to learn new behaviors or **coping skills** if we are to remain well adjusted.

### Early Childhood

Children develop most rapidly during the first few years of their lives (Figure 10-2). They develop gross motor skills such as walking, running, and jumping and fine motor skills such as holding a pencil or fork. They learn to use language to communicate their wants and needs, and they practice basic social skills such as table manners and sharing.

Children are constantly learning about the world around them. They feel secure when they know what to expect from others, but they often find new people and places frightening. A predictable routine provides security, while chaos or unexpected changes can cause anxiety. Changes in the family schedule, bedtime routine, or childcare provider should be introduced gently and gradually.

Infants and preschoolers may experience **separation anxiety** when they enter a new daycare or school. For days or even weeks, they may cry, claim to be sick, or beg to go home. Some elementary school students experience anxiety when coming to a new school or returning after a long vacation. To resolve separation anxiety, parents, care providers, and health

**FIGURE 10-1** Adjustment is a relative state that shifts according to life experiences. *Delmar/Cengage Learning*

**FIGURE 10-2** School-age children like to play in peer groups. *Delmar/Cengage Learning*

professionals should work together to help the child get used to the new situation and should be understanding of the child's feelings without giving in to demands to go home.

## Middle Childhood

For children who have developed physical, intellectual, and social skills during the early years, facing new situations becomes easier as they enter and progress through elementary school. Each year brings a new class, new friends, and new experiences. These changes pose only a minor threat to adjustment.

For students who lack basic skills or are developmentally delayed, entering school can create new fears and problems. For many students, difficulties in school can be traced to a lack of school readiness skills. Poor social skills may lead to conflicts with classmates, while delayed intellectual development can create a pattern of school failure. Daily situations such as school assignments and interacting with peers can pose major threats to a child who is already poorly adjusted. The earlier parents, educators, and health care providers can intervene to help such children develop needed skills, the more likely the child will be successful.

## Adolescence

As young people enter the teen years, they struggle to establish an identity separate from that of their parents. Adolescents are inclined to worry about appearance, self-worth as a person, the future, and—very important—the opinions of others. Relationships with peers become extremely important (Figure 10-3). Teens need to feel accepted and a part of the group. Disappointment or rejection by members of their peer group can pose a major threat to a teen's adjustment. Peer pressure—the feeling of having to go along with the group in order to be accepted—can influence teens' choices about clothing, about using tobacco and alcohol, or about sexual relationships. Mood swings and variable adjustment are typical of the adolescent period.

Romantic relationships form an important part of many teens' lives. Because many young people choose to become sexually active during the teen years, sexual relationships and pressures can create additional stress. Teens may worry about pregnancy or sexually transmitted diseases. Health care providers may find that teens turn to them with questions the teens are uncomfortable asking a parent.

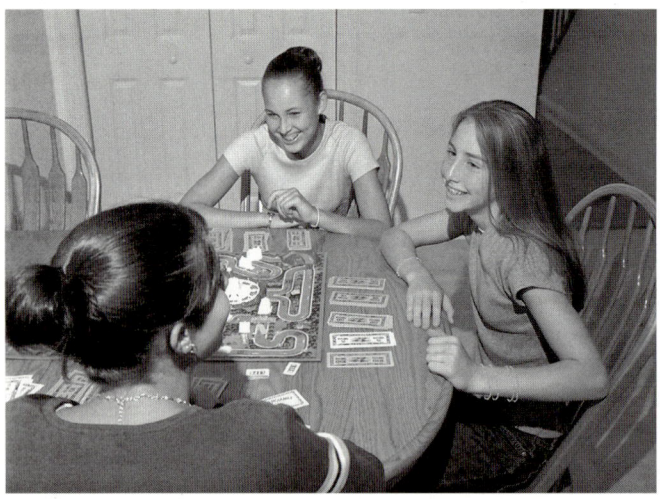

**FIGURE 10-3** Acceptance by the peer group is especially important during adolescence. *Delmar/Cengage Learning*

The teenager who has a positive self-concept and relatively good adjustment is likely to adapt to the challenges of the adolescent period. If one enters adolescence with a negative self-concept, poor interpersonal skills, ineffective behavior patterns, and/or inability to adapt to change, the problem may become more intense. If adolescence proceeds at a favorable pace, childhood patterns are gradually replaced by more mature patterns of behavior. If such growth does not occur, then childish patterns of behavior may continue into adulthood.

## Young Adulthood

Young adults face many changes as they establish their independence from their parents. Common changes include completing high school and beginning college or a job, setting up a home of one's own, marrying, and starting a family. Each of these changes brings new experiences and responsibilities. Young people who have already developed good coping skills will usually adapt to each of these changes. However, young adults with a pattern of school and family problems may see similar problems develop in their jobs or their own families unless they learn more effective ways of coping. Young adults' decisions about careers, having children, and whether to marry or divorce will influence the rest of their lives.

## Middle Adulthood

Middle-aged adults may become painfully aware of the passing of time. They may not have reached their earlier ambitions or found satisfaction in their jobs and may wonder whether it is too late to start again. Middle-aged adults who have achieved their earlier goals may find that life seems empty or lacking in challenge. Children are growing up and leaving home, leaving parents with an "empty nest." Parents who devoted their early years to their families may now feel unneeded. Physical changes, especially in women, can affect one's moods and emotions. A man's physician may tell him to give up some activities, to slow down. Many adults have difficulty accepting these signs of disappearing youth. The popular term "midlife crisis" describes an adult who is having trouble adjusting to the changes of middle age.

## Older Adulthood

Older adulthood brings many frightening changes. Losses of friends and relatives require frequent funeral attendance. Employers may encourage older adults to retire before they are ready to withdraw from work that has been a major part of life for many years. The widow or widower may find it necessary to change homes. Sometimes family and friends rush an elderly person, just bereaved of a life partner, into a decision to give up the home and move in with one of the children or into a long-term care facility. Such radical changes should not be made until the widow or widower has worked through the grief process (one to three years).

Older adults may face a number of fears: losing their independence, not having enough money, becoming physically or financially dependent upon others, becoming ill, or dying (Figure 10-4). The uncertainties of these years can affect attitudes, feelings, relationships, and total behavior. Many elderly persons view the future as dismal, offering only the prospect of increasing losses and, eventually, death.

On the other hand, some older adults experience this portion of life as "the golden years." For those who are financially secure, remain in reasonably good health, and enjoy close ties to friends and family, the later years can be rewarding. These adults enjoy opportunities such as retirement, travel, socializing, and spending time with grandchildren. As with every other age, effective coping skills and supportive relationships help a person deal with life changes and maintain a good state of adjustment.

## SOCIAL AND CULTURAL STRESSORS

As an individual grows up and grows older, he or she must also cope with the pressures of society. Stressors such as peer pressure, drugs, and **discrimination** can become serious threats to a person's adjustment.

**FIGURE 10-4** During senescence, illness is a serious threat to adjustment. *Delmar/Cengage Learning*

## Stressors of Childhood

Many children feel tremendous pressure to do well in school and/or sports and to be accepted by peers. For some children, success in these areas seems to come naturally. For slow learners, shy children, or those with behavioral difficulties, school becomes a major source of stress. Some children may also have difficulty fitting in with others and making friends. As a child moves into the older elementary and middle school years, peer relationships become increasingly important.

## Stressors of Adolescence

All the sources of childhood stress continue through adolescence—accompanied by additional sources of stress: the pressure of competition (athletics, extracurricular activities, school politics), pressure to excel (especially if college-bound), the need to belong, the need to be attractive to members of the opposite sex, eagerness to finish driver education and get one's own car. These are the familiar pressures of adolescence.

There is also the threat of school violence. Gangs exist in many schools; by belonging, there is safety in numbers, but one must conform to the gang's practices and beliefs. Initiation rites may include having sex (or committing a rape), shoplifting, car theft, "beating up" someone of a different race or ethnic group, or mugging. The initiate who fulfills this assignment then "belongs" to the gang, but not just as a member; any attempt to leave the gang may result in blackmail—gang members could provide testimony about the crime, resulting in a prison sentence for the would-be defector. Thus, the gang leader has power and control over members of the gang.

Those who are not gang members may live in fear of gang activity or reprisals following any dispute with a gang member. Weapons, once unheard of in a public school, are now prevalent. Some schools have electronic devices to detect weapons; but weapons are present in the parking lot. Assaults do occur, with both teachers and students as victims.

**Peer Pressure** Adolescence is a period when peer approval is extremely important. It is a time of life when family influence is challenged by the peer group because of the individual's need to belong. For that reason, each adolescent must choose between participating in certain practices that are widespread through the student body and the risk of being the outsider. Those who resist may experience pressure from their classmates to get involved, or to "just try it."

**Drugs** Drugs are a major problem, sometimes being sold and used in school restrooms and the parking lot. At social events there is peer pressure to use drugs such as marijuana, crack, cocaine, and heroin. "Just say 'No!'" is not easy advice to follow; by saying, "No," the student risks disapproval of the peer group. By saying "No" to someone who wants to sell the drug, a student risks some type of reprisal by the disgruntled dealer, especially if the dealer is a gang member.

**Sexual Activity** When the adolescent begins to date, there may be pressure almost immediately to engage in sexual activity. This may conflict with beliefs about morality the adolescent has learned in the home and at church. The adolescent experiences an internal conflict: the need for acceptance by the peer group and the need to uphold one's standards and maintain self-esteem. Today's trend toward becoming sexually active during the teens has serious health implications: pregnancy, sexually transmitted diseases, and the emotional effects of abandonment by a partner to whom one has become emotionally attached. In many communities, sex education remains a controversial subject. Providing information on self-protection or distributing prophylactic materials through a school program is emphatically opposed by many adults. A health care provider is very likely to be approached by a teenager who needs information or help in regard to sexual activity.

Fortunately, not every adolescent is exposed to some of these stressors, but many are exposed to all of them. Numerous stressors experienced by adolescents today did not exist, or were not prevalent, when their parents were in high school. Many parents therefore do not understand or accept the problems today's adolescents face at school. Every adolescent needs to be able to discuss these problems regularly with an adult who understands the problems, encourages the expression of feelings, and helps identify appropriate ways to deal with these difficult situations.

## Stressors of Adulthood

Many of the stressors and serious traumas of childhood and adolescence continue into adulthood. Some that are discussed below also occur during childhood or adolescence. But certain stressors, such as discrimination, rape, and domestic violence, seem more appropriate for discussion within the framework of adulthood.

**Discrimination and Sexism** Members of minority groups in all cultures and throughout time have experienced discrimination. There seems to be an innate human need for perceiving people in "us/them" terms, favoring those who are members of the "us" group. But this tendency does not excuse discrimination that violates the rights of others because of sex, race, nationality, ethnic group, age, or religion. It required many years of campaigning by a group of courageous women before American women finally gained the right to vote. Until about 40 years ago, it was illegal in some states for a Caucasian to marry an Asian American. African Americans have gained many rights as a result of the civil rights movement of the 1960s. Heightened awareness on the part of many Americans and a series of congressional acts have brought about numerous changes.

Federal laws pertaining to equal employment opportunities and prohibiting discrimination on the basis of race, sex, and age have been passed only in the past 40 years. Such laws do make it illegal to continue certain long-standing policies and practices. But laws do not change attitudes or beliefs. It is relatively easy to find examples indicating that discriminatory practices still exist, in educational settings as well as in the marketplace. As a new generation that grew up with civil rights and feminist activities assumes decision-making positions in business and government, fairness and equal opportunities may prevail. In the meantime, discrimination continues as a serious stressor to those who are victimized by such practices.

Discrimination may be practiced against anyone because of a specific attribute, such as race, sex, religion, age, weight, or other physical attribute. The most common basis for discrimination, however, is either race (racism) or sex (**sexism**). Other traumas related to sex include harassment, rape, and domestic violence.

**Sexual Discrimination** As more and more women become part-time homemakers and full-time workers, there is increasing awareness of the extent to which discrimination against women is practiced. The male teacher is more likely to be encouraged to move into administration than a female teacher. A male health care provider is likely to be "promoted" to a supervisory position after a few years of work experience, while female colleagues with more experience are not considered for the position. In the business world, women who rise to relatively high positions in a corporation may encounter a "glass ceiling" in their organization; everyone above that ceiling is male. Until recently, women who experienced discrimination on the job had no recourse; now, because of federal legislation, there are procedures for protesting discriminatory practices. Those who protest are at risk of losing their jobs; but that, too, provides a basis for filing charges of discrimination.

**Sexual Harassment** A more serious example of sexism is *sexual harassment,* which is the most frequently reported complaint in the workplace today. It may also occur in an educational setting. Usually the victim is someone with limited power (student, secretary), whereas the perpetrator (teacher, supervisor, customer) has some degree of power over the victim. The victim of sexual harassment is usually female, but may be male. The harassment may be verbal, may consist of inappropriate touching, or may involve requests or demands for sexual acts. Sometimes the victim perceives the harassment as including the threat of being fired; sometimes the promise of favorable treatment (a good grade, a promotion, a "business" trip) is implied or stated directly. Some women enjoy the attention and use these "offers" as opportunities for self-advancement; some who make that choice later regret it when the male turns his attention to his next victim. The majority of women, however, consider these unwanted sexual advances as harassment and see themselves as victims. The person who believes that he or she is being harassed should consider several questions:

- What can I do about this situation?
- How can I protect myself?
- What options are available to me?
- What is the best way to stop these unwanted advances?

Emotional reactions to sexual harassment include anger, fear, and guilt; the threat to self-esteem is obvious. The male who is accused of sexual harassment usually either denies that it occurred or blames the woman. At one time the female victim of sexual harassment had no recourse. If she reported the incident to a supervisor, she risked being fired, accused of lying, or worse. All too often, the perpetrator would be the supervisor. Today, however, it is possible to take legal action, since sexual harassment is covered by federal laws against discrimination. The woman who chooses to file a complaint should have some type of evidence, other victims who are willing to join the complaint, and/or witnesses who have heard or seen examples of harassment. The complaint probably will not be handled in the woman's favor if it becomes a matter of "her word against his."

The best approach is to stop harassment when the first incident occurs. Using "I" statements, the victim can express feelings and then in a matter-of-fact way establish limits on behavior. If this does not stop the harassment, then the employer's procedure for filing a complaint should be followed. A complaint can be filed with the proper federal agency if the employer does not take action to stop the harassment. If the victim does decide to file a complaint, she should be aware that there is risk of reprisal from the accused, from the employer, or even from colleagues who choose to side with the accused.

## MAJOR CHANGES

In addition to facing developmental changes and societal pressures, people of all ages must occasionally cope with major changes such as new experiences, illness, divorce, or death. These changes may require a person to give up old behaviors and learn new ones. Some changes considered particularly stressful include:

- Change in marital status (marriage, separation, divorce, or reconciliation)
- Change in employment status (being fired, retiring, or starting a new job)
- Death of a spouse, family member, or close friend
- Injury or illness (one's own or that of a family member)

Each of these changes can threaten a person's adjustment for a time while new behaviors are being learned.

### New Experiences

Even when they are positive, new experiences can be stressful. An adult beginning a new job must learn how to function in a new environment and get to know new coworkers. A student who graduates from high school and begins college must adapt to living away from home and assuming a greater amount of responsibility. A new parent may become exhausted and overwhelmed by the demands of caring for a young child. Adapting successfully to a new situation requires patience and often the support of family and friends.

For the person who is not ready for a new experience, a major change can become a crisis. The bride who is not ready to assume the role of a wife may try to cling to her role as a daughter, or even transfer the daughter role to the relationship with her husband. For the new mother who is frightened by the responsibilities of motherhood, the birth of her baby is a real crisis. The person who is not ready for the responsibility of being a health care provider may find that the ethics and job requirements of the health care field create a need for adjustments beyond those the individual is willing or able to make. Any crisis in regard to a vocational decision is a serious threat to adjustment. For people who have not learned to adapt to change, every life problem can add to poor adjustment (Figure 10-5). Any life event can become a crisis that creates anxiety and unhappiness for one who has not learned to deal with change.

### Illness

Illness is always a threat to adjustment. It interferes with the usual pattern of living, is accompanied by discomfort, may involve doubt as to the outcome, and often creates financial problems. Patients and their families react to illness according to the degree of threat it represents. Adjustment is always poorer during illness. Sometimes behavior patterns that are not typical of a person appear during illness. Someone who is usually easy to please, for example, may be very difficult to please during an illness. A person who is usually quite well adjusted may show signs of poor adjustment during the period of illness. The patient may react with anger

FIGURE 10-5 How do you approach a new experience? *Delmar/Cengage Learning*

or fear to feelings of helplessness or being dependent on others. Interestingly, the poorly adjusted person may react with positive feelings if the illness provides an escape from having to deal with daily problems.

The person who is self-reliant and has learned to deal with life problems usually finds illness frustrating. Familiar techniques for solving problems do not cure the illness. Perhaps the patient is accustomed to giving orders; now, the physician, nurse, laboratory assistant, radiology technician, and other personnel seem to be in charge. The shift from being independent to a state of dependency seriously threatens adjustment. The behavior of a patient may be markedly different from that person's usual behavior.

## Divorce

Divorce is almost always a traumatic experience for everyone involved, especially the children. Even if both parents agree that divorce is preferable to continuing the marriage, children are affected emotionally as they see their home and family breaking apart. Their daily life changes in many significant ways. The adults are dealing with their own emotional reactions to the trauma of marital discord. They may be unaware of the child's reactions: anger toward one or both parents, belief that the parent who is moving out "doesn't love me any more," or possibly guilt, believing that he or she is the cause of the family breakup. If the divorce is hostile, there may be a custody battle. Then the child has a serious conflict of loyalties and may witness numerous hostile encounters between the parents. The child experiences emotional turmoil: a mixture of love and hate, anger and grief, guilt about divided loyalty, and negative feelings toward one or both parents.

When either parent remarries, a step-parent enters the picture, further complicating the child's emotional life. If the parent who remarries is the custodial parent, and the new step-parent also has children, the result is a "blended family." A period of turmoil may last for months, because each person must adapt to new family relationships and establish new patterns of interaction. Ideally, these adaptations occur with minimal trauma, and family dynamics eventually become positive. It is unrealistic to expect this to happen immediately after the wedding. Family counseling can assist blended families in making these adaptations.

### Death

The death of a family member or friend can be very traumatic. Children especially need help in understanding death, accepting the permanence of death, dealing with feelings associated with the deceased, and coping with the sense of loss or abandonment. Effective grieving is very important. If grief is not processed, the suppressed emotions can affect future attitudes, emotional expression, and behavior when another loss is experienced. Unit 22 discusses the effects of grief in greater detail.

## CHRONIC STRESSORS

Change is not the only stressor that can threaten one's adjustment. Some difficult situations develop gradually and persist for a long time. A person with ongoing financial problems, family difficulties, or learning disorders may find it especially difficult to remain well adjusted. Often, difficulty in one of these areas affects an individual's performance in other areas of life. For example, a woman in an unhappy marriage may find it difficult to concentrate at work. A child whose parents fight constantly may misbehave at school. A parent who is struggling to make ends meet may snap at the children. Health care providers may be able to refer patients to appropriate community agencies for financial help, counseling, or educational evaluation.

### Financial Problems

Financial problems have many causes. Some individuals may be unemployed or lack the skills needed to earn a comfortable living. Others may have a reasonably good income but find themselves faced with overwhelming medical or legal expenses. Many people lack money management skills and find themselves in financial trouble because they do not know how to budget and set priorities. One family could not afford telephone service but spent $30 per week on a rent-to-own large-screen TV. A young mother who could barely pay the rent spent about $5 per day on prepackaged lunchbox items for her sons even though they were eligible to receive free lunch at school.

Other individuals face overwhelming credit card debts. Many community agencies offer free financial counseling. Health care providers should also be aware that out-of-control spending sprees are one symptom of bipolar disorder. For their own protection, individuals diagnosed with this disorder should not have access to checks or credit cards.

### Family Difficulties

Family is an important part of most people's lives. Healthy families provide emotional support, unhealthy or dysfunctional families can create anxiety and distress in a person's life. Put simply, a healthy family is one in which all family members are kind, caring, and respectful toward one another. Effective families function like a team, each person doing his or her part but also helping other members when needed. All families have conflicts and disagreements, but healthy families work to resolve their problems in a way that protects each family member's dignity.

A dysfunctional family may fight often or just not communicate at all. Members of an unhealthy family may not trust one another and may feel that other family members do not respect or care for them. Winning and being "right" become more important than working together. For adults, unhealthy **family dynamics** often lead to separation and divorce. What begins as poor communication and unhealthy dynamics often grows into feelings of unhappiness with the relationship, a lack of love for the spouse, and the desire to be with someone else. Some children in dysfunctional families misbehave or do poorly at school. Some use drugs or alcohol. Still others turn to relatives and friends for support and understanding. Unfortunately, unhealthy family dynamics are often learned and passed on to the next generation.

Being part of an unhealthy family is a tremendous threat to one's adjustment. Unfortunately, many of the families depicted in movies and on television are dysfunctional. Because the media portrays family difficulties as humorous and commonplace, viewers may come to accept fighting, insults, and infidelity as normal. In reality, these behaviors are symptoms of an unhealthy family. Counseling is available in most communities and can help families learn more appropriate ways to interact with one another.

## Learning Problems

In recent years it has become common for parents to seek medical advice when their child has difficulty in school. These difficulties may include poor grades, failure to learn new concepts, trouble completing assignments, or behavior problems. Today attention, learning, and behavioral disorders are most often diagnosed during the elementary school years. However, older students and even adults may suffer from undiagnosed disorders. These disorders can pose a threat to a person's adjustment at any age. Health care professionals should be aware of the signs of some common disorders and should encourage the child's parents or affected adult to seek professional evaluation. Warning signs of learning problems include:

- Slow development in speaking and writing
- Difficulty expressing ideas or understanding directions
- Difficulty with forming letters, writing, and spelling
- Difficulty memorizing and remembering information
- Clumsiness, poor handwriting, or poor coordination
- Difficulty paying attention and completing tasks
- Sloppiness, carelessness, or lack of organization
- Tendency to misinterpret others' behavior and become upset
- Sudden mood changes, frequent frustration

These behaviors may indicate a variety of learning problems. Some of the more common are described in the following sections.

**Attention Deficit Disorder and Attention Deficit Hyperactivity Disorder** Attention deficit disorder (ADD) and attention deficit hyperactivity disorder (ADHD) describe a pattern of inattentive, impulsive, and hyperactive behaviors. Students with ADD/ADHD may appear disorganized and have difficulty remembering information and completing tasks. They may show aggression and have poor relationships with their peers. Other common behaviors include daydreaming, staring into space, constantly moving or getting up, and blurting out. ADD/ADHD is a medical diagnosis, but health care professionals often seek input from a student's parents and teachers before making a diagnosis. Treatment of ADD/ADHD usually includes behavior modification and medication. Treatments such as hypnotherapy and neurofeedback have also proven successful for many individuals.

**Learning Disorders** When a student's academic achievement is significantly lower than one would expect given the student's level of intelligence, he may have a learning disorder. The three primary types of learning disorders are reading disorders (also called **dyslexia**), mathematics disorders, and writing disorders. A student with a learning disorder isn't "dumb" but has difficulty with a particular subject area. Students with identified learning disorders are entitled by federal law to receive special educational services, so health care providers should encourage parents to have their child evaluated if a learning disorder is suspected.

## Developmental Disorders

As their name suggests, **developmental disorders** affect an individual's mental or physical development. The two most prevalent developmental disorders in the United States are mental retardation and autism spectrum disorders. These disorders are usually diagnosed in the preschool or elementary school years.

**Mental Retardation** When most people hear the term *mental retardation*, they imagine a severely handicapped individual. In fact, mental retardation can be mild, moderate, severe, or profound. Retardation is typically identified through tests of intelligence and adaptive behavior skills, or skills needed to care for oneself and function in everyday situations. Mild retardation may not be identified until the school years, when it becomes clear that a child is learning at a rate slower than that of classmates. In older adults, mild retardation may never have been formally identified. Like individuals with learning disorders or physical disabilities, mentally disabled persons are protected against discrimination by federal law.

**Autism Spectrum Disorders** **Autism spectrum disorders** include classic autism, pervasive developmental order—not otherwise specified (PDD-NOS), and Asperger syndrome. Individuals with these disorders process and respond to information differently than typical individuals, causing difficulty with communication, behavior, and social interactions. Autism affects each individual differently, and the degree to which daily functioning is impaired can be mild to severe. Persons with autism can have low, average, or high levels of intellectual functioning. For example, Sue Rubin is a woman with autism who wrote a documentary about her experiences. Although she is unable to communicate through spoken language, she has an above-average level of intelligence and communicates through writing and the use of assistive communication devices.

Over the past few years, more and more children are being diagnosed with autism spectrum disorders. Treatments include special educational programs, occupational therapy, speech therapy, medication, and modified diet. Current estimates suggest that more than 1 in 150 children in the United States will be diagnosed with some form of autism.

**Behavior Disorders**

While most children misbehave at times, some develop a pattern of problem behaviors that can severely disrupt the school or home environment. Students with oppositional defiant disorder routinely defy the authority of parents or teachers. When told do to something, they may intentionally do the opposite. Students with a conduct disorder may not only disobey parents and teachers but also threaten or harm others, steal, or vandalize school or public property. These students may be treated with behavioral modification, therapy, and/or medication. Whenever possible, families of affected students should also seek counseling, since living with a family member's disorder is stressful. Likewise, many experts believe that family dynamics influence or even create behavior disorders. Improving family interactions can improve the problem behaviors.

**Discipline and Home Environment** While it is important to detect and treat legitimate disorders, families often find that children's behavior and academic performance improve when parents learn more effective discipline techniques. Contrary to popular opinion, *discipline* does not mean *punishment*. Discipline means teaching children the difference between appropriate and inappropriate behaviors and guiding them to choose behavior that is appropriate to the situation. Effective discipline includes the following techniques:

- Develop a warm, caring relationship with children.
- Explain and model socially appropriate behavior.
- Keep rules and expectations clear, simple, and age appropriate.
- Enforce rules calmly and consistently.
- When necessary, punish a child with time out or loss of a privilege, not by hitting or yelling.

In addition, children learn and behave better when they receive good nutrition and when parents monitor television and video games. Exposure to violent TV programs and video games has been linked to aggressive behavior.

Resolving a negative family situation can also improve behavior. One second grader developed a serious problem with aggressive and defiant behavior at school. Upon investigation, it was found that her mother used harsh punishments and often told the girl, "You're no good." Shortly after her father gained custody, the girl began to behave appropriately at school.

## COPING SKILLS AND RESILIENCE

Surprisingly, well-adjusted people are not always those who have led lives free of difficulty or trauma. Ultimately, it is not what happens to us that determines our level of adjustment but how we cope with it. Good coping skills and resources can help a person regain a good level of adjustment even when faced with difficult circumstances. The following coping skills and resources help individuals deal with problems as they occur:

- Eat a healthful diet and exercise regularly.
- Get a full night's rest.

- Talk to a friend or family member about emotions and problems.
- Set goals and work toward them one step at a time.

A similar concept is **resilience,** the ability to bounce back or recover from problems. Factors associated with resilience include having a positive attitude, believing one has the power to change one's circumstances, and developing strategies to reduce stress. Being part of a support network such as a caring family or a church or community group can also help a person recover from difficulty.

Coping with a difficult situation takes time. During the period of readjustment, a person may find counseling or a support group helpful. These resources are especially important for a person who has experienced a trauma. Unit 11 examines different types of trauma and the reactions a victim of trauma is likely to experience.

## REFERENCES AND SUGGESTED READINGS

Covey, Sean, & Curtis, Stacey. (2008). *The 7 habits of happy kids.* New York: Simon and Schuster.

Faber, Adele, & Mazlish, Elaine. (2005). *How to talk so teens will listen and listen so teens will talk.* New York: HarperCollins.

Rubin, Sue (Writer), & Wurzburg, Gerardine (Producer). (2005). *Autism is a world.* [DVD]. United States: CNN.

## SOURCES OF ADDITONAL INFORMATION

Autism Society of America, http://www.autism-society.org

LD Online (information about learning disabilities), http://www.ldonline.org

## REVIEW AND SELF-CHECK

1. What are six stages of life that can challenge a person's adjustment?

2. Identify one significant change that occurs in each of the six life stages.

3. How does peer pressure affect adolescents?

4. What are three examples of sexism?

5. What are three learning problems that can make school difficult for a student?

6. How do healthy family relationships differ from unhealthy family relationships?

7. What are two cultural stressors that can occur in childhood? Adolescence? Adulthood?

8. What are three strategies parents can use to improve a child's behavior?

9. Describe possible symptoms of an autism spectrum disorder.

## ASSIGNMENTS

1. Consider several of your life experiences that involved new situations. Try to recall how you felt during the early days in the new situation. Which of your familiar behaviors were inappropriate in the new situation? What changes did you make in your behavior patterns as you adapted to the new situation?

2. Consider the most uncomfortable experience you have had since entering this health occupations program. Why were you uncomfortable? What was your behavior? List changes in behavior that helped you return to a state of adjustment.

3. Make a list of rules to guide you in future situations of the following types:

    a. A radical change in your life situation

    b. A new job in which many of the techniques used are somewhat different from those you learned as a student

    c. A new job in the health field for which your present learnings provide a foundation, but your job responsibilities require that you learn many new techniques

4. A mother consults you about Joey, a second grader. She tells you that Joey has trouble remembering what his teacher said in class. Homework takes him hours to complete, and he often cries with frustration because he doesn't understand. She says, "One day Joey can do the work, and the next day it's like he's forgotten everything." What might you suggest to her?

5. Sarah, a fourth grader, has developed a behavior problem at school. She blurts out comments in class, hits others, and occasionally steals pencils and other small items. Her parents ask you what they should do to help Sarah. What factors might you consider in discussing Sarah's behavior with her parents?

6. Adele asks if a male colleague has ever said anything "inappropriate" to you. He has not, but you realize that he sometimes comes up behind you and runs his hand down your back. When you tell her this, she suggests he is checking to see if you are wearing a bra. What would be an appropriate action on your part the next time he runs his hand down your back?

UNIT 11

# Effects of Traumatic Events

## OBJECTIVES

Upon completion of this unit, you should be able to:

- Name three reasons a victim of a traumatic experience may need psychological counseling, in addition to treatment for physical injuries.
- State two reasons a health care provider should be aware of the various effects of traumatic experiences.
- List five normal reactions to a traumatic experience.
- Describe the symptoms of the following psychological disorders: anxiety disorder, panic disorder, post-traumatic stress disorder (PTSD), phobias, and depression.
- List three traumatic effects of each of the following: war or terrorism, rape, domestic violence, and child abuse.
- Explain the phrase "blaming the victim."

## KEY TERMS

Abuse
Heterosexual
Homosexual
Incest
Neglect
Pedophilia
Perpetrators
Sexual variation
Sexually transmitted disease (STD)

The preceding unit describes threats to adjustment that are experienced by everyone. Some people are fortunate in that they have never experienced severe trauma, but today more and more people, of all ages and from all walks of life, are having some type of traumatic experience. In addition, various types of abuse, once closely kept secrets, are now being exposed. Discrimination continues in schools, the workplace, and the community, in spite of federal laws that were intended to guarantee equal opportunities and protection for everyone. Health care providers need to be aware that such experiences are serious threats to adjustment and have implications for the physical, mental, and emotional health of victims.

You, as a health care provider, are more likely to encounter victims than perpetrators. The purpose of this unit is to help you be fully aware of the effects of traumatic experiences on victims. You also need to have a high level of suspicion about the possibility that a patient is actually a victim, even if the patient does not volunteer information to that effect. Any suspicion that you have should be reported to your supervisor and/or the physician for further evaluation and possible legal action. *Follow the policies and procedures of your employing agency; do not attempt to handle such a matter yourself.* Just as important, *do not ignore the indications that aroused your suspicion.*

## WHAT IS TRAUMA?

A trauma is an event that poses a serious threat to one's life or well-being. Trauma includes experiencing, witnessing, or learning of a crime, act of aggression, accident, natural disaster, or act of war. Physical, emotional, and sexual abuse are also considered traumas. Experiencing a trauma poses a serious threat to a person's adjustment. Even people who are normally well adjusted will develop physical and emotional reactions following a traumatic event.

A traumatized person may require medical attention immediately after the event. In other cases, the person may seek medical advice days or weeks later when secondary symptoms develop. In addition to treating physical injuries, health care professionals should inform patients about normal reactions to trauma and refer them to a mental health professional if these reactions become severe.

## TRAUMATIC EXPERIENCES

While any difficult situation may be perceived as a trauma by the person who experiences it, the following discussion focuses on events that are commonly recognized as traumatic. By understanding the most common types of trauma, health care providers will be better equipped to assist trauma victims in understanding their own reactions and seeking the help they need.

Victims of a single event, such as a mugging, experience intense emotional reactions in addition to their physical injuries. After the physical injuries have healed, professional counseling may be needed for processing the emotional trauma. Victims of recurrent trauma, such as long-standing **abuse,** need help in escaping their situation; these victims always benefit from professional counseling—to develop new insights and resolve deeply rooted emotional trauma.

### The Perpetrator

In reading the following paragraphs, remember that there are traumatic *events* (i.e., accidents), there are **perpetrators** (i.e., persons who inflict the trauma), and there are *victims* (persons suffering from the event). The behavior of a perpetrator may be the result of one or more of the following: early learnings in the home or on the street, cultural patterns, uncontrolled emotional expression, criminal tendencies, psychiatric disorder. The perpetrator's behavior may fall within the "normal" range of behavior (i.e., acceptable behavior within that particular culture) or may fall into the category of psychiatric disorder or criminal behavior. Discussion of the "causes" of a perpetrator's behavior is beyond the scope of this book; the study of such behavior falls within the disciplines of sociology, psychology, psychiatry, and criminology.

### Blaming the Victim

The trauma experienced by the victim is magnified when others choose to blame the victim. Those who would defend a rapist are likely to claim the victim "was just asking for it," citing her manner of dress or her presence in a particular location. If the victim was a child, someone may comment that she was often "flirtatious" or note that she would sometimes climb into a male relative's lap. Thus, an innocent child's natural ways of seeking attention and affection may be used to imply that she was responsible for an adult's sexual behavior.

This tendency to blame the victim sometimes extends even to those who are the victim of a criminal act or are involved in an accident:

*Why were you out at that time of night?*

*Why did you go to that place? You should have known better!*

*How many times have I told you not to drive so fast?*

Being blamed for what happened adds to a victim's emotional trauma. It is only natural to feel anger when being blamed at a time when one's need is for expressions of caring and emotional support. Although blaming may actually be a friend's or relative's expression of concern, it is inappropriate and not what a victim needs to hear. Also, blaming may be an example of displaced anger, from the cause of the event or the perpetrator, to the victim; this too is inappropriate. The health care provider sometimes has an opportunity to point out to relatives a victim's need for expressions of caring, emotional support, and protection from being blamed.

## Crimes and Accidents

Muggings, carjackings, burglaries, gang beatings, and other types of violence are all too prevalent. Once considered to be dangers characteristic of big cities, these crimes are now commonplace in the suburbs and in small cities and towns. Even more common are automobile accidents, a leading cause of death, especially for males under the age of 25. In addition, thousands of people each year sustain disabling injuries. Complete safety from crime or accidents does not exist.

Anyone who is the victim of a crime or who survives a serious accident has emotional trauma in addition to any physical injuries sustained. The health care system tends to focus on physical injuries, however. Once victims have been treated in the emergency room or discharged from the hospital, they usually receive follow-up treatment primarily for their physical injuries.

Fear and anger inevitably accompany the physical trauma of crimes and accidents. Some people can process these feelings over time; others need professional counseling to deal with the intensity of the feelings and any disabling effects, such as panic attacks or chronic anxiety. It is appropriate, within the role of some health care providers, to suggest to victims that they may benefit from counseling to deal with the emotional effects of their traumatic experience.

## Natural Disasters, War, and Terrorism

We often hear news reports of floods, hurricanes, tornadoes, and earthquakes that have taken lives and left many people without homes. A natural disaster can be devastating for both the community and the individuals affected. Damage to or loss of one's home, school, or workplace threatens one's sense of security and normalcy. An individual who has experienced a natural disaster may experience any of the reactions to trauma described earlier. In addition, some people may develop anxiety or phobias related to the experience. For example, a person who lived through a hurricane or tornado may become distressed during thunderstorms or high winds.

Experiencing or witnessing war or terrorist acts also causes trauma. Individuals often feel overwhelmed by fear, helplessness, and vulnerability. They struggle to understand what has happened and why. Scenes of destruction or suffering may play through a person's mind over and over. For those who lose friends, family, or homes, there is a tremendous sense of grief as well. War and terrorist acts can breed distrust among different nations or ethnic groups, planting the seeds for further aggression in the future.

Military personnel in combat face traumatic situations constantly. For some, the psychological effects are so devastating that they never regain their previous level of adjustment even after returning to civilian life. Many veterans find themselves unable to function after returning home. These veterans suffer from post-traumatic stress disorder.

Natural disasters, war, and terrorism affect not only individuals but entire communities. These large-scale traumas provoke many of the same reactions as other traumas. However, a trauma experienced by many has some noteworthy differences. Because many people have been affected, finding someone to talk to about the experience may be easier. Some survivors may find comfort in the feeling that, "We're in this together. I'm not alone." On the other hand, friends and family who are also traumatized may not be able to provide much emotional support. Ongoing media coverage and community discussion become constant reminders of the event.

## Bullying

Many children experience teasing and bullying in the home, on the playground, and at school. The child who is noticeably different (e.g., has a physical handicap or a tendency to stutter) is especially at risk for teasing by the peer group or bullying by larger children. School policies regarding children with behavioral disorders or learning difficulties set these children apart, a practice that often results in a child being labeled and possibly rejected by classmates. Bullying, however, is a more serious problem.

Bullying includes several aggressive behaviors, including name-calling, put-downs, threats, taunting, physical assault, taking or damaging property, and forcing a person to do something he or she does not want to do. A bully may be aggressive or passive. Aggressive bullies may instigate a bullying situation, while passive bullies rarely "start the fight" but join in once an aggressive bully has set the stage. Bullying can be described as follows:

- The behavior is intended to harm or disturb a less powerful victim, one who is smaller, weaker, or unable to defend him- or herself.
- The behavior occurs repeatedly over a period of time.
- The bully chooses a time when winning is almost certain, such as when there is no one present with the authority to intervene.
- The bully often has one or more allies present.

By choosing a weaker victim and surrounding him- or herself with allies, the bully, who lacks real courage, gains a sense of power by overpowering the victim.

Many parents and teachers view bullying as a normal part of growing up and therefore do little to intervene. Boys who fight are often described as "tough" or "standing up for themselves." Some parents of aggressive bullies are secretly proud of their child's tough reputation or blame other children for starting the fight.

Unfortunately, bullying often occurs more in schools than in any other single place. Research suggests that much bullying could be prevented by clear and consistent school discipline policies and close adult supervision on playgrounds before and after school. All students who report bullying should be taken seriously, and their anonymity should be protected.

Children who bully others need both firm discipline and understanding. Bullying behavior is often an indicator that a child comes from an unhealthy family. Researchers suggest that failure to bond with parents in the early years, lack of love, and ineffective discipline increase the likelihood of bullying. Some aggressive children are copying aggressive behavior they have learned from parents. For example, one father told his son, "Don't let anyone walk all over you." While bullying behavior should not be excused on the grounds that a child came from a difficult home, attempting to change the behavior without addressing its cause is unlikely to stop bullying. Many community mental health centers offer family counseling, parenting classes, and anger management sessions that can help bullies and their families learn more acceptable behaviors. It has been suggested that students who repeatedly assault others could be court-ordered to take violence prevention classes, much as men who assault their partners are often ordered to take anger management classes.

Victims of bullying require help in several areas. First, they need adult intervention to end the bullying or at least avoid bullying situations. Victims of bullying often develop low self-esteem and a feeling of powerlessness as a result of being repeatedly threatened or overpowered. They also need to learn how to protect themselves physically and emotionally in the future. When bullying is not adequately addressed, the effects can be devastating for the individuals involved and their community. Young people who have been threatened, taunted, and assaulted can develop the attitude, "No one cares about me. Everyone's against me." For some, this attitude leads to depression; for others, it creates a desire to strike back. Investigations into several school shootings in recent years revealed that the shooters had been the targets of bullying or felt rejected by their peers.

Adults may experience bullying in the workplace, the community, or in personal relationships. Anyone who routinely uses intimidation and manipulation to get his or her way at the expense of the rights of others is a bully. Standing up to a bully takes strength and courage. It is important to set limits and let the bully know in no uncertain terms when he or she has crossed the line. The bully must be told that the behavior is unacceptable and will not be tolerated. While "I talk" (discussed in Unit 8) helps improve most relationships, it may be necessary to use more assertive "you talk" with a bully. "You talk" includes statements such as "You need to back off," or "Keep those comments to yourself."

With the popularity of the Internet, text messaging, and other technological forms of communication, a new variation of bullying has developed—*cyberbullying*. Cyberbullying has been defined as "willful and repeated harm inflicted through the medium of electronic text" (Patchin & Hinduja, 2006), or more simply, "online cruelty." Examples include spreading vicious rumors, insults, threats, or hate messages through electronic messages. Cyberbullying occurs most often, though not exclusively, among adolescents. Victims of cyberbullying may experience fear, depression, lowered self-esteem, or even become suicidal.

The child who has positive emotional support in the home survives teasing and some degree of bullying without serious damage. The child who does not have opportunities for processing feelings about these experiences is likely to suppress anger and fear, develop a negative self-concept, and have problems with interpersonal relations. These experiences, though not as dramatic as some types of trauma, can have lifelong effects.

## Child Abuse

Child neglect and abuse are serious problems today. **Neglect** includes leaving young children unsupervised or failing to provide adequate food, clothing, shelter, hygiene, and medical care. Abuse includes harming a child emotionally or physically. Verbal abuse consists of put-downs, cursing, or making repeated comments like "You're no good. I wish you'd never been born. You're going to end up in jail just like your father (or mother)" (Figure 11-1). Emotional abuse includes "mind games," manipulation, or using fear to control the child. Physical abuse can include inappropriate discipline such as harsh beatings or locking a child in a closet. Any physical assault upon a child can be considered abusive, particularly if marks or bruises are visible afterward.

Sexual abuse occurs when an adult or older child forces a child to take off his or her clothes or perform any sexual act. While the act itself is physical, the damage to the victim is emotional, mental, and physical.

Both boys and girls can be victims of sexual abuse, but two out of three victims are girls. The perpetrator is most often a close family member, but may be a family friend or authority figure. If the perpetrator is a parent or sibling, the sexual encounter is **incest.** If the child is under 13 years old and the perpetrator is 5 to 10 years older than the child, it is **pedophilia;** the abuser is a *pedophile*. Studies of pedophiles indicate that many were themselves sexually abused as children. Some mental health professionals now believe that pedophilia is a third sexual orientation and is unlikely to be changed even with treatment. Sexual abuse of girls is almost always **heterosexual** (i.e., male/female). Sexual abuse of males is most often **homosexual** (i.e., male/male). Because the majority of sexual abusers are male, the pronoun "he" is used for the remainder of this discussion. There are, however, cases of sexual abuse of a male by a female.

With the rise of the Internet, there has been increasing public concern about "sexual predators" who meet young people online and engage them in inappropriate online or in-person sexual activities. A 2009 study by the University of New Hampshire Crimes Against Children Research Center found that arrests of offenders soliciting young people for sex online did increase between 2000 and 2006. However, arrests for online solicitations accounted for only 1% of arrests for sex crimes against young people in 2006. Only 4% of those arrested were

**FIGURE 11-1** "Can't you do anything right?" *Delmar/Cengage Learning*

registered sex offenders. The study found only one case of abduction resulting from online sexual solicitation. These results suggest that while young people should certainly be taught Internet safety precautions, the threat posed by online predators may be relatively small.

Health care providers, teachers, law enforcement officers, and other professionals are legally required to report suspected cases of abuse and neglect to their local Child Protective Services office. Community members and relatives may also make reports. The U.S. Department of Health and Human Services reports that each year, about three million such referrals are made throughout the United States. In 2007, over 1,700 children, most under the age of 4, died as a result of abuse or neglect. Many professionals believe that for each case that is reported and substantiated, there are several more that are never reported or that would be difficult to prove.

**Traumatic Effects** The effects of sexual abuse on a child are profound and can affect adjustment throughout life. Sexual abuse is not limited to physical sexual acts; it includes mental and emotional abuse. The perpetrator uses various devices to keep the child from exposing him. The act may be presented as "our secret" and the child made to feel that she or he is being given very special attention. If the child reacts negatively, the perpetrator may use threats to keep the child from telling anyone. Some perpetrators convince their victims that they are to blame, thus using shame and guilt to control the child. This enforced silence results in suppression of intense feelings: anger, fear, grief, and guilt.

Unfortunately, many adults refuse to believe a child who does try to tell them about being sexually abused. It is very difficult for a mother to believe such a report, especially if a little girl is saying that the father, stepfather, brother, uncle, or grandfather committed such an act. For example, little 5-year-old Edette told her mother repeatedly what the big brother was doing to her, and repeatedly she was punished for "telling lies." Even when she developed a recurrent bladder infection, neither the mother nor the urologist believed her story.

It is especially difficult for parents to believe that a respected authority figure, such as a teacher, coach, or member of the clergy, would sexually abuse their child. Yet abuse is most likely to occur in a dominant/submissive relationship, in which the child is powerless. Many adult survivors of child sexual abuse tell of seeking help from an adult, only to encounter disbelief and accusations of lying. Parents, teachers, ministers, adult friends and neighbors, and especially health care providers must *listen* when a child tries to tell what some adult did to them. Although the child may not have the vocabulary to describe the event in adult terms, it is important to *let the child tell what happened in his or her own words*. Do not suggest words you think might help the child's description, since that could be construed legally as having "planted the idea in the child's mind."

The damage of sexual abuse is physical, mental, and emotional. These victims grow up with low self-esteem, suppressed anger and fear, feelings of guilt and distrust, and perceptions of the world as a hostile place. They may contract a **sexually transmitted disease** (STD) or sustain other physical injuries. As adults, many survivors of childhood sexual abuse have difficulty forming an intimate relationship. Many have one relationship after another; others avoid intimacy altogether. Failed marriages are common. The lifelong effects of child sexual abuse are now acknowledged by the mental health community. Through psychotherapy and techniques such as hypnosis, many adults have been able to bring repressed memories to the conscious level, a necessary step in order for therapy to proceed. Support groups for survivors of abuse and incest have been established in many communities.

While enduring abuse is traumatic for a child, reporting the abuse and ending the situation can be traumatic as well. One 10-year-old girl told her mother that her stepfather had sexually abused her. As a result, the mother took the children and moved out. The abuse had ended, but now the girl faced the trauma of losing her stepfather and stepgrandparents. She had to adjust to a new home, a new neighborhood, and a new school. Some abused children who are "wise to the system" choose not to report being abused because they fear being taken from their parents. Enduring abuse is the price they pay to protect their families and avoid confrontation.

Appropriate action depends on the situation. Criminal charges may be filed against the perpetrator, but adults should not let that possibility prevent them from protecting the child against further molestation. Pedophiles tend to repeat their behavior, so every child within range of a pedophile is at risk.

The sexually abused child enters the adolescent period having already experienced some type of sexual activity. Some behaviors, emotional patterns, attitudes toward sex, levels of trust in others, and interpersonal relations differ from those of their sexually inexperienced classmates. Some children try various forms of escape: alcohol, drugs, food, sleep, or withdrawal. Those who have strong guilty feelings may inflict physical pain on themselves by head banging, beating hard objects with the fists, cutting or mutilating themselves, or even attempting suicide. These behaviors may be exhibited during adolescence or adulthood, years after the sexual abuse stopped or the individual escaped from the abuser.

## Rape

The use of threats or force in order to engage in a sexual act is *rape*. It is a crime and should be reported, even if the perpetrator is a relative, friend, date, or coworker. *Rape is not a sexual act; it is an act of aggression that violates the victim physically and emotionally.* Rapists tend to have a hostile attitude toward women. They may also have an intense need to experience a feeling of power over others. Some rapists want to inflict pain and enjoy the woman's fear. Because the experience satisfies the rapist's need for power and control, he is likely to rape repeatedly and to have more than one victim. The rapist who does not feel powerful enough to force himself on an adult woman may choose a child as victim. Rape is one of a number of acts included in the legal term "sex offender."

The rape victim often is victimized further by family members and/or "the system." If the rapist is a relative, family members may not believe the victim's report; some may actually side with the accused rapist. If the victim reports the rape to police, she may be subjected to dehumanizing procedures by officers who do not understand the significance of rape. Comments made about a rape or a rape victim often show total lack of understanding that *rape is a violent act of aggression.*

In many communities, the concerns of rape survivors, health care providers, and law enforcement personnel have led to educational efforts to sensitize officials to the needs of a rape victim. Every rape victim should have professional counseling to help her deal with intense emotions and the serious threat to self-esteem. Counseling and a support group can help the victim regain confidence in her ability to go about her daily routine without fear.

## Stalking

The U.S. Department of Justice estimates that in a 12-month period, 3.4 million people are victims of stalking. Stalking may take the form of unwanted letters, phone calls, emails, or gifts, or it may include following or spying on the victim. Posting inappropriate or negative information on the Internet or in a public place can also be considered stalking. While many people occasionally find themselves the object of unwanted attention, these behaviors can be considered stalking if they cause victims to fear for the safety of themselves or their family members. The highest rate of stalking occurs among 18- to 24-year-olds.

## Adult Abuse

Adult abuse has received growing media attention. Adult abuse occurs when disabled or elderly adults are neglected or mistreated by adult children, spouses, or other caretakers. For adults with developmental disabilities such as mental retardation, the risk of being physically or sexually assaulted may be 4 to 10 times greater than it is for other adults. Disabled women are assaulted, raped, and abused twice as often as nondisabled women. Elderly adults are also at risk for neglect, emotional abuse, and physical abuse. Abusers may include nursing home staff, adult children, spouses, or other relatives. Just as health care providers have a legal duty to report suspected cases of child abuse, they have an ethical duty to report suspected elder abuse to the authorities. Current laws do not require health care providers to report elder abuse because elders are assumed to be able to speak for themselves. In reality, not all are able to do so.

# DOMESTIC VIOLENCE

Abuse by one's spouse or partner is now recognized as a public health problem in the United States. According to the National Domestic Violence Hotline, one in four females and one in nine males will experience domestic violence at some point in their lives. Spousal abuse is found in all cultures, races, occupations, income levels, and ages.

Spousal abuse can take various forms, including physical aggression (assault), emotional trauma, "mind games," deprivation of needs (including access to money), and isolation from relatives and friends. Employers lose billions of dollars every year because of lost workdays, medical costs, and other problems associated with domestic violence.

## The Abuser Personality

Abusers have two personalities: the public personality, that of "a really nice guy," and the private personality, controlling and demanding. Few women would enter knowingly into an abusive relationship. The abuser initially is charming and shows care and concern, so the woman enters the relationship expecting romantic love and a "warm, cozy relationship." Gradually the abuser begins to make demands that lead up to isolating the victim from family and friends, getting control of the money (including the victim's paycheck), controlling the couple's activities (eliminating her activities and interests), requiring explanations for her behavior or comments, demanding a report on any time spent away from the abuser, and making decisions that any adult woman should make for herself. These demands are first made within an acceptable, and possibly flattering, context:

- I can't stand to be away from you.
- I want you to spend more time with me.
- You spent all afternoon with your sister when I needed you to be with me.

- I want you to be here while I watch the ball game.
- I want you to be home when I get back from the ball game.
- You know how important you are to me.

Initially the abuser makes the woman feel important and loved, but comments such as the above are leading up to controlling not only the relationship, but also all aspects of her life. The abuser's objective is *power*—total control over the other person.

The following statements illustrate the increasing degree of control:

- What did you and your sister talk about all afternoon?
- What did you do while I was at the ball game?
- I'll take care of paying the bills; I handle money better than you do.
- Wear the red dress; you really look great in it.
- Don't wear that short skirt to the party.
- What were you and Joe laughing about?
- Why did you stay in the kitchen with Amy so long?
- What did you mean when you said . . . ?

Next, the abuser begins to chip away at her self-esteem, then he works on making her feel guilty as well as inadequate:

- Why did you say (. . .)? That was stupid!
- Why can't you be more fun when we party?
- I don't like it when you dance with Jim.
- Why can't you be a better wife (mother, girlfriend)?
- You can't do anything right.
- You made me angry (jealous).
- You caused us to run out of money.
- You had me so upset I ran a red light; it's your fault I got this ticket.
- Yes, I drink too much, but it's because you make me so (. . .).
- I didn't get the promotion; you should have been nicer to my boss at the Christmas party.

## Effects on the Victim

Once the woman begins to believe that she really is the cause of his (and their) problems, he has tremendous power over her (Figure 11-2). With low self-esteem and overwhelming feelings of guilt, she is less able to evaluate the relationship and definitely less able to free herself from it. Once the man's power over her is established, he feels safe expressing his feelings through physical actions. After hitting the woman, the abuser points out that she is to blame: she didn't do as she was told, she didn't have dinner ready on time, she was late getting home from work, or whatever excuse he can think of at the moment. The physical abuse may escalate until the woman sustains serious injuries or is killed.

Women who grew up in a home where domestic violence was a way of life may simply accept abuse as part of a woman's role. At some point, a woman may realize she does not

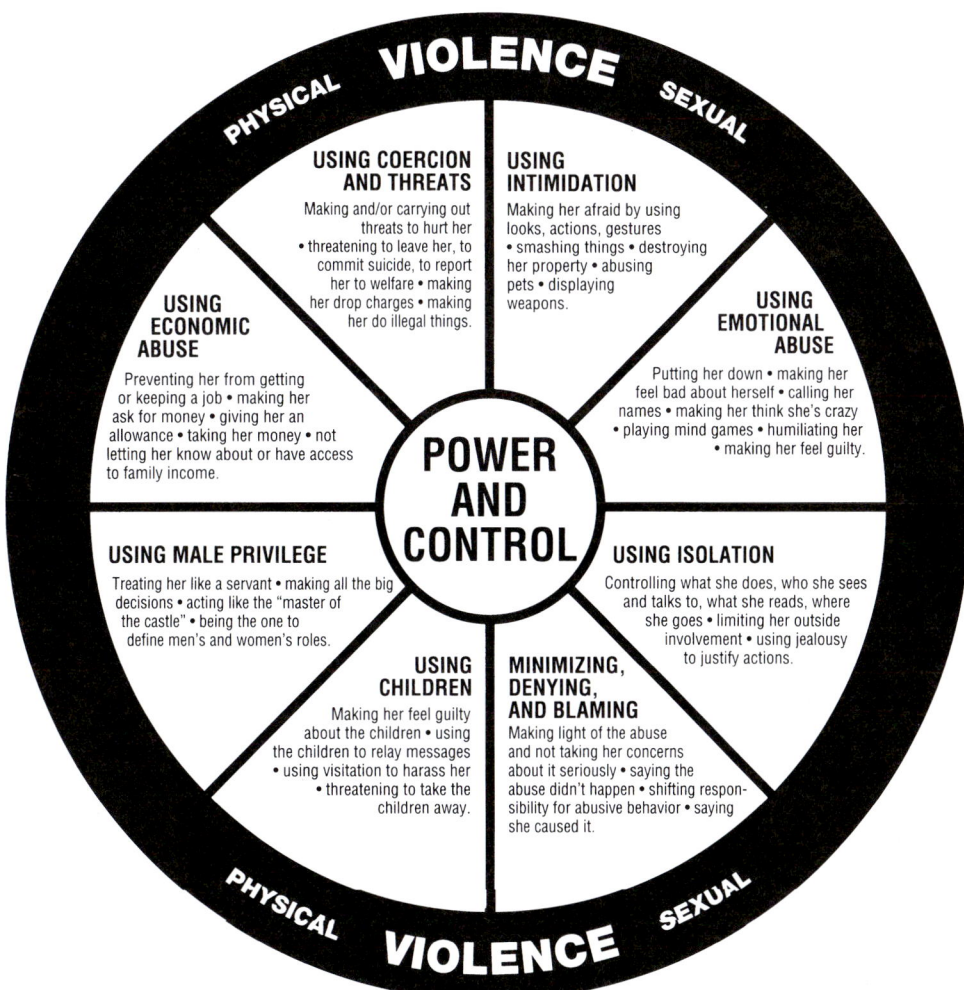

**FIGURE 11-2** Abusers have a strong need for power and control.
*(Source: From Minnesota Program Development, Inc., Domestic Abuse Intervention Project, 202 East Superior St., Duluth, MN 55802. Courtesy of Coral McDonnell.)*

have to submit to abuse. She may seek escape, but if she has no money and no job skills, escape requires help from others. If her family is supportive, she may seek their protection. In some cases, the wife's family has been so charmed by the abuser that they side with him and refuse to help her escape the abuser. Sometimes religious beliefs are a factor: "You are his wife for better or worse."

Even well-educated women, some with positions that would enable them to support themselves, find it difficult to leave an abusive relationship. The abuser maintains control by alternating periods of abuse with periods of proclaiming his love and promising "never to do it again." Survivors of abusive relationships refer to these periods as the "honeymoon" time; the woman, thinking each time that the abuse is a thing of the past, stays in the relationship. Sometimes a woman accepts the abuse in order to have the "honeymoon" periods, during which she is treated well (Figure 11-3). Any woman who has a negative self-concept and believes herself to be unlovable may become dependent on an abuser for love and approval. ("He's the only one who'll put up with me.") Some women stay in an abusive relationship rather than risk the uncertainties of being alone.

**FIGURE 11-3** Domestic violence: The cycle of abuse. *Delmar/Cengage Learning*

## Escaping Abuse

Most victims of domestic violence need outside help to escape the abusive relationship. Since an abuser takes control of the family's finances, the woman has no financial resources to aid in her escape. Sometimes the abuser tries to ensure that she remain financially dependent on him by interfering with her efforts to keep or obtain a job. He may assault her just before a job interview or hide the clothes she planned to wear to the interview. If she has left him, he may stalk her at work or at a training site.

Personnel in women's shelters report that many women who appear ready to become self-reliant actually go back to the abuser. Sometimes it takes several attempts before the woman finally frees herself. Many of these victims need several types of help:

- The belief that a woman does not have to submit to abuse
- Financial assistance
- A separate place to live
- Childcare
- Job and/or job training
- Child support
- Legal protection

As soon as arrangements are made for physical survival, it is important that the woman receive counseling to counteract the destructive effects of the abusive relationship. The damage to self-esteem may take years to overcome. Processing her fear, anger, and guilt may

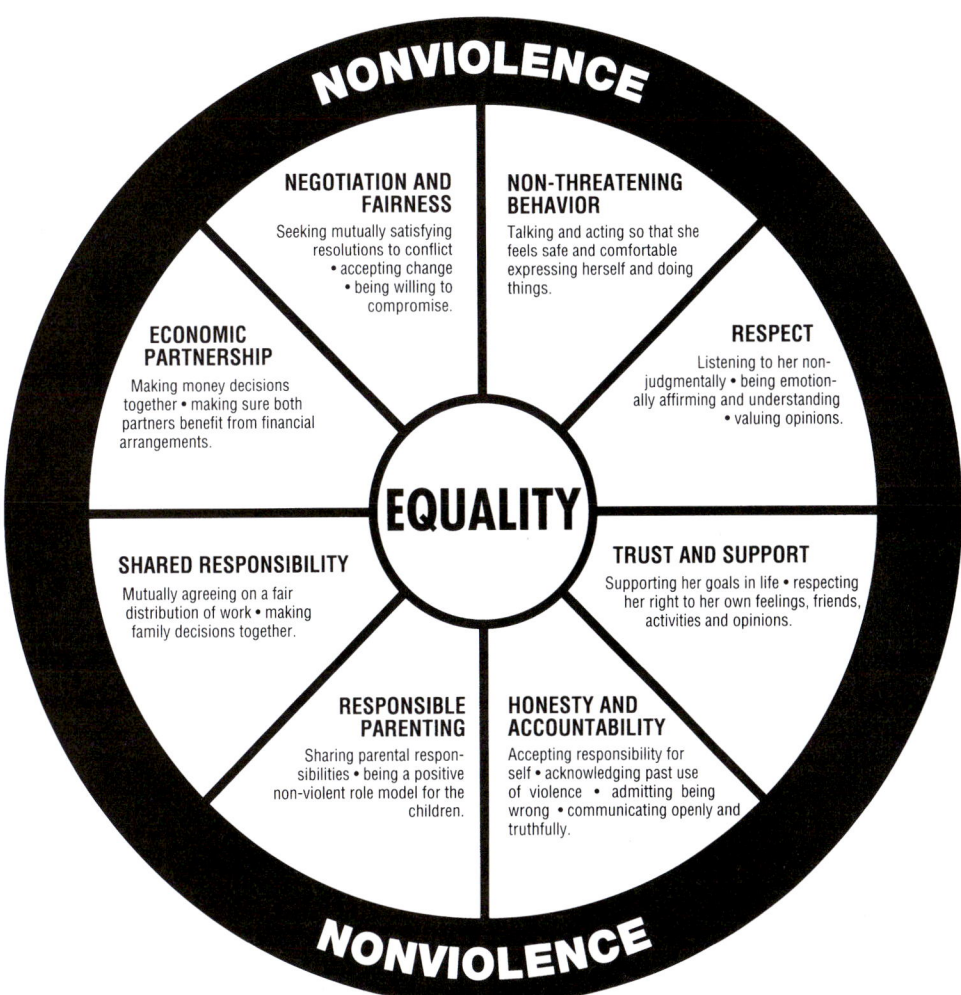

**FIGURE 11-4** A healthy relationship is characterized by equality and an absence of violent behavior. *(Source: From Minnesota Program Development, Inc., Domestic Abuse Intervention Project, 202 East Superior St., Duluth, MN 55802. Courtesy of Coral McDonnell.)*

require many months. Without effective counseling, the woman may not be able to trust other men or establish an intimate relationship based on equality (Figure 11-4).

## Hopeful Signs

The problem of domestic violence in American society has finally gained legal recognition. In 1995 the U.S. Congress passed the Violence Against Women Act (VAWA). The VAWA was reauthorized in 2000 and again in 2005, providing more funding for sexual assault treatment, education, and prevention programs. A third reauthorization is scheduled for 2010. This is the first federal law that recognizes and attempts to stop violence against women. The VAWA contains a civil rights remedy for victims of violence to file charges through a federal court and seek monetary compensation, court-ordered protection, and costs of legal expenses.

The effectiveness of the VAWA will depend on changes in the attitudes and procedures of law enforcement agencies and the court system. Also, there remains a need for widespread educational efforts to improve family relationships and parenting skills. Most important, there is need for change among those male groups who perceive women and children as "property" and believe a male is entitled to subject wives and children to any treatment he wishes.

## REACTIONS TO TRAUMA

Normal reactions to a traumatic experience vary by individual. Immediately following the event, an individual may experience shock, a feeling of being stunned or dazed. A similar reaction is denial, or not accepting what has happened. At first, trauma survivors may feel numb or disconnected from the world around them. Once these initial reactions pass, individuals experience a variety of feelings. They may become moody, irritable, or anxious. Sometimes these emotions are accompanied by physical symptoms such as sweating or a rapid heartbeat. Sleep and eating patterns can change. Individuals may have repeated memories of or dreams about the traumatic event. These reactions can develop immediately after the traumatic event, or they can be delayed for months or years.

Some people recover quite quickly from trauma, while others suffer for a long time. Friends may tell an individual, "Just get over it, Stop dwelling on the past." But some trauma survivors are not able to return to their prior level of adjustment on their own. Health care providers can assist these individuals by assuring them that their feelings are normal reactions to trauma and that they aren't "crazy." Counseling or a support group may be particularly helpful for these individuals.

The severity of reactions can also vary. For some individuals, reactions can be so powerful that they appear similar to mental illness. Health care providers should be familiar with common reactions to trauma so that a traumatized person will receive an appropriate diagnosis and referral for help. In the recovery process, trauma survivors need the support of friends, family, or trained professionals. Maintaining a routine is important in regaining a sense of normalcy. Because the emotions one experiences after a trauma can be overwhelming, it is wise to avoid major decisions and life changes, such as moving or ending a relationship.

The sooner after a trauma a person can talk about the event and receive emotional support, the less likely it is that long-term problems will develop. Some communities have organized teams of trained volunteers or professionals that debrief groups who have witnessed a traumatic event. Group leaders invite trauma survivors to tell what they witnessed and to describe their thoughts, feelings, and physical symptoms. Survivors receive information on normal reactions to trauma and referrals to community agencies if needed. While group debriefing is not available or appropriate in some situations, such as a trauma involving only one person, it is still important that the trauma survivor have someone to talk to about what he or she has experienced.

As with any negative experience, trauma survivors who employ the coping skills described in Unit 10 will find it easier to recover from their experience. Many trauma survivors attribute their recovery to strong relationships with family and friends, a positive attitude, and the ability to find meaning in the difficult experience.

Anyone who has experienced a trauma can benefit from talking to a counselor or therapist. But it is particularly important for an individual to seek help if the reactions just described become so severe or persist for so long that they interfere with daily living. In addition to the normal, albeit disturbing, reactions just described, individuals who have experienced trauma may develop one or more psychological disorders. Health care providers should be familiar with some of the more common disorders described in the following sections.

## Anxiety

A person experiencing generalized anxiety may worry most of the time, have trouble sleeping, and appear shaky or nervous. A patient with anxiety may say, "Doctor, I need something for my nerves." The anxious person may or may not recognize a connection between the trauma and the anxiety. More specific conditions associated with anxiety include panic disorder, post-traumatic stress disorder, and phobias.

**Panic Disorder** Some individuals experience recurring, unexpected anxiety or panic attacks. During these attacks, the person can have a pounding heart, chest pain, difficulty breathing, numbness or tingling, and a dizzy or faint feeling. The skin may become pale and cold. A patient may say, "I thought I was dying," or "I thought I was having a heart attack." While a single panic attack does not necessarily indicate panic disorder, recurring panic attacks or fears of having more attacks are signs that a patient needs treatment.

**Post-traumatic Stress Disorder** When a person continues to re-experience a trauma for weeks or months after it occurs, he or she may be experiencing post-traumatic stress disorder (PTSD). The term *PTSD* was coined following the Vietnam War when large numbers of soldiers returning from combat were unable to recover from the horrifying situations they had witnessed. Some were unable to function in jobs or in their families, and they felt they had no one to talk to since friends and family back home could not imagine the traumas they had endured. Soldiers in other wars had had similar reactions, referred to as "trench fever" in World War I and "shell shock" in World War II. After the Vietnam War, PTSD was recognized as a serious psychological disorder that could result not only from war but from almost any trauma.

Symptoms of PTSD include reliving the event through nightmares or flashbacks. The person may have strong reactions to or avoid anything that serves as a reminder of the event. She may be irritable or jumpy, feel in danger, or need to be "on guard" at all times. On the other hand, some people experiencing PTSD may feel numb, have difficulty remembering details of the event, and show a lack of interest in work or leisure activities.

**Phobias** A phobia is an intense, irrational fear that lasts for six months or more. Phobias may develop in response to a traumatic experience, or they may develop spontaneously. For example, one young girl developed a fear of the dark after her mother's car hit and killed an animal while driving at night. The girl feared that she would see a wounded animal if she looked out the window when it was dark. Some common phobias include fear of snakes, lightning, or speaking in public. A person with a phobia usually avoids the feared situation and experiences extreme anxiety if forced to enter it. Some individuals are unable to leave home because of their phobias. Treatments include therapy, hypnosis, and desensitization, in which the person is gradually exposed to the feared situation while in a state of relaxation. Ultimately, overcoming a phobia involves helping the person lower her anxiety until she is able to enter the feared situation more calmly.

## Depression

Depression is characterized by a feeling of sadness that won't go away. A depressed person may feel tired all the time and show a lack of interest in work, school, or leisure activities. She may have trouble concentrating and making decisions. Low self-esteem or even thoughts of suicide may be present. Additional symptoms of depression include restlessness, trouble sleeping, and sudden changes in appetite or weight. A person experiencing depression may appear to be very emotional, negative, or pessimistic, making comments like, "Nothing seems to matter anymore," or "It doesn't matter what I do. Nothing will help anyway." He or she may withdraw from social activities and avoid interactions with others. Trauma is only one cause of depression; other possible causes include genetics, poor coping skills, or ongoing conditions in a person's life, such as an unhappy relationship.

## THE SURVIVOR ROLE

Each victim reacts to trauma in accordance with her established patterns of behavior. For some, the role of victim provides certain benefits that she does not want to give up, and so "I am a victim" becomes part of the self-concept. Some refuse to work through the emotional effects, choosing instead to hold onto their anger, fear, or hatred. For these individuals, sharing their traumatic experience becomes a way to gain sympathy and support from others. Others find valuable lessons in their traumatic experience and make significant lifestyle changes to improve the quality of their lives.

One woman who was the victim of sexual harassment filed complaints through appropriate channels, with no results. She later filed a lawsuit and eventually received a substantial financial settlement. Instead of simply enjoying her financial gain, she chose to set up a nonprofit organization to provide assistance to others in dealing with sexual harassment. She also serves as a consultant to businesses and provides on-site seminars to help employers establish safeguards against sexual harassment in the workplace. This is an example of how a person can learn from a bad experience and eventually use that learning for a constructive purpose.

## THE CHALLENGE

Achieving a state of adjustment after having a traumatic experience is more difficult for some victims than others. When a victim finds it difficult to fulfill job or family responsibilities several weeks or months after a traumatic event, even though physical injuries have apparently healed, what sort of help is needed?

- Is the person now in a state of clinical depression?
- Has the victim developed a phobia?
- Is the person having panic attacks, nightmares, or flashbacks?
- Is the person unable to resume daily activities because of a pervasive distrust of other people?

Or is the person's prolonged inability to resume her daily routine a severe, but still normal, reaction to trauma? It is difficult to differentiate a "normal" from "not normal" reaction in many such situations. Psychological trauma can be just as disabling as physical injuries.

The victim is usually discharged from health care once the physical injuries have healed. But members of the family, friends, and coworkers may notice that the victim "just isn't the same since . . ." or comment that "he just can't get his act together." The victim does not need criticism or judgmental attitudes. Rather, such a person needs understanding and emotional support. If improvement does not occur within a reasonable period of time, the victim should have the benefit of professional counseling.

Health care providers should encourage victims and relatives to understand the serious nature of psychological trauma and help them recognize the need for professional assistance. Although the disabling effects of physical trauma are obvious, psychological trauma is less likely to be understood or acknowledged. With encouragement from a health care provider, the victim may accept that he or she needs professional assistance in dealing with the psychological effects of the traumatic experience. With therapy, the victim may regain a healthy state of adjustment within a few weeks or months. Without therapy, the victim may remain in a state of poor adjustment for months or years.

## REFERENCES AND SUGGESTED READINGS

Child Welfare Information Gateway. (2008). Child abuse and neglect fatalities: Statistics and interventions. Retrieved from http://www.childwelfare.gov/pubs/factsheets/fatality.cfm#children

National Domestic Violence Hotline. (n.d.). Violence Against Women Act (VAWA). Retrieved from http://www.ndvh.org/get-educated/violence-against-women-act-vawa/

Patchin, J. W., & Hinduja, S. (2006). Bullies move beyond the schoolyard: A preliminary look at cyberbullying. *Youth Violence and Juvenile Justice, 4*(2), 148–169.

U.S. Department of Justice. (n.d.). About domestic violence. Retrieved from http://www.ovw.usdoj.gov/domviolence.htm

U.S. Department of Justice. (n.d.). Stalking victimization in the United States: Special report. Retrieved from http://www.ovw.usdoj.gov/aboutstalking.htm

Wolak, Janis, Finkelhor, David, & Mitchell, Kimberly. (2009). *Trends in arrests of "online predators."* Durham, NH: University of New Hampshire Crimes Against Children Research Center.

## SOURCES OF HELP

Childhelp USA National Child Abuse Hotline, 1-800-4-A-CHILD (24 hours a day), http://www.childhelp.org

Cyberbullying Research Center, http://www.cyberbullying.us

National Institute of Mental Health Outreach, http://www.nimh.nih.gov/health/index.shtml

Office on Violence Against Women, http://www.ovw.usdoj.gov/

## REVIEW AND SELF-CHECK

1. Discuss three reasons that someone who has experienced a trauma may need psychological counseling as well as treatment for any physical injuries.

   _____

   _____

   _____

2. What are two reasons that health care providers should be familiar with the effects of traumatic experiences?

   _____

   _____

3. What are five normal reactions to trauma?

4. What are the symptoms of each of the following psychological disorders: anxiety disorder, panic disorder, post-traumatic stress disorder (PTSD), phobias, and depression?

5. What are three traumatic effects of the following: war and terrorism, rape, domestic violence, and child abuse?

6. What does "blaming the victim" mean?

## ASSIGNMENTS

1. Obtain the name of the agency and the emergency phone number for obtaining help in your community or state for the following situations:

    a. Reporting child abuse

    b. Reporting a rape

    c. Reporting domestic violence

    d. Obtaining emergency shelter for a battered woman

e. Obtaining legal aid for a battered woman

f. Filing a complaint about sexual harassment in the workplace (after the employer's established procedures have been followed, without results)

2. Consider any life experience that was emotionally traumatic for you. Did you receive any encouragement and support from friends and relatives? Did any health care personnel who cared for you show concern about the emotional effects of your experience? Do you experience fear, anger, or other strong emotions when you think of that experience? If so, consider the possibility that you could benefit from professional counseling. If the instructor schedules time for class discussions related to Unit 11, consider whether or not the class could learn from your sharing of this experience. Discuss it with the instructor first, however.

3. In reading the sections on domestic violence, did you recognize the behavior of anyone in your family? If so, what would be appropriate actions on your part?

4. Consider the following situations in terms of the trauma experienced by the victim and appropriate action by you as a friend or a health care provider:

   a. A child is brought to the emergency room by both parents, who report that the child fell down the stairs. After determining that the arm is broken, the physician asks you to take the child to the cast room and directs the parents to the waiting room. En route to the cast room, the child whispers to you "I did *NOT* fall down the stairs." What is an appropriate action for you?

   b. Your best friend has been married almost a year. At first you and she continued your custom of having lunch and going to a movie once a week. Then, she began to cancel at the last minute; once, she didn't cancel but failed to meet you. Today, she arrives at the restaurant wearing dark glasses. She says she cannot stay for the movie, as her husband expects her home in an hour. When she adjusts her glasses, you notice bruises on her arm. What are some appropriate statements you could make to her? Or should you just ignore what you have seen?

   c. Your coworker tells you she has a problem and asks if you will meet her after work. She reveals that, as a child, she was sexually abused by her father. She left home as soon as she finished high school and visits her parents (in a nearby city) only on special occasions. She is divorced and has custody of her 10-year-old daughter. Now, her parents are insisting that she allow the daughter to spend one weekend a month with them. The daughter is excited about this, but has told you that Grandpa kissed her on the lips during their last visit. What factors should influence the coworker's decision?

   d. Sylvia, a recently divorced nurse, occasionally mentions that her ex-husband would beat her about once a week. She always follows such comments with, "But I know I deserved it." What would be an appropriate response for you, the next time you hear her make that statement?

5. For homework, watch one of the following movies: *The Little Princess* or *What's Love Got to Do with It?* Then discuss the following questions with your classmates.

   a. What bullying or abusive behaviors did you see in the movie?

   b. How did the main character respond to these behaviors?

   c. How did the main character finally stand up to the bullying or abuse?

# UNIT 12

# Defense Mechanisms

## OBJECTIVES

Upon completion of this unit, you should be able to:

- State three purposes of defense mechanisms.
- Name six common defense mechanisms.
- Define rationalization, projection, displacement, daydreaming, escape into illness, repression, and withdrawal.
- Explain how occasional use of a defense mechanism can contribute to good adjustment.
- Compare escape into illness and malingering.
- Compare substance dependency and defense mechanisms.
- State three guidelines for improving adjustment by modifying one's use of defense mechanisms.
- Define alcoholism, addiction, tolerance, drug dependency, and codependency.

## KEY TERMS

| | | |
|---|---|---|
| Aberrant | Enabler | Malingering |
| Abstinence | Fantasy | Perception |
| Addiction | Fetal alcohol syndrome (FAS) | Psychoanalysis |
| Alcoholism | Habituation | Psychotherapy |
| Codependency | Hallucinogenic | Self-deception |
| Dependency | Hypnosis | Withdrawal |
| Dysfunctional | Imminent | (drug related) |

There are certain mental devices that all of us use at times in order to feel more comfortable and make our behavior seem reasonable to ourselves and others. These devices are known as *defense mechanisms*.

## THE PURPOSE OF DEFENSE MECHANISMS

When we find ourselves in a situation that we cannot handle effectively, feelings of threat are aroused: fear, anxiety, hostility, frustration, or other negative feelings. Inability to handle the situation is a threat to one's self-esteem, in addition to the possibility of physical or

**176** Section III: Behavior and Problems in Living

psychological harm. When an individual feels unable to deal with a situation, a defense mechanism may be used.

Defense mechanisms are attempts to protect against loss of self-esteem. They help us handle feelings of discomfort, make it possible to "save face," provide an *apparently* logical reason for the behavior used, and enable us to maintain self-respect in spite of the outcome. Obviously, defense mechanisms are useful—provided they do not become habitual devices for avoiding reality. Defense mechanisms can help us, or they can become crutches that substitute for more effective ways of dealing with difficult situations (Figure 12-1).

As a health care provider, being able to recognize common defense mechanisms is a tool that will help you understand behavior. It is also desirable that you recognize your own use of defense mechanisms in order to develop effective ways of dealing with difficult situations. This unit explains seven common defense mechanisms: rationalization, projection, displacement, daydreaming, escape into illness, repression, and withdrawal. The remainder of the unit addresses substance dependency. You will encounter friends, perhaps family members, and patients who have some type of substance dependency.

## RATIONALIZATION

In the ancient fable of the fox and the grapes, a fox found he could not jump high enough to get some grapes. So he announced that the grapes were sour, and therefore he did not want them. Thus, the fox avoided admitting to himself that he had tried but failed. This is one type of rationalization—the "sour grapes" approach to handling failure or disappointment.

**FIGURE 12-1** Overuse of defense mechanisms can indicate poor adjustment. *Delmar/Cengage Learning*

**FIGURE 12-2** Rationalization. *Delmar/Cengage Learning*

Rationalization involves offering an apparently reasonable, socially acceptable explanation for behavior, when the true reason would be too painful for the individual. Thus, rationalization helps to relieve disappointment, provides a means for avoiding a situation perceived as threatening, and avoids admitting an inadequacy that would be damaging to self-esteem (Figure 12-2). Unfortunately, rationalization is a form of self-deception. Frequent use of rationalization is self-defeating because it displaces efforts to improve one's competence in dealing with life situations. Consider an example of a young girl using rationalization.

Mary has been invited to a party. The other girls know the latest dance steps. Mary does not dance. Although Mary wants to be a part of the group and have a good time, she thinks this party will place her at a disadvantage in relation to the other girls. To Mary, this is a very big problem. She believes her acceptance by members of this group will be affected when they discover she does not dance. To Mary, missing the party is preferable to being embarrassed. Mary's mother is in poor health, but she is not so sick that Mary should stay home with her and miss the party. Yet her mother's health provides a graceful way to avoid the party.

By rationalizing, Mary has avoided admitting to herself the degree of fear she feels at being unable to "hold her own" at the party. She has also given her hostess a socially acceptable reason for her absence. Perhaps Mary even feels somewhat proud of making a sacrifice in order to be a dutiful daughter. No conscious decision making is involved in this situation. Mary's fears lead to seeking an escape, and her mother's poor health has provided an easy, socially acceptable way to avoid the party—and the threat it represents to Mary.

When rationalization is used habitually, it becomes an *unconscious* mechanism. Friends of the habitual rationalizer may be unaware of the fears and anxieties that are the basis for hard-to-understand behaviors. They may regard the habitual rationalizer as a person who always makes excuses.

## PROJECTION

Projection is a device for placing blame for one's own inadequacies on someone else or on circumstances. Projection is also used to attribute one's own unfavorable characteristics and desires to someone else; a person who is often critical of other people may be exhibiting projection. When projection is used to an extreme, the individual develops distorted perceptions of life situations and of people.

James is a health occupations student who is not making satisfactory grades. In discussing his academic standing with the counselor, he says that he cannot study at home because his mother wants him to help around the house. When one of the instructors corrects James on his technique in performing a procedure, he complains that the instructor does not like him. When hostility develops between James and a classmate, James explains the situation by saying that his classmate is jealous because James is dating Joanne.

Every undesirable situation in James's life is explained as the fault of something or someone other than himself. His use of projection is preventing an honest appraisal of his problems and how he himself helps to create them. Other people may be saying, "Why doesn't James wise up?" But James is more comfortable projecting blame than looking at himself. He avoids having to admit to himself that he has some shortcomings.

Some people blunder through life using projection and other defense mechanisms instead of learning to see themselves and situations realistically (Figure 12-3). Each of us makes a mistake at times. It is no disgrace to be wrong, but to be unable to admit being wrong is not so good. *Being able to recognize how we contribute to an undesirable situation and being able to learn from our mistakes lead to growth as a person.* Frequent use of projection interferes with such growth. Projection is self-deception and a distortion of reality.

**FIGURE 12-3** Projection. *Delmar/Cengage Learning*

**FIGURE 12-4** Displacement. *Delmar/Cengage Learning*

## DISPLACEMENT

Displacement is the redirection of strong feelings about one person to someone else. Displacement occurs when there is fear or inability to direct the feeling toward the object or person who aroused the feelings. Usually, displacement involves negative feelings, but it can also occur with positive feelings.

Bob is a health care provider with hostile feelings toward his supervisor. He is well aware that the supervisor makes out the assignments and the schedule; also, the supervisor must recommend any member of the staff for a raise. It would be unwise for Bob to be openly hostile to one who has so much control over his daily work and over progress in his career. Bob recognizes this and is always pleasant to the supervisor, even doing a little "apple polishing" at times. Whenever Bob has a conference with the supervisor, the next person he sees is likely to become the object of his hostility. Sometimes Bob carries his hostility home and is irritable and short tempered with his family or the family pet. Bob is displacing the hostility he feels for the supervisor to others who did nothing to create his negative feelings.

Obviously, displacement creates interpersonal problems. Family and friends may be tolerant for a while, especially if they recognize that the hostility has been aroused by someone else. They may even take sides with the individual and attach unflattering names to the person who aroused the anger. Usually, however, the person who habitually displaces negative feelings is perceived by others as irritable and "hard to get along with."

You have learned that the energy generated by negative feelings needs to be worked off, preferably through physical activity. Displacement is an *unhealthy* method of using negative energy (Figure 12-4). It is an undesirable pattern of behavior, both because of the self-deception involved and because of unfavorable effects on relationships.

## DAYDREAMING

Daydreaming is a device that provides escape. It is a useful mechanism if it creates dissatisfaction with things as they are, inspires the setting of goals for the future, and leads to a course of action designed to attain those goals. Daydreaming may lead to invention or inspiration for a creative activity.

If daydreaming provides an escape by substituting **fantasy** for reality, then it contributes to poor adjustment. When habitually used as an escape, daydreams can become more satisfying than life experiences. In the extreme, this escape from reality is a symptom of illness—adjustment so poor that the individual substitutes escape for dealing with life situations.

Lou, Ed, and Sue were all in high school together. None of them planned to go to college, yet all did well in their science courses and had an interest in health careers. They all tended to daydream at times, as most young people do. Lou dreamed of himself as a famous surgeon, acclaimed the world over for unusual and startling medical accomplishments. Ed and Sue also dreamed of themselves as physicians, but their dreams were more in line with things they had seen physicians doing. Ed's daydreams enhanced his interest in health science, and he began to save the money from his after-school job. Eventually, he entered a program for orthopedic technicians and obtained a job that enabled him to work closely with orthopedic surgeons. Sue got a job after high school and continued to daydream occasionally about herself as a physician. Soon, family responsibilities increased until she could not afford to enroll in an educational program. She continued to think of herself as a person who could have been a physician if circumstances had permitted, but she never made any real effort to achieve such a goal (Figure 12-5).

Meanwhile, Lou found his daydreams highly satisfying. He began to neglect his schoolwork. Occasionally, he imagined himself to be a famous surgeon as he performed his daily activities. Lou's first job lasted about a year: his employer said he could not keep his mind on his work. Lou's next job was quite distasteful to him; the unpleasantness of his workday made his daydreams more important than ever. Since daydreams had become Lou's main source of satisfaction in life, he was very irritable if something interrupted his daydreaming. Lou had retreated into a world of fantasy to such an extent that he could not function as a responsible adult. Escaping from reality through daydreams leads to increasingly poor adjustment, because it substitutes escape into fantasy for achieving satisfaction from real life experiences.

**FIGURE 12-5** Daydreaming. *Delmar/Cengage Learning*

## ESCAPE INTO ILLNESS

Escape into illness involves periodic illnesses that serve a definite purpose, but the individual is not aware of the purpose. Illness as an escape usually has its beginnings in childhood. Parents tend to be especially attentive when a child is sick, even if the illness is a minor one. Sometimes busy parents do not give children much more attention than is necessary for the daily routine, until a problem arises involving the child. Then the child becomes the center of attention. When the problem has been taken care of, the busy routine may be resumed, with the child again receiving only necessary attention. Thus, the child learns that illness is rewarded with parental notice and concern.

If illness during childhood is rewarded by special attention, gifts, permissiveness, sweets, or other things desired by children, then illness serves a definite purpose—the reward of being "special" and of having privileges *not usually allowed when well*. If the parents permit a child to use illness to avoid a dreaded situation and/or to gain advantages available only during an illness, then these early learnings can become an unconscious mechanism that will influence behavior throughout life. Once the child has learned that a headache, a cold, or other minor physical complaint can serve a purpose, illness may be used to get special attention or to avoid certain situations. Eventually, the purpose is no longer in the conscious mind and periodic illnesses have become "real."

Escape into illness must be distinguished from malingering. Escape is a defense mechanism, protecting the individual from threatening situations, but operating below the level of conscious thought. **Malingering,** on the other hand, is *deliberate pretense of illness* when there is none.

Many people habitually use escape into illness as a means of avoiding some of their life problems (Figure 12-6). When the stress of accumulating problems reaches a certain point, or

**FIGURE 12-6** Illness can provide escape from an unpleasant situation.
*Delmar/Cengage Learning*

when an anticipated event arouses fear or anxiety, a minor illness can conveniently provide temporary escape. The symptoms experienced are real; the misery the individual feels is real. There may even be great annoyance at the inconvenience caused by this illness, yet the pattern of behavior is based on the individual's inability to face certain situations. Let us look at Joe, who is enrolled in a program for surgical technicians.

Joe is 19, a high school graduate. He likes sports and has high ideals about team spirit and fair play. He can hold his own with his age group, whether in sports or in standing up for his beliefs.

The surgical technician program proved very interesting to Joe—until the class went into the operating room. Suddenly Joe had some feelings he did not understand. Patients on stretchers, containers of body organs, hospital staff members with masks and floppy gowns—it was a frightening and unreal world to Joe. After several days, Joe's negative feelings about the operating room were stronger than on the first day. Increasing familiarity did not relieve his intense feelings, whereas most of his classmates had become accustomed to the sights and smells of the operating room suite.

Over the weekend, Joe could think of nothing but the operating room and its effect on him. He went bowling with the gang, but he made a poor score and could not get into the jolly mood of his friends. Monday morning he could not eat breakfast. When his mother anxiously inquired about his health, he said he must have hurt his back when he was bowling. Joe, with his mother's encouragement, went back to bed and slept all day.

Joe was not pretending to be sick. His doubts and fears had mounted to the point that stress was manifested as physical symptoms. Joe really did feel terrible! His retreating into illness was an unconscious escape.

At this point, Joe's early learnings will influence the behavior pattern of the next few days. If he has learned to use illness as an escape, his back pain will become worse and he will withdraw from the surgical program because of a "bad back." If Joe is able to face life realistically, he will eventually recognize that his emotional reactions to the operating room are affecting him unfavorably. An honest and realistic appraisal of himself in relation to the job requirements of a surgical technician should be made. If Joe is not temperamentally suited to the operating room, he should feel free to withdraw from the program on that basis, without the need to project blame on his "injured back."

Sometimes a person develops insight into tendencies to use escape into illness and, through determination and effort, learns to face problems rather than trying to escape them. Many people, however, have used this device for years and are unable to develop insight into the purposes of the illnesses without professional counsel.

## REPRESSION

Repression is the forcing of an unpleasant memory into the subconscious mind. Once a memory has been forced into the subconscious mind, it cannot be recalled at will. Although deeply buried, the memory is still a powerful influence on behavior. Repression occurs most often with painful experiences of childhood, but it can also occur with an adult experience. Anyone who has had a traumatic experience may repress the memory because the experience is too painful to keep within conscious awareness. Family members may, at some future time, be surprised to hear that individual say, "I don't remember that," or actually deny that such an experience ever occurred. Repression is less susceptible to conscious control than the defense mechanisms discussed previously.

Repressed memories usually come to light only during **psychotherapy.** A therapeutic method aimed at reaching these deeply buried memories is **psychoanalysis.** Many therapeutic sessions are necessary to bring repressed memories back into the conscious level. **Hypnosis,** possibly with age regression, is sometimes used to identify and/or help a patient "relive" a traumatic experience that has been repressed. This is usually accomplished with only a few hypnosis sessions. These methods require the skills of a psychiatrist or psychologist with specialized training.

You, as a health care provider, should be aware of the influence of repressed memories on behavior. A traumatic experience, especially during childhood, may exert a powerful influence on adult behavior, even though the adult does not recall that experience. As a health care provider in contact with pediatric patients, try to prevent the child's experience with the health care system from being psychologically traumatic.

## WITHDRAWAL

Withdrawal as a defense mechanism involves either shutting off communication or removing oneself physically from a situation that is perceived as threatening. Withdrawal may be the strategy of choice in a situation in which defeat is **imminent,** as in a disagreement when the other person becomes physically threatening. Extremes of withdrawal are characteristic of some psychiatric conditions. A less extreme, but quite serious, example of withdrawal is the desertion reaction of some pediatric patients if no member of the family stays with the child. Lying in the fetal position, a tendency of some chronically ill patients and many geriatric patients, is also an example of withdrawal. If your role as a health care provider will involve caring for patients who exhibit these types of withdrawals, you will study these conditions in other courses. But in every health care role and in your personal life you will see examples of withdrawal used as a coping strategy in difficult situations.

If a discussion becomes unpleasant and you refuse to participate further, you are using withdrawal. If a conference with the supervisor arouses anger and you excuse yourself from the conference, then you are withdrawing physically. If you do not do assignments and have made low grades on the tests, then drop the course the week before exams, you are withdrawing to avoid the threat to your self-esteem that a failing grade represents.

Suppose your first position as a health care provider requires that you work with someone you dislike. Every day you have one or more contacts with this person, and each encounter leaves you angry or unhappy. Except for this one person, you like your job very much. Should you resign? Should you keep the job in spite of these daily annoyances? This situation requires a decision between "fight" or "flight." You can stay on and try to cope with your reactions to this person, or you can "flee" to another job.

There are times when it is a better strategy to withdraw physically from a situation than to put up with the problems it involves. There are other times when the satisfactions of a situation can balance the unpleasantness. Decisions about whether to withdraw or remain should be made on a *rational rather than emotional basis;* but the probable long-range effects of the alternatives should enter into the decision.

Sometimes a situation can be changed or one can develop a better attitude toward it. If there is interpersonal conflict, open and honest talk may lead to improved understanding. But if a situation cannot be improved and one's feelings cannot be changed, then staying in the situation can only have unfavorable effects—the rational approach is to withdraw from that situation. If similarly unhappy experiences occur in the new setting, then a close look at oneself is indicated. Perhaps the source of the problem is the self, rather than others.

## SUBSTANCE DEPENDENCY

Defense mechanisms involve mental tricks—the use of the mind to deal with uncomfortable situations. Another approach to dealing with difficult experiences is the use of substances that have physical effects, thereby providing some relief from stress or diminished awareness of discomfort. Like the defense mechanisms, these substances—tobacco, alcohol, and drugs—provide an escape. With repeated use, one may develop addiction to one or more of these substances.

### Nicotine Addiction

It is now known that nicotine, contained in all tobacco products, is highly addictive. During 1996, the tobacco companies were accused of purposely adjusting the levels of nicotine in their products. Many lawsuits have been filed, charging tobacco companies with creating serious health problems, including death from lung cancer and long-term disability due to emphysema.

Evidence that tobacco is a major threat to health has been increasing for several decades. As a result, many public buildings and most hospitals have been declared smoke-free environments, smoking is prohibited on airlines, and restaurants have a nonsmoking section. Many smokers refuse to give up their habit until they experience a major health problem, such as a heart attack. Others choose to give up smoking as part of a larger plan for a more healthful lifestyle. But for those smokers who choose to continue their habit, current societal restrictions are sources of frustration and anger.

Why do people smoke? The usual reason is that smoking provides relief from feelings of stress. For many people, the primary reason is social; this is the appeal to teenage smokers, for whom conformity to group behavior patterns is important. For an individual whose parents were smokers, the smell of a cigarette, cigar, or pipe may arouse pleasant childhood memories and feelings of comfort and security. Once a person has become addicted to nicotine, smoking is a response to subtle signals from the body that it needs a nicotine "fix."

The decision to give up tobacco may be made voluntarily or under pressure from one's physician, family, or friends. Many smokers are able to give up their habit simply by deciding to do so. When an addictive substance is no longer available to the body, physical symptoms of **withdrawal** occur. (This meaning of "withdrawal" is different from its meaning as a defense mechanism.) Nicotine withdrawal results in nervous agitation and intense craving for a cigarette (or whatever form of tobacco the individual uses). People who cannot tolerate withdrawal symptoms may use nicotine chewing gum or a skin patch. Psychotherapy also can provide assistance through hypnosis or relaxation with guided imagery.

As a health care provider, you will encounter people who either continue to smoke or are trying to quit. These people may be patients, coworkers, family, or friends. Learn about the dangers of tobacco and the various approaches to giving up tobacco products, so you can be a source of information for anyone who seeks your help.

### Alcohol Abuse/Alcoholism

Alcohol is a drug with specific physiological effects. The use of alcohol, like tobacco, may begin as a social activity and a desire for peer approval and acceptance. It is readily available, more affordable than most drugs, and present in many homes, making it accessible to children and adolescents. The use of alcohol is so pervasive that "drinking" and "having a drink" are synonymous with "having an alcoholic drink."

Social use of alcohol can provide quick relief from stress, anxiety, guilt, insecurity, and other uncomfortable feelings (Figure 12-7). These effects may lead to occasional abuse—overindulgence to the point of becoming intoxicated. Regular use of alcohol over a period of time can result in psychological **dependency** and, eventually, physiological addiction—**alcoholism.** The distinction between occasional abuse and alcoholism is clear cut:

1. An alcoholic's drinking is compulsive (i.e., cannot stop after a reasonable number of drinks).
2. After a period of **abstinence** (hours), the alcoholic experiences withdrawal symptoms that can only be relieved by taking a drink.

Intoxication and alcoholism carry a high price tag. The Center for Disease Control and Prevention reports that in 2008, over 11,000 people were killed in alcohol-related traffic accidents. The same year over 1.4 million drivers were arrested for driving under the influence of alcohol or narcotics. In industry, high rates of absenteeism, errors, low productivity, and occupational accidents are attributed to alcohol. Alcohol is involved in a large percentage of crimes, especially murders, and in domestic violence, child abuse, and sex offenses. Alcoholism is now recognized by the courts as a disease (not punishable), but the individual (alcoholic or not) can be prosecuted for any crimes committed while under the influence of alcohol.

Why do people drink? Alcohol provides *escape.* Although classed as a central nervous system depressant, alcohol is considered by many people to be a stimulant, because it lowers inhibitions and releases muscular tension. Unfortunately, these relaxing effects are accompanied

**FIGURE 12-7** Alcohol and drugs provide escape—from the "black abyss" of depression, intolerable stress, and problems in living—but the escape is only temporary. *Delmar/Cengage Learning*

by diminished judgment, thinking skills, and memory—effects that make the drinker a danger to self and others. The use of alcohol to escape the feelings of despair and hopelessness that characterize clinical depression and the depressive phase of manic depressive illness is common. If such patients have also developed alcoholism, their clinical status is "dual diagnosis." Alcoholism must be treated before the psychiatric problem can be addressed.

Why do some people progress from social drinking to dependence on alcohol? Many factors have been implicated: physiological, metabolic, nutritional, genetic, emotional, and social. Certain personality traits seem to predominate: the individual tends to be dependent on others, harbors hostility, is somewhat egocentric, and has unrealistic expectations that result in frustration and feelings of failure. Regardless of causative factors, the condition is treatable, but only when the individual can admit to needing help. This may occur only after numerous arrests, hospitalizations, and various losses (job, spouse, home) have occurred. Whereas medical treatment is required for acute phases, especially during withdrawal, the support and encouragement of family and friends is crucial to long-term recovery of an alcoholic.

Effective treatment includes helping the individual learn to face reality and deal with life problems, instead of trying to escape them. This learning can be facilitated by counseling and participation in group therapy. Alcoholics Anonymous (AA), whose membership consists of recovering alcoholics, has proven to be effective for many people. AA emphasizes *total abstinence* from alcohol; newcomers are encouraged to avoid having a drink and to cope one day at a time. Making it through one day is achievable for many people, but vowing to "never take a drink again" is a promise too easily broken.

The sharing of experiences at AA meetings and the encouragement and support of fellow members, all of whom "have been there and know what you're going through," enables a new member to achieve sobriety and become a recovering alcoholic. Once the alcoholic is sober and his or her body is free of alcohol, attention shifts to healing mind and emotions by following AA's "Twelve Steps to Recovery." The Twelve-Step program has been so successful during the 60 years of AA's existence that organizations devoted to other specific problems (i.e., gambling) have adapted the 12 steps to their own purpose.

Anyone may attend an open AA meeting, but closed meetings are for alcoholics only. In recognition that alcoholism is a family affair, support groups for family members have been established. Al-Anon is a self-help group for all family members; Alateen, for adolescent children of an alcoholic parent, is sponsored by Al-Anon, as is a group for adult survivors of alcoholic families. Adult Children of Alcoholics (ACOA) is a separate group, specifically for adult children of an alcoholic parent.

One tragic consequence of drinking has emerged during the last two decades: **fetal alcohol syndrome (FAS).** This disorder is the result of a woman's drinking during the prenatal period. *Even one or two glasses of wine per day during early pregnancy increases the probability that the baby will be born with FAS, since alcohol penetrates the placental barrier and enters the fetal bloodstream.* Serious damage to the brain results, so the baby is born with an *untreatable disability.* The newborn infant is small, has characteristic cranial and facial features, and may have deformities of the limbs. Growth and development will be inhibited; mental retardation may be diagnosed when the child is old enough for testing. This condition is so definitely related to drinking during pregnancy that the National Institute on Alcohol Abuse and Alcoholism issued a statement in 1980 that *pregnant women should totally abstain from alcohol consumption.* In some states, establishments that serve alcohol are required to display warnings about the relationship of alcohol to birth defects.

## Drug Abuse

The use of drugs is so pervasive in modern society that few people are unaffected. A *drug user* is any person who takes drugs, regardless of the purpose or type of drug, so that term applies to almost everyone at times. *Drug misuse* refers to taking doses that exceed the prescribed amount or taking medication prescribed for someone else. *Drug abuse* occurs when someone uses a drug for a nonmedical purpose. Drug abuse usually involves a class of drugs referred to as "recreational drugs," because they are often used in a social setting. That phrase is unfortunate, because it gives the false impression that these drugs are fun and harmless.

Any drug can be abused, but those most likely to be abused are drugs that relieve pain, alter one's mood, have a stimulant effect (provide a "high"), relieve anxiety, or have a **hallucinogenic** effect. Regular use of these types of drugs leads to **habituation,** which is psychological dependence on the drug. If usage continues over a period of time, *tolerance* may develop, meaning that larger and larger doses are required to get the desired effect. *Addiction* exists when there is a physiological need for the drug at regular intervals. *Drug dependency* and *chemical dependency* are now the preferred terms, without concern about whether the patient's condition is habituation or addiction. *Withdrawal,* when used in relation to drug dependency, refers to the symptoms that occur when a drug is withheld. These symptoms range from nervous agitation and anxiety to psychotic behavior and convulsions, depending upon the specific drug being withdrawn.

Table 12-1 lists some commonly abused types of drugs, with the symptoms and dangerous effects of each. Although the table lists inhalants as a group, certain examples deserve comment. Children, boys especially, may build model cars, planes, or boats, a hobby that requires the use of model plane glue. "Sniffing" this glue can produce effects the child perceives as pleasant. This common practice related to an educational hobby may introduce the child to inhalants as a source of exhilarating experiences. Continuation of this practice can lead to serious physical damage, as detailed in Table 12-1.

Cocaine is an extremely addictive drug that is not included in Table 12-1. Cocaine is a white powder that is also known as "snow" and "coke." Its freebase form is "crack," cheaper than other forms of cocaine and even more addictive. As the drug of choice for young, lower-income drug users, the use of crack is now pervasive, even among pregnant women. The term "crack baby" has emerged to describe the newborn infant who is already addicted because of the mother's drug use during pregnancy.

Methamphetamine is another drug that is commonly used among some populations. This drug can be smoked, injected, snorted, or taken orally and is a central nervous system stimulant. Because it can be manufactured from common ingredients, methamphetamine is sometimes created in users' homes in makeshift "meth labs." Ongoing abuse of this drug is associated with impaired motor skills, cognition, and ability to learn.

Drug use may be legal or illegal. The use of a prescription drug in accordance with the physician's directions is legal. The appropriate use of over-the-counter (OTC) drugs is legal. Misuse of a prescription drug or OTC may or may not be illegal, but is certainly unwise, unethical, and immoral. Drug abuse usually involves drugs that fall into one of the 11 categories of "controlled substances" as defined in the Controlled Substances Act of 1970. Certain controlled substances are prescribed for management of pain, anxiety, mood disorders, and other medical conditions. Other controlled substances, used for nonmedical purposes, are most often obtained illegally; these are known as "street drugs."

## TABLE 12-1

### Abused Drugs: Symptoms and Effects

| DRUG | STREET NAME | SYMPTOMS | ADVERSE EFFECTS |
|---|---|---|---|
| **Hallucinogens** | | | |
| marijuana | grass, weed, maryjane, tea, pot, reefer, joint, hemp, hashish, hash, rope | sense of well-being; possible anxiety; talkative; relaxed; exhilarated; happy; altered time sense | reduced memory recall; impaired coordination and moral judgment; easily distracted; highly suggestible; long-term effect not known |
| LSD | 25, acid, cubes, sunshine, the big D, trips, the chief, the ghost, the hawk | heightened and distorted perceptions; euphoria; altered time perception; dreamy, floating state; enlarged pupils; bizarre sensations | chromosomal damage; loss of control over normal thought processes; violence, self-destructive feelings; highly unpredictable behavior; slowed reaction time and reflexes; personality changes; paranoid symptoms |
| PCP | angel dust | lapse of memory; difficulty concentrating; convulsions; partial paralysis | effects highly unpredictable |
| **Inhalants** | | | |
| glue, gasoline, spray paint, aerosols | | similar to alcohol intoxication; sense of floating or spinning; blurred vision; confusion; staggering gait; slurred speech | brain damage; lead poisoning; damage to liver, heart, kidneys, and bone marrow; death |

*Source:* From Waughfield, Claire G. (2002). *Mental health concepts* (5th ed.). Clifton Park, NY: Delmar, Cengage Learning, p. 367.

The most commonly abused drugs are some that are socially acceptable and completely legal: caffeine, nicotine, and alcohol. Most people do not think of these three as drugs, but each has physiological effects, each is addictive, and each is subject to misuse and abuse. The coffee drinker who decides to forgo caffeine knows all too well the severe headache that lasts for several days—a symptom of caffeine withdrawal. The smoker who decides to quit knows well the symptoms of nicotine withdrawal. For an alcoholic, withdrawal of alcohol can have

**FIGURE 12-8** Treatment approaches for drug dependency.
Source: From Waughfield, Claire G. (2002). **Mental health concepts** (5th ed.). Clifton Park, NY: Delmar, Cengage Learning.

such serious consequences that it should be accomplished only under medical supervision, preferably with the patient hospitalized. And these are legally, socially acceptable drugs!

The treatment of dependency is complex and long term. The individual must become drug-free, known as being "clean," and then must learn the coping skills required for dealing with life situations, rather than using drugs as a form of escape. For persons with a dual diagnosis, dependency must be treated and then a treatment protocol developed for the psychiatric condition. Such patients present an especially difficult situation, since the psychiatric condition often involves noncompliance with the physician's prescribed therapy. Figure 12-8 shows various approaches used in treatment of drug dependency.

The problem of drug abuse is now so pervasive that it has become a societal issue; full discussion is beyond the scope of this textbook. Yet every health care provider should be informed about drug abuse, both from the standpoint of health care and legal/societal concerns. The "Assignments" section of this unit will suggest activities to help you become better informed.

## CODEPENDENCY

**Codependency** is a situation in which the dysfunctional behavior of an alcoholic or drug abuser meets some need of the spouse or other close family member. The role of rescuer or protector becomes such an important part of the codependent's life that the possibility of giving up that role is quite threatening. Family members may have spent years "rescuing" the addict and pleading for a change in behavior. They cling to the belief that life would be good if and when the addict takes control and gives up the addictive substance. Eventually this interaction becomes an important part of life activities; the rescuer role fulfills an important need. At that point, family members *unconsciously* encourage and support the addiction. If the addict undergoes treatment, family problems increase because family members who are codependent cannot cope with the new behavior of the former addict.

A codependent's *conscious* belief is that the family's problems will be resolved when the addiction has been treated. The reality is that a codependent *unconsciously* functions as an **enabler** by facilitating the addiction. Enabling takes many forms, such as "lending" the addict money that the enabler knows will be used for drugs, even though the addict promises to use the money for food and rent. In the case of alcoholism, the enabler may insist on going to parties where alcohol will be served or continue to keep liquor in the home for personal use, knowing that its presence is a temptation for the alcoholic. In the mental health field, codependency is itself considered an addiction that requires intensive psychotherapy.

Obviously, where codependency exists, treatment of the addict must include treatment of the codependent person also. Ideally, the entire family will be involved in therapy, so that any dysfunctional family dynamics may be corrected. The addict must learn to cope with life problems effectively, without escaping into a drug-induced euphoria or relying on the codependent for solving his or her problems. The codependent must learn to encourage the addict to be self-reliant and must be willing to give up the role of rescuer, protector, and caregiver. *Effective treatment of an addict must involve family members.* Otherwise, the "cured" addict will return to a dysfunctional family situation that does not support being drug-free. A difficult adjustment for the recovering addict is giving up old friends and associates who continue to use drugs. New relationships must be developed that include a drug-free lifestyle and ongoing support and encouragement as the recovering addict struggles against the temptation to resume the use of drugs. The desire to experience that drug-induced state of euphoria may remain, even after years of being drug-free.

## DEFENSE MECHANISMS AND ADJUSTMENT

All of us need to use adjustment mechanisms of many types, including defense mechanisms. At one time or another we all have unhappy experiences, problem situations to face, and obstacles to overcome. We all experience disappointment and failure at intervals. We all need to feel good about ourselves, but our self-esteem is always at risk—vulnerable to negative experiences. When circumstances threaten self-esteem, we tend to become defensive.

A situation that you perceive as threatening may not bother your best friend. Conversely, you may be puzzled about your friend's defensive reaction to a situation you consider to be ordinary. Some of us become defensive whenever we are criticized. Some of us become apprehensive when we are expected to show achievement. Some of us become uncomfortable in the presence of an authority figure. Some of us distrust others, always expecting a put-down or criticism. Threat, then, is quite personal. It is based on our own specific areas of sensitivity, the psychological scars that are the result of hurtful experiences in our past.

### The Patient

As a health care provider, keep in mind that illness and hospitalization represent a threat to most people. Therefore, you are likely to see many examples of defense mechanisms as you work with patients. If you work with psychiatric patients, you will need to learn about other mechanisms and about behavior deviations that psychiatric patients manifest. In the meantime, observe behavior and learn to recognize defense mechanisms.

When you become aware that someone is using a defense mechanism, realize that the person feels threatened by a situation. It is *not your role to point out the defense mechanism*. Your role is to *reduce the degree of threat the individual feels.* Through reassurance, acceptance, and sincere interest in the patient's well-being, you can usually reduce a patient's need for defensive behavior.

## The Health Care Provider

How can you use knowledge about defense mechanisms to improve your own adjustment? First, keep in mind that defense mechanisms can be useful in relieving discomfort or negative feelings. Suppose a friend drops in just as you are about to leave home for a movie. At first, you feel quite irritated, but then you tell yourself, "I didn't really want to see that movie anyway." Having thus rationalized, you disposed of the angry feelings toward your friend and are free to enjoy the unexpected visit.

*The key to healthful use of a defense mechanism is awareness.* If you are aware of using a defense mechanism and of your reason for using it, then you are probably using it healthfully.

Suppose, on the other hand, your supervisor criticizes your performance frequently, but each time you place the blame on someone else or on circumstances. For example, the supervisor comments that you should have explained a procedure to your patient before carrying it out, but your reaction is, "I didn't have time." For every criticism you have an excuse. Then your use of projection is an obstacle to improving your performance as a health care provider. *Self-deception and distorted* **perception** *of situations are incompatible with learning and improved performance.*

In striving to improve your own adjustment, be aware of the frequency and purposes of the defense mechanisms you use. As you learn to recognize your use of each defense mechanism, you will be able to identify the types of situations that are threatening to you. Then you can seek ways of effectively dealing with such situations. If you have a habit of projecting blame, you may have to force yourself to admit a shortcoming now and then. Eventually, you will find it easier to admit being wrong or having made an error. By discarding the defense mechanism, you open the way to learn from experience.

As you become more aware of your tendencies to use defense mechanisms, you will begin to recognize those you have previously been using unconsciously. This awareness will not come overnight, nor will it come without some effort on your part to study your behavior patterns.

With increased understanding of yourself and your use of defense mechanisms, you will be ready to eliminate **self-deception,** learn to face reality, and use appropriate behavior in a variety of situations. Through practice in dealing with problems rather than "fleeing" from them, you will improve your skill in solving problems—even those that involve some unpleasantness. At that point, you will have less need for defense mechanisms.

## REFERENCES AND SUGGESTED READINGS

Beattie, Melody. (2009). *The new codependency: Help and guidance for today's generation.* New York: Simon & Schuster.

Centers for Disease Control and Prevention. (2009). Impaired driving: Fact sheet. Retrieved from http://www.cdc.gov/MotorVehicleSafety/Impaired_Driving/impaired-drv_factsheet.html

Fine, Alain. (2005). Flight into illness. In *International Dictionary of Psychoanalysis* (Vol. 1, p. 590). Gale Virtual Reference Library. Farmington Hills, MI: Gale.

Kuhn, Cynthia et al. (2008). *Buzzed: The straight facts about the most used and abused drugs from alcohol to ecstasy.* New York: W.W. Norton.

National Institute on Drug Abuse. (2009). NIDA infofacts: Methamphetamine. Retrieved from http://www.nida.nih.gov/InfoFacts/methamphetamine.html

Waughfield, Claire G. (2002). Alcoholism; drug dependency. In *Mental health concepts* (5th ed., pp. 323–350, 351–378). Clifton Park, NY: Delmar, Cengage Learning.

## SOURCES OF ADDITIONAL INFORMATION

**Alcoholics Anonymous,** http://www.aa.org
For over 50 years, AA has offered community support for alcoholic individuals.

**Al-Anon/Alateen,** http://www.al-anon.alateen.org
Al-Anon and Alateen provide support for family members of alcoholics.

**Narcotics Anonymous,** http://www.na.org
Narcotics Anonymous offers community support for individuals recovering from drug addiction.

## REVIEW AND SELF-CHECK

1. State three purposes of defense mechanisms.

    _____

    _____

    _____

2. Name six commonly used defense mechanisms.

    _____

    _____

    _____

    _____

    _____

    _____

3. Define each of the following terms in your own words, based on information in Unit 12:

    a. rationalization _____

    b. projection _____

    c. displacement _____

    d. daydreaming _____

    e. escape into illness _____

    f. repression _____

    g. withdrawal _____

4. Explain how occasional use of a defense mechanism can contribute to good adjustment.

   _____
   _____

5. Compare malingering and escape into illness.

   _____
   _____

6. Compare substance dependency and the use of defense mechanisms.

   _____
   _____

7. Develop three guidelines for modifying one's use of defense mechanisms as a means of improving adjustment.

   _____
   _____
   _____

8. Define each of the following terms in your own words:
   a. alcoholism _____
   b. addiction_____
   c. tolerance_____
   d. drug dependency _____
   e. codependency _____

## ASSIGNMENTS

1. Explain the difference between daydreaming as used by Lou, Ed, and Sue in the example earlier in the chapter.

2. Use the following as a checklist to set objectives for modifying your use of defense mechanisms. The first item is explained to show you how to think through an item before applying it to yourself.

   a. I tend to use rationalization when I must choose between duty and pleasure.

   *Explanation:* This is true of me to a large extent. When I want to watch television, I convince myself that I have studied enough and understand the material. The next day, I wish I had studied. Therefore, I shall check this item as an example of a habit I need to modify.

*Or:* This is not particularly true of me. I like to do my work and fulfill my responsibilities. Then I can enjoy my free time without worrying about what I should be doing. I will not check this item.

    b. I think of myself as a very capable person, yet I become anxious when a test is scheduled (or substitute another type of threatening situation). If I do not do well, I tend to rationalize. I do not like to admit that I did not do something well.

    c. I do not like to be criticized, even when I know the criticism is true.

    d. I am easily hurt by other people's remarks. It seems to me that people are too ready to be critical or to say unkind things.

    e. I have a lot of trouble with teachers (parents, supervisors, etc.) because of things other people did. I also have a lot of bad luck.

    f. Other people often make me angry (or unhappy), but I usually do not let them know it. I wait until I am home and then "let off steam."

    g. Sometimes my daydreams are more pleasant than what is going on around me. Then I have trouble keeping my mind on my work.

    h. It seems as though my colds always come when we have a big test scheduled (substitute some other type of threat if it is more applicable to you).

    i. I don't believe in getting upset. When the going gets rough, I leave.

    j. Some people irritate me, so I don't talk to them unless I have to.

3. Select one item you checked in activity 2 (or substitute a specific defense mechanism that you tend to use). State how you will modify your use of this defense mechanism.

4. Select a defense mechanism you have used in the past week.

    a. Explain the defense mechanism in your own words.

    b. Describe the situation in which you used this defense mechanism.

    c. Explain why that situation elicited defensive behavior.

    d. Consider the situation from your own viewpoint and, as best you can, from the viewpoint of other people who were present.

    e. List two or more ways you could have dealt with the situation without using a defense mechanism.

5. Participate in a class discussion on the topic: "Watching television serves as an escape for many people."

6. Your Uncle Bob was an alcoholic. The family often expressed sympathy for "poor Mary Lou," who put up with his drinking for many years. When Uncle Bob died unexpectedly, the family believed Mary Lou could now enjoy life, free of the problems Uncle Bob had created. Several months later the family was amazed to learn that Mary Lou had married Joe, who was known to be an alcoholic. Explain Mary Lou's behavior.

7. You work at Community Hospital. A family friend, Joe (who married your Aunt Mary Lou in activity 7), often seeks your company at family gatherings. Today he says to you, "I really want to stop drinking. I've tried several times, but sooner or later I fall off the

wagon. Can you help me?" Describe three things that must happen in order for Uncle Joe to become a recovering alcoholic.

8. What will be your first step in helping Uncle Joe?

9. What role could you play over the next year as Uncle Joe works on controlling his drinking? List specific actions you could take and indicate whom you could involve.

10. List five dangers of alcohol abuse.

11. Consult your local telephone directory and obtain phone numbers for each of the following:

    Alcoholics Anonymous

    Alcohol abuse 24-hour helpline

    Drug abuse 24-hour helpline

    Your local community agency for alcohol and drug abuse

> **Note:** Some toll-free (800) numbers provide information, some provide a local phone number for obtaining assistance, and some are private organizations seeking clients. Optional activity: Call each toll-free number and determine which ones offer guidance for locating community services and which ones are for-profit agencies. If they ask about your health insurance, they are a for-profit agency.

12. Using the Internet, locate and visit Web sites for the agencies listed in assignment 11 above. Using any search engine, locate other Web sites related to substance abuse.

13. Participate in a class discussion on one or more of the following topics:

    Why health care providers should be free of addictions

    Effective ways to stop smoking (or give up coffee, alcohol, drugs)

    Indications that an adolescent is using drugs

    Indications that a coworker is using drugs (illegal)

    Examples of the destructive effects of alcohol

    Examples of the destructive effects of prescription drug abuse

    Examples of the destructive effects of drug abuse (illegal)

# UNIT 13

# Inner Conflict

## OBJECTIVES

Upon completion of this unit, you should be able to:

- Define inner conflict and explain how it differs from interpersonal conflict.
- List five influences on inner conflict.
- List and explain three types of inner conflict.
- State one requirement for dealing with inner conflict.
- List seven steps for resolving inner conflict.

## KEY TERMS

| | | |
|---|---|---|
| Alternative | Incompatible | Prognosis |
| Analgesic | Manipulative | Prosthesis |
| Debilitating | Narcotic | Vacillate |
| Digital | Proficient | |

You have learned that habitual use of defense mechanisms can cause poor adjustment. Another common cause of poor adjustment is inner conflict.

## THE MEANING OF INNER CONFLICT

Perhaps you are accustomed to thinking of conflict as a fight or argument. Such conflicts involve two or more people and are *interpersonal* conflicts. This unit is concerned with inner conflict—that which exists *within one person*. Other people may contribute to a person's inner conflict and others may be affected by the behavior resulting from inner conflict, but it is the individual with the conflict who is most affected.

Inner conflict creates inner discomfort. It is difficult to understand. It may arouse strong emotions. Until the conflict has been resolved, the individual may experience a variety of emotions, especially negative ones. Inner conflict, then, may cause much unhappiness unless one learns to recognize it, use a rational approach to identifying the needs that are in conflict, and then use good judgment in resolving the conflict.

Inner conflict exists when an individual has two **incompatible** needs or goals, or when the individual must choose between two or more **alternative** means for meeting a need or achieving a goal (Figure 13-1). The conflict arises because of the incompatibility of these needs,

**FIGURE 13-1** Inner conflict exists when one must choose between alternative means for meeting a need. *Delmar/Cengage Learning*

goals, or means, but other behavior influences may also be involved. One's value system, standards of behavior, beliefs, interests, personality traits, character traits, and self-concept may all contribute to inner conflict.

The person who has an inner conflict is usually aware of the need to choose between two goals or two courses of action. However, the individual may be unaware of the basic needs, values, interests, beliefs, and other factors that contribute to the conflict.

## Conflict between Needs

Adolescents are often faced with a conflict between the need for acceptance by the peer group and the need for maintaining their beliefs about "right" and "wrong" behavior. Suppose someone in Bill's crowd proposes a risky adventure involving behavior Bill believes to be wrong. Bill must choose between participating in the adventure or refusing to participate. His need to belong, feel accepted, and be approved by members of his peer group is in conflict with his need for maintaining his standard of behavior, beliefs, and self-concept—"I am a person who does not do things that are wrong." Going along with the adventure requires lowering his standards of behavior, which is a threat to his beliefs, values, and self-concept. Opposing the proposed adventure involves risking his status with the group, which is a threat to his need to belong. Through no fault of his own, Bill is in a situation that requires a decision between two alternative actions, both of which threaten something he values.

## Conflict between Means

Conflict also exists when a goal can be reached in two or more ways. Mrs. P. has a chronic condition that causes her much discomfort. She usually relies on **analgesic** drugs, but more and more often she must have a **narcotic** to obtain full relief from pain. Her physician now warns her that continued use of drugs will have undesirable effects. He recommends surgery to correct her problem.

Mrs. P.'s goal of restored health requires choosing between habitual use of drugs and surgery. To be free of pain, she must use one means or the other. When Mrs. P. was a child, her oldest brother died during an operation. Since then, she has heard numerous stories about unsatisfactory surgical results, each one adding to her fear of surgery. Now, the thought of going to the operating room terrifies her, yet she desperately wants to be free of pain. To Mrs. P., with her deep-seated fear of the operating room, this conflict between two remedies for her health problem may be far more distressing than the physical discomfort associated with surgery.

## TYPES OF INNER CONFLICT

Regardless of whether a conflict is between needs, goals, or the means for achieving them, the individual must choose between alternatives. These alternatives may be positive (desirable) or negative (undesirable). Even in a choice between two positives, unhappiness may result from giving up one alternative. The degree of difficulty in making a decision is often influenced by whether the alternatives are both positive, both negative, or positive accompanied by a negative outcome.

### Approach-Approach Conflict—Two Desirable Goals

Approach-approach conflict involves two needs or goals that are incompatible. Al is working in the local hospital as a nursing assistant. He enjoys his work and is especially good with elderly patients. His supervisor calls him into the office and states that he has been recommended to the director of the practical nursing program. The supervisor points out the advantages of being a licensed nurse and indicates belief in Al's potential for succeeding in the program. Al is proud that the supervisor has so much faith in him. He is suddenly fired with ambition to improve himself through educational preparation for a career.

When Al tells his girlfriend about his exciting opportunity, she says, "But how can we get married if you are not going to have any income for a year?" Al is eager to get married and has been saving for the costs of setting up a home. Any delay in these plans will be just as disappointing to him as to his girlfriend.

Al has two goals, each of which he would like to reach as soon as possible. He is eager to get married, but he is also aware of the advantages of educational preparation for his job. He cannot get married immediately and at the same time enroll in the practical nursing course.

Al has a conflict between two strong but incompatible needs—they cannot be met at the same time.

## Approach-Avoidance Conflict—Desirable Goal with a Negative Effect

Ryan is enrolled in a dental laboratory technology course. He is having difficulty developing some of the **manipulative** skills necessary for constructing dental **prostheses.** His teacher discusses the problem with him, emphasizing that he must spend more time on laboratory practice to develop the necessary **digital** skills. The only time Ryan has for this extra practice is the period the basketball team practices. Ryan is top scorer for the team.

Ryan wants to pass his lab course, but to do so he has to miss basketball practice. To achieve his goal of becoming **proficient** as a dental laboratory technician, Ryan has to accept the negative aspects of giving up his prized position on the team: feeling disloyal to the team and relinquishing an activity that gives him much satisfaction. Regardless of which choice he makes, Ryan will lose something that he values.

Approach-avoidance conflict is a special type of conflict involving a desirable goal with undesirable effects. The individual **vacillates** between trying to reach a certain goal and abandoning the goal. The decision to abandon a goal usually occurs as the individual approaches achievement of the goal or when the time for a desired event approaches.

Emily is a dental assistant who is engaged to Jake. Emily gets along well with her parents. She especially likes her room, which she decorated and furnished during her first year as a "career woman." When she comes home from her job, mother has dinner ready. Emily's only home responsibility is cleaning her own room. She is able to save a large portion of her paycheck. Getting married and moving into an apartment requires that Emily give up these benefits of living with her parents. On the other hand, she loves her fiancé, wants her own home, and wants to have a family.

Emily has set the wedding date several times. Repeatedly, when ordering the wedding announcements could not be delayed any longer, she has broken the engagement. Jake is persistent and has accepted each delay with good humor. But each time the date approaches for achieving her goal (getting married, having her own home, starting a family), Emily develops intense feelings (anxiety? panic?) that she relieves by breaking off the engagement. Thus, she avoids achieving the goal that would involve giving up the advantages of living with her parents.

## Avoidance-Avoidance Conflict—Two Negative Alternatives

Avoidance-avoidance conflict exists when an individual must choose between two alternatives, both of which will have a negative outcome. Carolyn is a student in a medical assistant program. Last week her best friend in the class broke an expensive piece of equipment and returned it to its storage case without reporting the breakage. Carolyn was present at the time, and her friend insisted that Carolyn promise not to tell anyone. Today, Carolyn learns that another student in the class has been blamed for the broken equipment and told to pay for it.

Carolyn has strong feelings about loyalty to friends. She also has strong feelings about keeping promises, honesty, truthfulness, and fair play. Carolyn knows who actually broke the equipment, but the guilty person refuses to report herself. Carolyn can break her promise to this friend and report the incident, or she can keep silent and permit an innocent person to take the blame. Carolyn's values are involved, yet either course of action will violate personal traits on which she places a high value. Carolyn's self-concept is also involved: she does not want to be a person who breaks promises, nor does she want to be a person who permits an injustice when she could prevent it. She has to choose between loyalty to her friend and her sense of fairness. She has to choose between telling the truth and breaking a promise. To maintain her self-concept, Carolyn needs to uphold these personal traits she values. Therefore, either alternative involves a threat to her self-concept. Regardless of which alternative she chooses, there will be negative effects.

How Carolyn handles this situation will probably be determined by her values. She must place a higher value on one set of traits than the other in order to select an alternative. If she reports the breakage, then honesty and fair play assume a higher place in her value system than loyalty to friends and keeping promises.

Carolyn's behavior patterns will affect how she works through this conflict. She may put off a decision and, by her inaction, allow the wrong person to be blamed. She may project blame by saying to herself that it is her friend's responsibility to tell the truth. She may rationalize by telling herself it is not really her business. Which choice she makes and how she justifies that choice to herself will result from many years of forming behavior patterns to deal with unpleasant situations.

## HOW TO DEAL WITH INNER CONFLICT

Inner conflict may be handled effectively *only by making a decision between alternatives* (Figure 13-2). Obviously, the choice will be better if the individual recognizes that a conflict exists and identifies the competing needs or goals. Insofar as possible, the feelings and values related to the conflict should also be examined.

**FIGURE 13-2** Inner conflict can only be resolved by making a choice. *Delmar/Cengage Learning*

### Exploring Emotional Aspects

Suppose Sarah has cancelled her plans for marriage several times because her mother has a health crisis each time Sarah sets a wedding date. Strong emotional factors are involved: Sarah's love for her fiancé, her love for her mother, her fiancé's feelings about the delayed wedding, negative feelings toward her mother for being an obstacle, guilty feelings about having negative feelings toward her mother, feelings of loyalty, sense of duty to her parent, resentment and indignation at being deprived of living her own life, and many other feelings. Sarah, in order to use a rational approach to resolve this situation, needs to explore these feelings honestly to avoid letting any one emotion or value dominate her decision.

### Thinking through a Conflict Situation

The following steps provide a rational approach to resolving a conflict:

1. Recognize that there is a conflict.
2. Identify the two incompatible needs (or goals).
3. Examine the situation in terms of interests, values, immediate needs, long-term needs, and other relevant factors.
4. Decide how each need could be met (or each goal achieved).
5. Think through the probable effects of each possible action: what will be gained, what will be lost, and whether or not the action would be in accord with your beliefs, value system, interests, goals, and needs.
6. After thorough consideration of the probable effects of each possible choice, make a decision.
7. *Fully accept your decision.* One alternative has been selected; the other has been discarded. Do not flounder in doubt about whether the right choice was made. Set out to prove that you made a good decision. Do not develop feelings of guilt or failure about the alternative that was discarded. Remember: *A choice had to be made.*

### Identifying Opportunity Cost

In business a concept known as "opportunity cost" may be used to assist in making decisions. This concept, when applied to inner conflict, can help the individual focus on presumed facts; by so doing, vague fears about alternative actions can be translated into information—the basis for a *rational*, rather than an *emotional*, decision. Opportunity cost refers to what one must give up (an opportunity) when choosing one course of action over another.

In resolving inner conflict, opportunity cost consists of what will be given up if action 1 is pursued, and what will be given up if action 2 is pursued. Opportunity cost may be the basis for anxiety about choosing either action. The cost of a specific decision, then, includes not only the obvious consequences of that decision, but also the opportunity cost involved in not following the other course of action.

Anna is working the night shift at Community Hospital; she needs to leave home by 10:15 to be on time for report. It is her birthday, but her husband still is not home at 9:00. She and her husband have only one car, and he knows she is scheduled to work tonight. She puts on her uniform so she will not have to dress after he does arrive. As she worries about why he is not home yet, she hears the car pull into the driveway. Her husband enters, laughing, accompanied by Donna (his coworker), Donna's husband, and a couple she does not know. They are carrying refreshments and exclaiming, "Happy birthday!" It is now 9:45.

Anna gets glasses and ice for everyone, then explains that she must leave for work. She is greeted by a chorus of, "Oh, no! It's your birthday. We came to party." When Anna explains that she cannot stay and party, that she is needed at the hospital, her guests suggest, "Just call in sick. They'll never know you are having a birthday party." Leaving aside the matter of her husband's behavior, let us look at Anna's inner conflict. Should she stay home and enjoy these guests who want to give her a birthday party? Or should she go to work?

The *reward* of choosing to call in sick and stay home would be that Anna has a birthday party, enjoys socializing with friends, and becomes acquainted with the new couple. The *cost* of staying home would be that Anna uses a sick day she might need later. The *opportunity cost* of this choice could be a sense of guilt for lying to the supervisor and leaving her coworkers short-handed. Anna is conscientious; her self-esteem would be affected negatively if she fails in her duty. Possibly, her supervisor would learn that she is not sick but stayed home to party.

The *reward* for choosing to go on duty as scheduled would be that Anna retains her self-respect, her self-esteem is not threatened; she does not harbor guilt about her behavior; she does not worry about the supervisor finding out that she lied about being sick; she does not feel guilty about her coworkers having to do double duty; and she does not risk hearing later that a patient did not receive some needed attention during the night. Also, Anna still has that sick day in reserve in case she needs it. The *cost* of not staying home to party was missing her own birthday party and the annoyance of her husband and the guests about her leaving. The *opportunity cost* was not having a chance to become acquainted with the new couple.

Note that identifying the rewards, costs, and opportunity costs of each alternative paves the way for a *rational,* rather than *emotional,* decision. So adding the concept of opportunity cost to your problem-solving method can facilitate the resolution of an inner conflict.

## INNER CONFLICT AND ADJUSTMENT

The approach just described illustrates the familiar saying, "You can't have your cake and eat it too." Even minor conflicts cause a certain amount of inner discomfort until they are resolved. If you put off doing an assignment in favor of more pleasant activities, you eventually reach the point of having to resolve the conflict. You must either decide to do the assignment instead of some preferred activity, or decide not to do the assignment and accept the consequences. You are probably a little uncomfortable as long as you continue to put off the decision.

Many people react to conflict with indecision, either procrastinating as long as possible or making one choice and then changing to another (Figure 13-3). Only a firm decision truly resolves a conflict. Sometimes the decision is necessarily accompanied by an unfavorable effect, either on oneself or on others. *The ideal result in handling conflict is to gain the desired goal with the least possible undesirable effect.*

Inner conflict contributes to poor adjustment in a number of ways. Some people are not able to recognize a conflict. They become upset over failure to gain some goal that actually is incompatible with other goals they are pursuing. Other people may be aware that a choice needs to be made but find it too difficult to face. Sarah, for example, knows she must choose between her mother and her fiancé: this is not an easy situation to resolve. She can choose to be the dutiful daughter and give up her plans for marriage, or she can choose to marry and

FIGURE 13-3 Many people react to an inner conflict with indecision. *Delmar/Cengage Learning*

hope her mother will accept this decision without permanent damage to their relationship. Sarah may continue to postpone her marriage repeatedly. Negative feelings may develop following either choice: guilt if she leaves her ailing mother or bitterness and resentment if she abandons plans for marriage.

## INNER CONFLICT AND THE HEALTH CARE PROVIDER

As a health care provider, you can make good use of your understanding of conflict and its effects on behavior and emotional states. Health care providers frequently have inner conflict. The responsibilities of being a health care provider are great. Health care providers often possess confidential information. People tend to put health care providers into conflict situations by asking about patients or seeking health advice. The necessity for providing many health services on a 24-hour basis requires that some health care providers have a schedule different from that of their families. Staffing problems give rise to occasional changes in time off, sometimes on short notice. Urgent situations require working overtime, being "on call," or returning to work unexpectedly after putting in a full day's work.

The health care provider who is dedicated to serving others and has a strong sense of duty is likely to experience conflict between loyalty to the job and loyalty to the family. There may be occasions when there is a conflict between responsibilities and "rights" as a person.

Medical ethics and the policies of your place of employment can help you with some of these conflicts. For example, when a close friend asks about a patient, your *ethical responsibility* to hold in confidence what you learn about patients in the course of your job helps you resolve the conflict between responsibility and desire to have your friend's approval. At times, you may have to justify your *sense of duty* when job requirements interfere with plans involving family or friends. Thinking about such possible conflicts in advance can help you resolve them if they actually occur.

## INNER CONFLICT AND THE PATIENT

Many patients have inner conflict related to their illness. Mr. B. has orders for strict bedrest, yet he feels capable of returning to work. He has a conflict between his need for self-interest (perhaps self-preservation) and his need to fulfill his job responsibilities. Ms. J., who is having diagnostic studies, may have a conflict between the need for relief from distressing symptoms and the fear of learning something unfavorable as a result of the studies.

Family members, too, have inner conflict when decisions must be made. It is difficult to agree to painful procedures on someone you love, yet refusing permission for the procedure may contribute to continued illness or the loved one's death. The decision on whether or not to consent to surgery involves many emotions, including the possibility of guilty feelings if the outcome is unfavorable. An emotionally wrenching conflict for family members is a decision to discontinue life support. Even if the patient's status fits the conditions specified in an advance directive, an inner conflict exists for each person involved in the decision. Some physicians try to protect families from decisions that may lead to guilty feelings. However, it is desirable that the family be involved in decisions about painful or **debilitating** treatments and the use of life-support systems for persons whose illness involves a hopeless **prognosis.**

## USING KNOWLEDGE ABOUT INNER CONFLICT

As a health care provider, be aware that some of the distress you see in patients and their families is due to inner conflict. With such understanding, you are better able to accept behavior that appears unreasonable and accept emotional reactions that seem out of proportion to the seriousness of the illness. Be aware, too, that sometimes the physician has given the family or patient information that you do not have, such as an unfavorable prognosis.

Applying knowledge about inner conflict to your personal life can help you resolve conflict situations rationally to achieve the best possible outcome for you and your family. Applying your knowledge of inner conflict to relations with patients can help you be more understanding and more accepting of your patients and their families.

## REFERENCES AND SUGGESTED READINGS

Bouckenooghe, Dave, et al. (2005, July). The prediction of stress by values and value conflict. *The Journal of Psychology, 139*(4), 369–383.

DiMarsico, Bruce. (2006). *Unlock your happiness with five simple questions.* Walnut Grove, CA: Dragonfly Press.

Evans, Mandy. (2005). *Emotional options: A handbook for happiness.* Garden City, NY: Morgan James Publishing.

Gureckis, Todd, & Love, Bradley. (2009). Short-term gains, long-term pains: How cues about state aid learning in dynamic environments. *Cognition, 113*(3), 293–314.

## REVIEW AND SELF-CHECK

1. Define inner conflict and explain how it differs from interpersonal conflict.

2. List five factors that influence inner conflict.

3. Describe the three types of inner conflict and explain the basic problem that characterizes each type.

4. State one requirement for dealing with inner conflict.

5. List seven steps a person could use to resolve an inner conflict.

## ASSIGNMENTS

1. Refer to the previously described conflicts experienced by Al, Ryan, Carolyn, or Sarah. Select one example and complete the following chart:

a. What *values* does the individual probably have that should be considered in resolving the conflict? What strong *needs* does the individual probably have that should be considered in resolving the conflict? What *beliefs* does this individual seem to have? What are the two conflicting needs (or goals or means)? Indicate which example you are analyzing: Al ___ Ryan ___ Carolyn ___ Sarah ___

| VALUES |
|---|
| NEEDS |
| BELIEFS |
| THE CONFLICTING NEEDS (GOALS, MEANS OF ACHIEVING A GOAL):<br>1.<br><br>2. |

b. List two or more alternative actions that might resolve the conflict. Then anticipate the possible effects of each.

| ACTIONS | EFFECTS | |
| --- | --- | --- |
| | DESIRABLE | UNDESIRABLE |
| | | |

2. Consider one conflict you have had during the past month.
    a. Analyze this conflict in terms of the following:
        - Your basic needs
        - Goals that were incompatible
        - Emotions you were experiencing

- Values involved
- Beliefs involved

b. Describe how you handled the conflict.

c. Describe the effects of your handling of this conflict.

d. State two possible alternatives for resolving the conflict.

e. In the light of your knowledge about inner conflict, how do you *now* think you should have handled this particular conflict? Justify your answer in terms of basic needs, value system, emotional effects, and short-term or long-term goals.

3. Refer to Carolyn's conflict situation and put yourself in Carolyn's place. You decide to talk to your coworker about the broken equipment and your own feelings, including regret that you agreed to the promise your friend wanted from you. Describe the conditions under which you will initiate this conversation—certainly not during lunch! Next, write out what you will say:

- Your opening statement
- Key points you want to make
- How you will respond if the coworker insists you should keep your promise not to report her
- Statements you could make to encourage the coworker to take responsibility for the broken equipment

**Note:** Your instructor may choose to schedule this situation for role-play during class time.

4. Identify the opportunity cost involved in each of the following situations:

    a. Al decides to enter the practical nursing education program.

    b. Ryan chooses to spend extra time in the lab.

    c. Emily chooses to marry and move into an apartment.

    d. Carolyn chooses to report the coworker.

    e. Sarah's sense of duty to her mother controls her decision, and she cancels her wedding plans.

5. You are on night duty; one of your patients, Mr. R., has an advance directive and a do not resuscitate (DNR) order on his chart. Suddenly his wife rushes out of the room saying, "My husband has stopped breathing!" You automatically reach for the phone to call a Code. Then you remember the DNR; should you make the call?

# UNIT 14

# Frustration

## OBJECTIVES

Upon completion of this unit, you should be able to:

- Name four sources of frustration.
- List four environmental factors that could be sources of frustration.
- List five factors that could influence a person to obstruct another's goal-seeking efforts.
- Explain prejudice as a source of frustration for members of certain groups.
- Describe emotional reactions to frustration.
- Describe a general approach to dealing with frustration.
- List five guidelines for preventing unnecessary frustration in one's life.
- Use a systematic approach to study a situation in which frustration is occurring and make a rational decision about how to deal with it.

## KEY TERMS

| Aspirations | Capabilities | Perfectionism |
| Attitude | Frustration | Subtle |

You are now aware that everyone experiences threats to adjustment at intervals and reacts to such threats according to learned patterns of behavior. A type of threat that tends to arouse negative emotions and evoke aggressive or defensive behavior is **frustration.** The effects of frustration on the individual and the tendency of the resulting behavior to be misunderstood by others can seriously interfere with interpersonal relations and adjustment.

Frustration exists when progress toward a desired goal is blocked. Frustration is a threat to one's feelings of adequacy and can be an obstacle to reaching a goal. It is a common experience for all of us. How we react to frustration determines to a large extent whether or not we reach the desired goal.

## DEGREES OF FRUSTRATION

Frustration may evoke irritation or a major emotional reaction. Minor frustrations occur almost daily. The car won't start when we are in a hurry; a pencil point breaks just as we begin a test; we miss the bus; someone keeps us waiting; a button pops off when we do not have time to sew it back on. Such experiences arouse feelings that range from annoyance to intense anger—these feelings are due to frustration.

Major frustrations involve larger aspects of living. A person whose job is not satisfying—who has many job-related problems or has been passed by repeatedly for promotion—has frustrations in the workplace. A mother who wants a career but feels "trapped" by home responsibilities experiences frustration involving almost her total life situation.

Minor frustrations cause annoyance for a relatively short period of time, though a frustration encountered in the morning often sets the pattern of the day. On such days we are likely to comment, "I should have stayed in bed today." Major frustrations, however, may affect the individual's total personality—behavior patterns, values, beliefs, moods, attitudes, and general outlook on life. Major frustrations of long duration are incompatible with good adjustment.

## CUMULATIVE EFFECTS OF FRUSTRATION

Minor frustrations are significant if they lead to a buildup of negative feelings, with sudden release over a seemingly minor incident. A series of frustrations during the day may be the underlying cause of Dad's explosion when Johnny asks for five dollars. Or Dad may show his annoyance on Friday after giving Johnny one dollar every morning. Unknown to Johnny, his requests for money are frustrating Dad's effort to make his money hold out until payday. Knowing that Johnny has to have lunch money does not help Dad with his own frustration.

People differ in their tolerance for frustration. Some react emotionally whenever their goals are blocked, and others show the effects of frustration only when it is major. Most people react to minor or moderate frustration with some type of action to resolve the problem; but when frustration is overwhelming, performance deteriorates.

Occasionally the news media report an incident of bizarre or violent behavior. A tobacco farmer who believed his livelihood was being taken away from him by government intervention in the tobacco industry drove his tractor to Washington, DC, and threatened to set off explosives. Workers who went to their workplace and shot colleagues, supervisors, or innocent bystanders have given rise to new terminology; "going postal" refers to this type of behavior because it has occurred several times in the postal system. Although each case of such behavior would require detailed study for a full understanding of the individual's behavior, it is likely that cumulative frustration and a sense of powerlessness for dealing with the sources of frustration were major factors.

## SOURCES OF FRUSTRATION

Blocking of progress toward a goal can arise from many sources: personal characteristics, the environment, other people, illness, or prejudice.

### Self

Frustration involves both needs and goals. Each of us is influenced by many different factors in setting our goals. Whether or not these goals are in accord with our own **capabilities** and the opportunities available to us has a bearing on the amount of frustration likely to occur.

As high school seniors, Jack and Paul shared an interest in the health field. Both boys discussed their futures with the guidance counselor, taking into consideration many types of information, including high school record, achievement and aptitude test scores, vocational interest surveys, personal interests, family finances, and other factors.

Paul's record indicated that he could probably be successful in college. Family finances were strained, and Paul did not like to think of four or more years of school. He liked the idea of becoming a laboratory assistant, so he enrolled in the nearby technical institute. After completing his course with honors, Paul accepted a position in the local hospital. Soon he asked the laboratory supervisor to teach him some of the complex procedures, but he was told that only the registered medical technologists were allowed to do these tests. Paul felt resentful and became increasingly hostile toward his coworkers. He felt he was quite capable of doing more than he was allowed to do. Paul had settled for objectives too low for his potential. As a result, he was frustrated in his job because he was not allowed to function like the more highly trained technologists. Yet, because of the expense and long-term preparation required to become a medical technologist, Paul did not set his goal in accordance with his abilities.

On the other hand, Jack applied to a college, even though he had difficulty with high school subjects. The school counselor had encouraged Jack to plan vocational goals rather than academic ones. Jack's mother always said she wanted her son to be a doctor, so Jack had grown up with the idea of attending medical school. He refused to recognize evidence that he probably would not be able to succeed in college courses. After failing three out of four courses at the university, Jack came home confused and upset about his failure. He had set his objectives too high, in spite of guidance that could have helped him plan more realistically.

Frustration, then, can result either from trying to reach what is unreachable or from achieving unchallenging goals. A career goal should be carefully selected on the basis of all information available about the individual and occupations in which the person is interested. Career goals are important to achievement, development of one's potential, job satisfaction, and, ultimately, to adjustment and happiness.

Goals are also involved in short-term aspects of living. To some youngsters, failure to make the Little League team is a shattering experience. Athletic ability is, to a great extent, based on physical characteristics and motor skills. If one's goal is to make the football team in spite of small physical build and limited stamina, then frustration is sure to occur. If one enjoys singing, the short-term goal of being accepted into the school chorus is probably realistic. On the other hand, the goal of becoming an opera star is realistic only for those few who have rare talent, resources to develop the talent, and the determination and perseverance to strive many years for that goal.

Goals are more realistic when related to what we enjoy and learn readily. Satisfaction is greater if goals continue to offer challenge. In measuring goal progress, it is better to compare yourself today with yourself in the past, rather than with other people. Thus, progress can be noted and a sense of achievement experienced. Aspiring to be "the best" in anything is more likely to lead to frustration than aspiring to "continue to improve."

## The Environment

Environment—either physical or social—can be a source of frustration because of a lack of opportunities or the presence of obstructions. The environment is less subject to control than one's goals and **aspirations.** Rain on the day of a picnic or lack of snow for skiing are frustrations one must learn to accept. The opportunities an environment offers should be considered in making long-range plans. If one elects to follow a career for which there is no locally available opportunity, frustration will occur unless resources can be made available or a move to another community can be arranged.

Sometimes the customs and practices of a community are the source of frustration. The health care provider who wants to improve health habits in a community must give careful consideration to the established beliefs, values, and customs of that community. Cultural aspects of the social environment may block efforts to change established practices.

## Other People

Many obstacles can be overcome through persistence, problem-solving techniques, or an approach that removes the obstacle or allows one to get around it. When the obstacle is a person, however, overcoming the obstacle is likely to be difficult.

Paul's laboratory supervisor was an obstacle to his learning advanced techniques, even though the supervisor was basing the decision on hospital policy, role differentiation, and Paul's lack of educational foundation for the judgments required by advanced procedures. For Sara, whose mother did not want her daughter to leave her, the mother was an obstacle to marriage. Suppose Jack had been refused admission to college. Then the admissions committee would constitute an obstacle to his attending college. If a man firmly believes "a woman's place is in the home," then his belief is an obstacle to his wife's having a career.

Many people who represent obstacles, and thereby contribute to someone's frustration, do so as a job responsibility. This is especially true of school admissions committees, personnel directors, teachers, supervisors, or anyone whose evaluation or judgment determines whether or not a person will have a specific opportunity.

In other cases, people are obstacles because of their beliefs, prejudices, attitudes, superior ability, dependency, and many other factors (Figure 14-1). When achieving a goal requires changing an **attitude** or belief of the person who is an obstacle, then the frustration is not likely to be overcome easily; people do not readily change their values and beliefs.

**FIGURE 14-1** This patient is frustrated; she feels powerless and lacks control over her life. *Delmar/Cengage Learning*

In competition, the abilities of other people determine whether or not an individual makes the team, wins a gold medal, or gets a promotion. When the obstacle is a competitor's superior ability, then personal effort to surpass such ability is necessary to reach the goal.

## Illness

Illness may cause either minor or major frustration, depending upon the duration of illness and the patient's life situation. A minor illness that lasts a few days may simply be an inconvenience, or possibly a welcome relief from the daily routine—a chance to stay home and take it easy. But even a minor illness can create intense frustration if it interferes with some important event.

If the illness is serious or life-threatening, the patient experiences numerous frustrations. There may be a feeling of losing control of one's life. Suddenly someone else (i.e., a doctor) is telling the patient what he or she must do. Often these mandates include major life changes: stop smoking, change jobs to minimize stress (or physical exertion or exposure to chemicals), stop playing tennis, eat fresh vegetables, do not eat red meat, stop drinking alcoholic beverages, stop drinking sodas, exercise at least 20 minutes every day, stay in bed a minimum of 10 hours a day, have at least two rest periods, stay out of the sun between 11 a.m. and 3 p.m., agree to a course of chemotherapy (or radiation), go to a medical center for special tests or treatment. Whatever the mandate includes, it will impact the patient's lifestyle. The significance of each thing that must be given up determines the degree of frustration. The specific treatment may also be a source of frustration, especially if there are side effects.

Frustration is experienced as anger. When you, as a health care provider, realize that a patient's behavior seems to be an expression of anger, consider what impact the illness is having on the patient's life. Show interest in the patient's life situation with an expression of caring and concern, such as, "I suppose this illness is really changing your life." If the patient is willing to talk about the effects, it will help to diffuse the anger. As you carry out your responsibilities for health care, be aware that the recipient of your services is a person who may be angry and/or sad about the losses involved as his or her life is disrupted by illness.

## Prejudice

Federal legislation has attempted to remove prejudice as an obstacle to educational and job opportunities. Unfortunately, the passage of a law does not change deeply rooted beliefs or the behavior patterns of a lifetime. Yet this legislation has increased awareness of the extent to which prejudice creates obstacles for women, minority groups, youth, elderly, handicapped, and those with low income. Such prejudices of employers and school officials continue to create obstacles for many people, but in more **subtle** ways than in the past. At this time, a person who has been discriminated against because of one of the conditions covered by equal rights legislation may petition the courts to remove the obstacle. Some professional groups and consumer advocate organizations provide legal assistance to people whose rights to equal opportunity have been violated.

Members of minority groups are familiar with the obstacle represented by prejudice. Perhaps with increasing opportunities for various groups to work and learn together, there will be greater readiness to accept each person as an individual and judge each on the basis of personal attributes, rather than the group (age, religion, nationality, race, sex) affiliation. This ideal can serve as a guide for us as we strive to better ourselves and our environment.

**FIGURE 14-2** Each person reacts to frustration in his or her own way. *Delmar/Cengage Learning*

## EFFECTS OF FRUSTRATION

Each of us reacts to frustration according to patterns we have learned throughout life. These reactions, therefore, vary from one person to another, but they usually involve either hostile behavior or withdrawal (Figure 14-2). Frustration arouses negative emotions: fear, anger, disappointment, anxiety, resentment, or a combination of these. Both behavior and emotional reactions to frustration are influenced by the importance attached to the goal as well as the individual's adjustment. A person who is insecure and inclined to perceive frustration as a threat is likely to feel a mixture of fear and anger. A person who is self-confident is likely to feel some degree of anger, with little fear. The person who is easily discouraged is likely to give up when there is an obstacle to success. Quitting, remember, is a form of withdrawal. The person who is stimulated to try harder in the face of difficulty is likely to react to an obstacle by increased effort or a change in strategy. Why should there be such extreme differences in reactions to frustration? The answer lies in early learnings that influence the formation of behavior patterns.

## FRUSTRATION AND BEHAVIOR PATTERNS

Everyone who has cared for a baby or young child has seen examples of behavioral responses to frustration. The pattern of response is learned behavior, largely based on how others react to the child's frustration. Ideally, an adult would recognize that the child is frustrated and take action to assist the child or remove the source of frustration. Frequently, however, the child's need is not recognized and the frustration is viewed as misbehavior. Thus, patterns become established based on whether or not the child's behavior led to satisfaction of a need.

## Early Learnings

Experience with frustration may begin almost with birth. The infant who is fed according to a rigid schedule, rather than when hungry, experiences frustration as well as the physical discomfort of hunger. Each developmental task (such as turning over, sitting, and standing) requires many efforts before success is realized. Early efforts to perform such activities are frustrating, but the infant persists until bodily control has been mastered. Many infants show distress when these early efforts result in failure.

Toddlers know what they want long before they can state their needs verbally. When a toddler is unable to make wants known, the reaction may involve falling to the floor, kicking, or crying. The child's frustration is due to inability to communicate verbally—a lack of competence for the task attempted. The parent who does not understand frustration may punish the child. Then the child feels anger as the result of frustration and fear as the result of punishment. Such experiences affect the child's learnings about frustration and also about the "right" to express feelings. The parent, without realizing it, is teaching the child that it is "wrong" to express negative feelings. This can be the beginning of ineffective patterns for dealing with frustration. It can also be the beginning of a pattern that you have already learned is undesirable—suppression of emotions.

## Childhood

During childhood, many frustrations result from the child's lack of competence for tasks being attempted, parental restraints, and rules at school, in clubs, and other organizations. Adults should make a conscious effort to help children understand the necessity for placing limits on behavior, especially where there are groups of children. Yet, even when the need for rules is understood, the child is frustrated when these limits interfere with a desired activity. If the frustration is great, the child may feel resentment toward the source of the rule—a parent, teacher, club sponsor, or whatever authority figure seems to be preventing a desired activity. If punishment is also involved, fear and distrust of authority figures may develop. Rebelliousness or hostility toward authority, beginning with such childhood experiences, may later interfere in relationships with authority figures, such as supervisors in the job setting.

## Adulthood

Adults experience frustration in many forms and in every aspect of living. For the majority of people, probably the most common frustration is lack of enough money to have the material possessions desired. The major adaptations required by marriage, parenthood, and a job all involve numerous frustrations. Even after one has learned to function within the various roles of adulthood, frustrations periodically occur in each role.

As a health care provider, you are likely to have patients who are experiencing frustration. Illness and injury interfere with one's life. Loss of income due to inability to work and difficulty in performing self-care tasks, such as buttoning a shirt, are common problems for patients. Some patients, however, have long-term frustrations. The amputee who must learn to use a prosthesis, the stroke patient who has lost the use of one side of the body, and the laryngectomee who cannot speak are examples of patients who live with frustration. Be aware that some of your patients are experiencing intense frustration; try to anticipate their needs and be sensitive to the feelings they are experiencing.

## PERFECTIONISM AND FRUSTRATION

A personal trait that ensures an individual will experience frustration rather frequently is **perfectionism.** This trait probably has its roots in childhood, with the child seeking parental approval through performance of assigned tasks, school work, or athletics. Parental efforts to motivate a child to improve performance may result in the child learning that no performance is ever good enough. "Well, it's good that you passed the audition for choral. Now, I expect you to be a soloist by the end of the year." In this type of situation, one child may give up hope of winning unqualified approval; another may become determined to please, to turn in the perfect performance that is sure to win approval. Thus, the seeds of perfectionism may be planted.

The perfectionist may direct expectations of perfection inwardly or may expect perfection from others, especially a spouse, one's children, or coworkers. When perfectionism is focused inward, the individual views any less-than-perfect performance as unacceptable, even humiliating. "You may make mistakes, but not me!" This person may agonize over a mistake or social blunder that others hardly notice. Self-forgiveness is not even considered.

The person whose perfectionism is directed outward is repeatedly disappointed in the performance of other people. Being intolerant of mistakes or poor performance by others, the perfectionist tends to be critical and irritable, leading to poor relationships within the family and on the job. These high expectations of self and others inevitably result in frustration for a perfectionist.

## COPING WITH FRUSTRATION

You will experience frustration at intervals throughout life. This is a good time to evaluate your behavior patterns and decide whether you need to find new ways of dealing with frustration. By learning to handle frustration effectively, you can spare yourself much unhappiness and increase the proportion of satisfying experiences in your living (Figure 14-3).

**FIGURE 14-3** Patience may be necessary to break through a patient's fears and frustration. *Delmar/Cengage Learning*

There are numerous ways of dealing with frustration. The most desirable method of handling one particular frustration may be inappropriate for handling another. The general approach requires three steps:

1. Expect a certain amount of frustration in living and avoid overreacting emotionally or using defense mechanisms to avoid dealing with the problem.
2. Recognize frustration when it occurs.
3. When experiencing frustration, evaluate the situation and use the systematic procedure described next to select an approach for dealing with the obstacle.

## Overcoming the Obstacle

There is no guaranteed way to overcome any and all obstacles. Recognize that the negative feelings of the moment are due to frustration, and then use a rational approach to solve the problem at hand. If dealing with the frustrating situation can be delayed, it is helpful to put it out of your mind for a while; take time to "sleep on it." You may then be able to return to the problem with a fresh viewpoint and with less emotional influence on your thinking. The following questions can help in planning to overcome the obstacle:

- Exactly what goal am I trying to reach?
- What is preventing my reaching that goal? (Identify the obstacle.)
- How can I overcome or get around this obstacle? List *all* possible ways to deal with the obstacle.
- How is each possible solution likely to affect my achieving the goal?
- How is each possible solution likely to affect the way I feel about myself?
- How is each possible solution likely to affect other people?
- Is this *my* goal? Or did someone else set this goal for me?
- Which solution is most likely to help me reach my goal?
- Is the goal important enough to me to justify the expenditures (time, effort, energy, money) required for reaching the goal?
- What other benefits (such as new competencies, widened experience, and future opportunities) am I likely to gain from continued efforts to achieve the goal?
- Shall I persist in striving for this goal? Or shall I substitute another goal?
- Make a decision.
  a. If you decide to continue to strive for that goal, select a means for dealing with the obstacle and follow through with it.
  b. If your first effort does not remove the obstacle, try another approach.
  c. If you decide not to continue to strive for that goal, modify the goal or substitute a different goal.

## Preventing Frustration

It is also desirable to use a preventive approach to frustration. As illustrated by Jack and Paul, unrealistic goals can be the source of much frustration. If one sets unreachable goals, major frustration is inevitable. If one sets goals that offer too little challenge, especially if reaching that goal limits future goals, then frustration is inevitable. Goals should be realistic and yet sufficiently challenging to provide satisfaction when they are achieved.

Long-term goals, such as preparing for a career, usually include numerous short-term goals. There may be many frustrating experiences before the long-term goal is reached. If the short-term goals provide stepping-stones to be reached one by one, then frustration is offset by achievement of these intermediate goals.

The philosopher Socrates once advised his students, "Know thyself." This is good advice to apply in setting one's goals. Striving to know yourself can also help you recognize sources of frustration within yourself. Does your behavior arouse negative feelings in others, which they then express by opposing you? Is your reaction to defeat so satisfying to others that they enjoy winning in a competition with you? In numerous ways, we create obstacles for ourselves. With a change in our own behavior, frustrations may be fewer.

Lack of a particular skill for achieving a goal is an obvious obstacle. Sometimes it can be corrected by personal effort, but in some cases assistance from others is necessary. Undertaking a new activity is almost invariably frustrating during a period of orientation. Your courses that were frustrating at first become satisfying, rather than frustrating, as you acquire basic knowledge and develop skills. If you fail to acquire the necessary basic knowledge, then course assignments become more and more frustrating.

The most important principle in preventing unnecessary frustration is to direct your living so that you succeed in achieving some of your goals. It is also desirable to know your environment and the people in it. You can change some things in the environment through your own efforts; others are beyond your ability to change. You can "win over" some of the people who obstruct you; however, a certain proportion will oppose you. When it is appropriate to make changes, and it is within your ability to do so, then make those changes in order to reach your goal. If you cannot change the situation, do not "burn out your bearings" trying to change what cannot be changed.

As indicated earlier, many people create a certain amount of frustration for themselves, resulting from what they attempt to do. Frustration is involved in the very process of achieving. Some frustration is involved in dealing with the everyday problems of living. Frustration cannot be avoided, but we can learn not to create *unnecessary* frustration for ourselves. In that sense, we have some control over the amount of frustration we experience. Ultimately, however, our skill in coping with frustration influences the degree of satisfaction and happiness we experience in life.

A prayer used in Alcoholics Anonymous meetings expresses a positive approach that is applicable to preventing frustration for anyone who adopts it as an approach to daily life:

> God grant me the serenity to accept the things I cannot change, the courage to change the things I can, and the wisdom to know the difference.

## REFERENCES AND SUGGESTED READINGS

Blair, Gary. (2009). *Everything counts: 52 remarkable ways to inspire excellence and drive results.* Hoboken, NJ: John Wiley & Sons.

Mayne, Brian. (2006). *Goal mapping: How to turn your dreams into realities.* London, England: Watkins Publishing.

Williams, Redford, & Williams, Virginia. (2006). *In control: No more snapping at your family, sulking at work, steaming in the grocery line, seething in meetings, stuffing your frustration.* New York: Rodale.

## REVIEW AND SELF-CHECK

1. Name four sources of frustration.

2. List four environmental factors that can be a source of frustration.

3. List five reasons one person might obstruct another person's efforts to achieve a certain goal.

4. Explain how prejudice can be a source of frustration for members of certain groups.

5. Describe several possible emotional reactions to frustration.

6. Describe a general approach to dealing with frustration.

7. List five guidelines for preventing, or at least minimizing, frustrating experiences in one's life.

8. List steps for systematically studying a frustrating situation and deciding how to deal with it.

## ASSIGNMENTS

1. Your goal for a particular course is a B grade. The examination is two weeks away. In the meantime, you have three laboratory reports and a term paper due. Develop a plan that will increase the probability of your feeling prepared for the exam and also completing the other assignments. Explain how your plan would minimize the frustration likely to occur.

2. Suppose you receive a D in that course, which means that you must make an A in the next course in order to graduate. Explain how each of the following might affect attaining that A:

   a. Projecting negative feelings about your grade onto the subject matter of the course.

   b. Conflict between your need to study and your need for approval from friends who expect you to participate in the usual social activities.

   c. Hostile feelings toward the teacher.

   d. Use of a problem-solving approach to completing course requirements.

3. You have a 2-year-old male patient who is to be hospitalized for about a month. During the first days in the hospital, the child tries to talk to those caring for him, but no one can understand him. He frequently throws himself down in bed and kicks violently; sometimes he bangs his head on the crib.

   a. Explain the child's behavior.

   b. How should you as a health care provider react to this behavior?

   c. How could those in frequent contact with this child best help him?

   d. Describe this child's primary need.

   e. List some possible long-term effects on the child if health care providers:

      (1) Label the child "spoiled" and avoid the child whenever possible.

      (2) Make a sincere effort to understand what the child is trying to say.

4. You have accepted a well-paid position in a large health agency. Job descriptions have been written for each position. The job description for your position lists the procedures you will be permitted to do, omitting several that you learned in your health occupations course. You resent not being allowed to perform these procedures.

   a. What are some possible approaches to dealing with this situation? Describe each approach fully in terms of your goals, possible actions, possible effects of each action, and the solution you believe is most likely to help you reach your goal.

   b. Contrast the probable outcome of each of the following actions:

   (1) Ignoring the job description and doing the procedures whenever you have a chance.

   (2) Accepting these restrictions without objection and functioning in a more limited role than that for which you are educationally prepared.

   (3) Functioning in a limited role but voicing your feelings about the restrictions at every opportunity.

   (4) Developing hostile feelings toward administrative personnel of the agency, who you believe are responsible for restricting your role.

   (5) Quitting your job in protest over the restrictions.

5. Hailey is a graduate of a two-year Medical Office Assisting program. She began work at a large clinic immediately after graduation. This clinic has family practice physicians plus eight different specialists, its own laboratory, and a physical therapy unit. As part of her orientation, Hailey worked for one week in each department and is now assigned to Patient Admissions and Intake. Her responsibilities include an interview and initial history, scheduling appointments with specific services, and setting up the new patient's chart. Most of the scheduling is done by telephone.

   There are frequent mix-ups in patients' appointments and other problems related to interdepartmental communications. Hailey is efficient and well organized, but noticed during her rotation that some departments did not function efficiently. Some of the clerical personnel were careless about messages and viewed the paperwork as a nuisance. Hailey believes that some relatively simple changes in procedure would improve communications and increase efficiency. She schedules an appointment with her supervisor and offers three suggestions; the supervisor nods and says she will "take care of it." A month passes with no changes in procedures. During her break today, a coworker comments, "I hear you don't like the way we do things." Hailey is increasingly unhappy with her job, as the same problems occur time and again.

   Participate in a class discussion dealing with the following questions:

   What is Hailey experiencing?

   What are some possible ways of dealing with her feelings?

   Why did the supervisor not implement the changes Hailey suggested? (Brainstorm to list all possible reasons.)

   What actions might Hailey take to prevent these problems?

   If conditions do not change and Hailey feels more and more unhappy about the problems, what are her options?

6. Consider the following beliefs and place a checkmark beside each that applies to you:

   It is humiliating to make a mistake.

   If I perform well enough, people will approve of me.

   If I do not perform well, people will look down on me.

   I'm not doing as well as I can; I must try harder.

   It is possible to be right all the time.

   It is inexcusable to make a mistake.

   There is a right way and a wrong way to do everything.

   Some people just don't seem to care if they make a mistake.

   Some people keep on doing things the wrong way, even after I point out the right way.

   I addressed someone by the wrong name last week; I am so embarrassed I want to avoid seeing that person.

7. Which statements in Assignment 6 might be true of a person who directs perfectionistic expectations inward?

8. Which statements in Assignment 6 might be true of a person who directs perfectionistic expectations outward?

9. If you checked more than two of the items in Assignment 6, consider how you might make your beliefs and expectations more realistic.

Section

# Becoming an Effective Health Care Provider

The technological advances of the health field tempt the health care provider to become absorbed in complex equipment and the details of technique. To the patient, however, the *social climate* that health care providers create has great importance. Each contact with a member of the health team affects the patient's peace of mind, emotional state, and outlook. *Scientific breakthroughs and sophisticated procedures cannot replace the human element in patient care.*

Section IV is designed to help you learn ways to promote a favorable outlook for the patient. Make it your aim to relate to each patient as a human being and develop your own personal technique for identifying patient needs. As you learn to select the behaviors that promote favorable reactions in others, you will also enrich your personal living. Thus, you can grow not only as a health care provider, but also as a thoughtful, self-directing person, gaining increased satisfaction in living and at the same time enriching the lives of others.

# UNIT 15

# Effects of Illness on Behavior

## OBJECTIVES

Upon completion of this unit, you should be able to:

- List six physical effects of illness.
- Name five possible emotional reactions to illness.
- List five indications of a patient's emotional reaction to illness.
- List seven influences on a patient's reaction to illness.
- State six guidelines for providing effective care for a hospitalized child.

## KEY TERMS

| | | |
|---|---|---|
| Desertion reaction | Lethargy | Separation anxiety |
| Disguised behavior | Mind-set | Verbalize |
| Incapacitated | | |

Illness is always a threat to one's sense of security. Even a minor illness or injury is a threat to physical and emotional well-being. The pattern of life is disrupted. There is discomfort and inconvenience. The threat arouses feelings—perhaps fear, anger, or grief. These feelings are often manifested through the patient's behavior, but are not verbalized.

In other courses you are learning about specific illnesses: symptoms, diagnostic procedures, therapeutic techniques. Such knowledge is essential to safe and efficient performance as you provide patient care. Your *effectiveness* as a health care provider, however, is dependent upon your skill in applying knowledge about human behavior to relationships with patients. An effective health care provider/patient relationship promotes the patient's well-being. For one patient, reassurance in large amounts is needed to counteract fear and anxiety. For another patient, you may need to build confidence in the health team in order to gain the patient's cooperation in following the therapeutic plan.

Trying to provide a therapeutic atmosphere that is favorable for each patient is a never-ending challenge. Human variability is so great that no one method will work for all patients. By applying your knowledge about human behavior and the effects of illness, you can become sensitive to patient behaviors and their possible significance in terms of mental and emotional needs.

## PHYSICAL EFFECTS OF ILLNESS

Patients not only experience the signs and symptoms of a specific illness, but also various physical effects related to emotional reactions, change in daily routine, drugs, and numerous other factors. Examples of such general physical effects are fever, pain, nausea, lack of appetite, urinary problems, and difficulty with elimination. The overall effect may range from extreme **lethargy** to extreme restlessness. These general effects may be just as distressing to the patient as the symptoms of a specific illness. *The patient's complaints about general or vague effects should be noted.* These general symptoms may indicate either physical or emotional needs. Since interpretation may be beyond the scope of your role, report such complaints to your team leader or supervisor.

## EMOTIONAL EFFECTS OF ILLNESS

Most people react to illness with negative emotions that vary in type and intensity. Some patients are mildly annoyed at being sick; others are quite angry. Some patients are apprehensive; others are almost in a state of panic. Some feel sorry for themselves, while others react with pronounced self-pity. Some people feel bitter about their misfortune; bitterness is a combination of anger and self-pity.

Some patients readily **verbalize** their feelings. The patient who says, "Why me?" is probably expressing anger. The patient who says, "It seems as though everything happens to me!" is probably expressing self-pity. Obviously, the words alone do not carry the full message. Be alert for additional evidence about the patient's emotional reaction to illness: facial expression, tone of voice, body posture, choice of words, and emphasis given to certain words.

Negative feelings may also be expressed through **disguised behavior**. The patient who is very talkative may be covering up fear. The patient who is eager to please may be covering up fear, hostility, or other negative feelings. Such patients are just as much in need of understanding and interest from health care providers as those who verbalize their feelings. Do not make the mistake of thinking that the patient who is pleasant does not have fears and anxieties; for these patients, too, illness is a threat. *Each patient reacts to threat in a very individual way* (Figure 15-1).

## GENERAL EFFECTS OF SERIOUS ILLNESS

During serious illness there is some depression of mental and emotional functioning. The individual's energy resources are being utilized to cope with the physical stress of illness. There is likely to be decreased awareness of surroundings and lessened concern about life problems. One exception to this is the patient with coronary occlusion. These patients often are alert, very much aware that life is hanging in the balance, and, therefore, extremely fearful. A calm, interested, and caring manner on the part of health care providers is essential to provide these patients with emotional support, reassurance, and, hopefully, some relief from fear.

Sometimes a patient who has been very cooperative during the serious stage of illness shows a marked change in behavior as convalescence begins. Energy resources are no longer fully required for coping with physical demands. The patient is now more aware of discomfort. There is energy for emotional reactions and for conscious attention to symptoms and life problems. You may find it difficult to cope with this change in behavior, because you probably believe the patient should now exhibit a positive emotional state. Accept a patient's

**FIGURE 15-1** People have various reactions to illness. *Delmar/Cengage Learning*

behavior as indicative of needs and problems, rather than condemning behavior because it is different from what you think it should be.

## INFLUENCES ON PATIENTS' REACTIONS TO ILLNESS

As a health care provider, you will see situations involving pain, discomfort, disability, and even death. The atmosphere of the health agency is your work environment. The equipment you use daily has meaning to you in terms of its purpose. The clinical sights, smells, and sounds that are so familiar to you may be frightening to other people. The strangeness of the health agency, equipment, protective apparel, and procedures contribute greatly to the emotional reactions of some patients. Most patients will benefit from your taking time to explain a procedure and to answer questions, no matter how routine that procedure has become for you (Figure 15-2). By dealing with the strangeness of a situation and by helping the patient understand, you can have a positive influence on patient behavior. Be aware that numerous other influences may affect the behavior of a specific patient.

### Childhood

Age influences patient reactions to illness, especially if the patient is at either extreme of the life span. The young child reacts to illness with all the characteristics of the stage of development, in addition to the child's fear of strange places, the discomfort of illness, and expectations developed from past experiences with health care providers.

Hospitalization may result in a "desertion reaction" or "separation anxiety," unless some member of the family stays with the child. **Desertion reaction** is a form of withdrawal in which the child retreats to a corner of the crib or curls up into the fetal position. The child is unresponsive when caregivers try to communicate. **Separation anxiety** is a type of panic reaction when the child realizes the parent is going to leave him or her in a strange place. Young children cannot understand the need for hospitalization; nor do small children

**FIGURE 15-2** Help your patient understand the situation by using appropriate vocabulary. *Delmar/Cengage Learning*

understand that they are not being abandoned and the family will return later. Because of these two common reactions of small children, most hospitals now allow, or even encourage, a member of the family to stay with a small child.

How to work effectively with sick children of various ages is a full course of study. By observing some general rules, however, you will improve your effectiveness with young patients. Accept each child according to their current stage of development. Allow the young patient to express feelings—do not suggest that a 3-year-old "be brave" and not cry when something hurts. Do not expect cooperation from those who are too young to understand. Be aware that the child does not understand what is happening. Accept that the child is afraid. Remember that children often sense the feelings of adults. If you have negative feelings, the child is likely to sense your true feelings. Some child behavior is actually a reaction to the feelings of an adult.

As a health care provider, it is your task to win the child's confidence. *When a treatment or diagnostic procedure must be done, indicate that you accept the child's feelings and are sorry that the child is having pain.* Be aware that any traumatic experience will influence the child's behavior throughout this illness, create negative feelings toward health care providers in general, and influence behavior in future illnesses.

## Senescence

Most elderly people fear becoming bedridden or otherwise losing their independence. For the senescent patient, any illness is especially threatening. This may be the illness that will render the patient helpless. An elderly patient may have greater anxiety than you think is justified by the particular illness. Such patients need your sincere interest and concern as they cope with the threat their illness represents.

In caring for an elderly patient, encourage independence insofar as it is reasonable. The need for help with buttoning a shirt may be due to arthritic hands—very different from a child who needs help with buttons! Do not assume that the elderly patient's need for help with some aspects of daily living also means that the patient is to be treated like a child. Allow the patient to make decisions whenever appropriate, rather than insisting that the patient conform to every routine of the facility. Keep in mind that some routines are for the convenience of the staff and may not be in the best interest of every patient. Above all, remember that this elderly person, now somewhat dependent on you, was at one time independent and self-reliant. The loss of one's independence is a difficult loss to accept.

## Life Role

One's life role assumes great importance during illness. The mother with small children has anxiety about their care while she is **incapacitated.** Possibly, there is also anxiety about her ability to fulfill her responsibilities as a wife and mother. Her reaction to illness may be quite different from that of a woman with the same illness whose family is less dependent on her.

Occupational role also influences the degree of threat. Illness can seriously threaten job security; even if one's job is secure, there may be loss of income. Sick leave, salary continuation plans, whether or not one works on commission, whether or not insurance will help with the costs of illness—all influence the amount of anxiety the patient feels. If there is permanent disability, a change of occupation may be necessary. For most of your patients, you will not know the details of their life situation; hence, you cannot know what their worries are. You can, however, be sensitive to manifestations of anxiety, and you can listen when a patient indicates a need to talk.

## Adjustment

The usual adjustment of a patient has much influence on reactions to illness. The patient who has a sense of security and usually copes with life problems effectively is very likely to cope with illness effectively also, even though adjustment will not be as good as usual. *Even for the well-adjusted person, illness is accompanied by inconvenience and discomfort, which alters the degree of adjustment.*

Those same personality traits and patterns of behavior that influence adjustment also influence how one reacts to illness. A person who is inclined to use defense mechanisms will continue this pattern during illness. The person who is inclined to find escape from unpleasantness will try to avoid facing the reality of illness. Sometimes the defense mechanisms fail the individual during illness; then the patient may be unable to cope with the situation. When the usual patterns of coping fail, the individual may become fearful and may even panic. Patients who seem overly anxious may not know how to cope with illness.

## Dependency

Some people are quite independent, in the sense of being self-reliant. Others are inclined to lean on someone else whenever possible. This trait is known as dependency. People who are extremely dependent may react to illness in a way that reflects this characteristic. It is expected that the sick be dependent on others; therefore, illness justifies dependency. During illness, *dependent persons* escape the self-reliance normally expected of adults. Therefore, *unconsciously* wishing to prolong an illness, they find it difficult to admit they are improving. New complaints may be offered as evidence that they are still sick.

It is easy to be critical of such patients. Yet if you had that patient's life problems, background, and patterns of behavior, then you would probably be using the same behavior pattern the patient is using. Instead of being critical, the health team should plan ways for such a patient to resume self-care progressively during convalescence.

## Cultural Background and Language Barriers

Another influence on patient reactions to illness is cultural background. The United States has experienced an influx of people from all over the world. They come from Central and South America, Asia, the Middle East, Africa, and Eastern Europe. Each culture has certain beliefs about sickness, death, and dying. In some cultures, members of the family and the community care for the sick. Hospitals and doctors may be viewed with suspicion and are consulted only if the situation becomes desperate. When a person moves from that type of culture to one where medical care is a common occurrence, admission to the hospital may be perceived as meaning the patient's illness is hopeless.

The patient with limited understanding of English presents a special challenge to health care providers. The patient may have difficulty describing symptoms or conveying needs—frustrating for both patient and health care provider. Such patients should be given careful explanations of procedures and routines to alleviate fear and prevent misunderstandings. Many hospitals now have a roster of community members who speak various languages and can serve as translators for foreign patients who do not understand English. These patients present an opportunity for the health care provider to learn about the patient's culture, perceptions of illness, and lifestyle.

Cultural differences also include religion and membership in one of the American subcultures. The patient whose religious beliefs influence diet and other practices needs assurance that the practices will be respected. Patients from a minority group may expect prejudice from caregivers. Efforts to show that they are accepted may even arouse suspicion. There is no room for prejudice in providing health care, however. Your philosophy of individual worth should guide you in providing quality care for each patient, regardless of cultural background.

## Past Experience

Experience creates in each of us a "mind-set" toward certain types of experience. **Mind-set** influences how we perceive a situation. How we perceive the situation influences how we react. The patient who has had unfavorable experiences with sickness, health care providers, or health agencies is likely to perceive greater threat than a person who has not had such unfavorable experiences. The patient who has a mind-set that health care providers are cold and impersonal may perceive coldness even in a friendly care provider. If the patient expects inefficient care, then examples of inefficiency will be found. Evidence of defensiveness, distrust, hostility, or fear toward health care providers may indicate traumatic past experiences.

You cannot undo past damage quickly. Mind-set is a fixed expectation that is not easily modified; it creates readiness to behave according to the *expectation*, rather than according to the specific situation. When you encounter a patient who seems to have had unfavorable experiences with health care providers, do not expect to establish rapport immediately. However, your efforts may be more effective than you realize and pave the way for new and more favorable attitudes in the future.

## THE CHALLENGE FOR HEALTH CARE PROVIDERS

As a health care provider, you will sometimes be extremely busy performing all the procedures required to complete your assignment. Both time pressure and work load can be quite stressful. At such times you may tend to focus on task completion, rather than identifying patients' needs, being aware of patients' emotional reactions to their illnesses, and understanding that certain behaviors are reactions to illness. Actually, *giving your attention to human relations as you perform various procedures* will help you manage your own stress. You will be able to enjoy interacting with each patient and be less aware of job pressures (Figure 15-3).

### Relating to the Patient

Practicing effective human relations is not time-consuming; it is a matter of *where you focus your attention*. Familiar procedures do not require a lot of concentration, so you can focus on relating to the patient while you carry out a procedure. If you do need to concentrate on the task, you can simply state to the patient, "I really need to focus on what I'm doing; we'll talk some more when I have finished."

Relating to your patients effectively requires certain attitudes: genuine concern for others, the belief that other people are important, and willingness to see a situation from the patient's point of view. Actually, these three attitudes are essential to feel empathy for another person. The caregiver who truly feels empathy for a patient is likely to be perceived by the patient as warm and caring (Figure 15-4).

Certain personal traits also contribute to effective relationships, especially sincerity, truthfulness, and honesty. In addition, behavior patterns affect relationships. Attentiveness, giving one's full attention to the patient, is absolutely necessary to convey caring and concern. Two health care providers who carry on a conversation with each other while performing a procedure on a patient are sending the message: "We are not really interested in you as a human being. We are just here

**FIGURE 15-3** A worried patient may be reassured by gentle touch. *Delmar/Cengage Learning*

FIGURE 15-4 Everyone needs intimacy and human touch. If in doubt about a patient's reaction, ask for permission to touch or hug. *Delmar/Cengage Learning*

to do this task." Making eye contact at frequent intervals also conveys attentiveness. Have you ever tried to have a conversation with someone who looked over your shoulder or kept glancing around the room while you were talking? If so, you probably felt that the other person was not really interested in you or what you had to say. Probably the most important of all caring behaviors involves just "being there" when someone needs comfort and emotional support. Being there may or may not include conversation. It may involve simply taking the patient's hand in yours for a moment, or simply asking, "Do you need anything?"

Attitudes, personal traits, and behavior patterns all influence your effectiveness in relating to others. Effective communication, the subject of Units 18 and 19, is another essential component of effective human relations. The following paragraphs present key aspects of effective communication within the context of effective patient care.

## Communicating with the Patient

Your purpose in communicating with a patient affects your communication style. Interviewing a patient to obtain information, instructing the patient in self-care, explaining a procedure or the patient's care plan, or conveying empathy are examples of different purposes that would require somewhat different approaches. Regardless of purpose, however, it is important to convey caring and concern for the patient. Communication includes both verbal and nonverbal messages, so you should become aware of your own communication style, especially your use of body language as you communicate verbally.

Spoken communication should make use of appropriate vocabulary for the patient's age, educational level, and linguistic skills—the patient's ability to understand the message you wish to send. Enunciate clearly and speak loudly enough for the patient to hear. Look directly at the patient while speaking; one who has hearing problems may use lip-reading to supplement hearing. Make eye contact at frequent intervals. Be sensitive to the patient's desire to respond or ask questions. Examples of statements that show concern for the patient are listed in Table 15-1.

**TABLE 15-1**

**Statements That Show Caring**

| ACTIVITY | EXAMPLES OF STATEMENTS TO PAIR WITH ACTIVITY |
|---|---|
| Bringing something for the client | "I brought you a book to read. It is one I thought you would like." |
| Covering the client with a blanket | "It feels chilly in here. Perhaps this blanket will help." |
| Assisting the client to dress | "I really like that robe. It brings out your color," or "I noticed you are having a little trouble getting your robe on. Perhaps I can help." |
| Feeding the client or serving a tray to the client | "It is time to eat. Your food arrangement is colorful." |
| Giving the client a drink of water | "Here is some fresh water for you," or "How would some cool water taste right now?" |
| Offering the client a chair | "You look tired. I'll help you with your chair." |
| Offering the client assistance | "Here, let me help you. Perhaps together we can arrange these flowers." |
| Leaving a room | "What else can I do for you before I go?" or "I am leaving now, but I will be back in 20 minutes." |
| Moving the client up in bed | "You look so uncomfortable. Let me move you up in bed." |
| Making the client's bed | "Now you have a nice fresh bed. I hope that will make you more comfortable." |
| Regulating the temperature of the environment | "It seems very warm in here. Perhaps if I turn the air conditioner up, it will help." |
| Rubbing the client's back | "A back rub sometimes helps to ease tension." |
| Turning the client in bed | "Changing position really makes a difference, doesn't it?" |
| Straightening a pillow | "Let me straighten your pillow for you," or "That ought to feel better now." |

*Source:* From Waughfield, Claire G. (2002). *Mental health concepts* (5th ed., p. 93). Clifton Park, NY: Delmar, Cengage Learning.

At times, you may feel that a miscommunication has occurred between you and the patient. Common causes of miscommunication are shown in Box 15-1. Clarifying any misunderstanding shows the patient that you care and can prevent additional problems. To minimize misunderstanding, when the patient does speak, *listen!* Look at the patient, not at

> **BOX 15-1**
>
> **Reasons for Ineffective Communication**
>
> - Senders may not send the message they thought they were sending.
> - Receivers may not hear the message the sender intended.
> - Verbal and nonverbal messages may conflict.
> - The message may be disguised by the sender.
> - Many English words have multiple meanings.
> - The message may be abstract and therefore confusing.
> - The receiver may be prepared to hear another message.
>
> *Source: From Waughfield, Claire G. (2002). Mental health concepts (5th ed., p. 85). Clifton Park, NY: Delmar, Cengage Learning.*

the chart in your hand. Allow plenty of time for the patient to finish speaking; do not interrupt and do not use this time for cleaning the bedside table or filling the water pitcher. Follow up on statements that seem to signal unspoken concerns of the patient:

- "I'm not sure I understand what you mean by that."
- "Are you saying that . . . ?"
- "I sense that you are feeling . . ."

In responding to the patient, convey respect for what the patient has said, but tactfully correct any errors or apparent misunderstandings. If the patient has a complaint, listen respectfully without becoming defensive. If you can resolve the complaint, do so; otherwise, assure the patient that you will inform the appropriate person of the complaint. Then check back with the patient after a reasonable period of time to see if the problem has been corrected. It is especially desirable to avoid the types of statements that tend to shut off communication, as shown in Table 15-2.

In talking with patients whose diagnosis is serious or life-threatening, avoid statements that offer false hope. It is very easy to say, "Now don't you worry. I'm sure everything will be all right." This type of statement may make you feel better, but it conveys to the patient that you do not want to hear his or her concerns and fears. This type of situation calls for effective listening, in which your comments encourage the patient to continue to talk. In Units 18 and 19, you will have the opportunity to practice communication skills, both nonverbal and verbal.

So the ongoing challenge throughout your career as a health care provider will be to practice effective human relations, including clear communication, as an essential part of your overall performance.

## TABLE 15-2
**Blocks to Communication**

| TECHNIQUE | EXPLANATION | EXAMPLE |
|---|---|---|
| Belittling | Statement that tends to make light of the client's beliefs or fears | Client: "I will not leave here alive."<br>Nurse: "That is ridiculous. You should not even think that way." |
| Disagreeing | Response that indicates that the nurse believes the client to be incorrect; it generally relates to the cognitive rather than the affective message | Client: "Why am I here? Nothing is being done for me and I am not getting any better."<br>Nurse: "You are getting better." |
| Defending | Statement used to repel a verbal attack | Client: "I had my light on for 15 minutes."<br>Nurse: "I am doing the best I can. You are not the only client I have." |
| Stereotyped statement | Common statement made without sincerity | Client: "I am really worried about the children. I came to the hospital so quickly and I did not get to see them. They just will not understand. I wish I could have talked to them."<br>Nurse: "I know exactly what you are going through." |
| Changing the subject | Different subject introduced to prevent talking about a topic that causes anxiety | Client: "They are doing a biopsy tomorrow. I hope it is not cancer."<br>Nurse: "Are these your children? That is such a nice-looking family." |
| Reassuring cliché | Reassuring statement that is not sincere | Client: "What will I do if it is malignant?"<br>Nurse: "Don't you worry. Everything will be all right." |
| Giving advice | Statement that tells the client what the nurse thinks the client should do | Client: "I broke my arm when I fell off a skateboard."<br>Nurse: "At your age, I would suggest you give up skateboards." |
| Agreeing | Statement that shows that the nurse believes the client's cognitive message is correct; it may not be the client's real concern | Client: "I am afraid the doctor will not discharge me tomorrow."<br>Nurse: "I am sure you are correct. I doubt the doctor will let you go home so soon." |

*Source:* From Waughfield, Claire G. (2002). *Mental health concepts* (5th ed., p. 89–90). Clifton Park, NY: Delmar, Cengage Learning.

## REFERENCES AND SUGGESTED READINGS

Munoz, Cora, & Luckman, Joan. (2005). Culture and cultural values. In *Transcultural communication in health care* (2nd ed., pp. 21–44). Clifton Park, NY: Delmar, Cengage Learning.

Tamparo, Carol D., & Lindh, Wilburta Q. (2008). The helping interview. In *Therapeutic communications for health professionals* (3rd ed., pp. 56–79). Clifton Park, NY: Delmar, Cengage Learning.

Waughfield, Claire G. (2002). Effective communication. In *Mental health concepts* (5th ed., pp. 83–107). Clifton Park, NY: Delmar, Cengage Learning.

## REVIEW AND SELF-CHECK

1. List six physical effects of illness.

2. List five possible emotional reactions to illness.

3. Name five behaviors that could indicate a patient's emotional reaction to illness.

4. List seven factors that influence a patient's reaction to illness.

5. State six guidelines for care of a hospitalized child.

## ASSIGNMENTS

1. Consider some past illness you have experienced. Describe your reactions to this illness in terms of the following:

    a. Perception of threat

    b. Emotional effects

    c. Physical discomfort

    d. Your behavior when you were uncomfortable

    e. Inconvenience of the illness

    f. Effects on your daily habits

    g. Effects on your state of adjustment

    h. Patterns of behavior you used to cope with the illness

    i. Influence of one or more personality traits on how you reacted to illness

    j. Expectations or mind-set that affected your relationship with those caring for you

> **Note:** Reactions to illness occur even if the illness is a minor one. If you have never had any illness that could provide a basis for this assignment, interview a friend or member of your family who has had a recent illness.

2. You have been having annoying symptoms for several months. Then a new symptom appears—one that you know is a warning sign of cancer. When you consult your physician, she recommends hospitalization for diagnostic studies. Picture yourself on admission to the hospital. Using parts a through j in Assignment 1, think through the reactions you might have under these circumstances.

3. As a health care provider, you probably would react somewhat differently from a layperson when you have a potentially serious illness. How is being a health care provider an advantage? How is being a health care provider a disadvantage?

4. It has been said that doctors and nurses make "poor" patients. Why?

5. Your neighbor comes to you to talk about her recent experiences with diagnostic studies. She states, "The doctor says there is nothing physically wrong. He says I should stop being so nervous. I don't know what he means." How could you help this neighbor understand what the doctor means, without exceeding your role as a health care provider?

6. A member of your family has a disorder that can only be treated by extensive lifestyle changes. List specific suggestions for helping this relative make the necessary changes.

7. A friend informs you that her husband has a malignancy and describes some changes in his behavior. How could you help her to understand her husband's behavior?

8. You are assigned to a patient whose treatment includes bedrest. As you prepare to give a bedbath, you put on gloves. The patient says angrily, "Am I so dirty that you can't touch me with your bare hands?" How will you respond?

# UNIT 16

# Coping with Patient Behavior

## OBJECTIVES

Upon completion of this unit, you should be able to:

- List and explain eight guidelines for improving health care provider/patient relations.
- List nine behavior patterns commonly manifested by patients and an appropriate reaction of a health care provider to each behavior.
- Name five behaviors that may indicate a patient's emotional reaction to illness.
- Explain and give one example of the following behaviors: egocentrism, regression, aggressive behavior, and hostility.
- List five communication techniques that can be used to make appropriate responses to patients.

## KEY TERMS

Covert          Overt          Passive aggression

Behavior is highly individualistic. Each person has typical patterns of behavior for various situations. Each person has specific patterns for reacting to stress, including the stress of illness. Do not expect to know exactly why each person behaves in a certain way. You can, however, be aware of *possible* reasons for behavior and thus be more accepting of whatever behavior the patient does exhibit. Through such understanding, you can avoid a judgmental attitude toward your patients, thus eliminating one big obstacle to effective relationships.

It is the purpose of this unit to provide guidelines for forming effective relationships. Recognize, though, that learning to form effective relationships does not come from reading a book or even from completing a course of study. Such learning begins with knowledge and understanding of human behavior, *but skill in interpersonal relations comes through a conscious effort to apply your knowledge and understanding to every relationship with another person—at work, at home, and in all activities involving other people.*

## GENERAL GUIDELINES

With experience, you can develop sensitivity to the feelings behind specific types of behavior. Once you begin to develop this sensitivity, you can strive to adapt your own behavior to each patient in an effort to provide the kind of relationship that promotes the patient's well-being. The following guidelines describe ways to improve your relationships with patients.

## Accepting the Patient

Each patient needs to feel approval and acceptance by providers of health care. Many patients are sensitive to any evidence of irritation, impatience, indifference, or hostility on the part of a health care provider. Accepting every patient may require effort, because each of us has some prejudice or lack of understanding toward those who are different from ourselves. Through increased experience with a variety of people, you can grow in understanding of others—provided you avoid a critical or judgmental attitude. This is the key to learning to accept others—*recognize that other people are like you in many ways, even though different in other ways.*

Accepting someone includes accepting that person's behavior—even if it is not pleasant. There may be good reason for a patient's irritability or criticism. It is not realistic to expect everyone to be pleasant all of the time; such an expectation is especially unrealistic in regard to people who are sick.

Occasionally, a patient's behavior *is* unacceptable. Then, without showing anger or fear, the health care provider can use an "I" statement to indicate that such behavior is unacceptable. If the behavior is repeated after limits have been set, the supervisor should be consulted. Obviously, with patients who are inebriated, confused, psychotic, or otherwise irresponsible, it is more difficult to obtain cooperation in observing limits.

## Showing Interest and Concern

While you are caring for a patient, give that patient your full attention. Address the patient by name, listen, respond appropriately, and show willingness to act on any requests (Figure 16-1). In many situations, hospital routine requires that things be done at a certain

**FIGURE 16-1** You can help patients cope with their illness by showing acceptance, caring, and concern.
*Delmar/Cengage Learning*

time; usually, an explanation will gain the patient's cooperation. In other situations, health care providers unnecessarily force patients into a routine. If a patient customarily bathes at bedtime, why insist upon a morning bath while in the hospital? Some patients deeply resent unnecessary interruptions or changes in their daily routine. Before insisting that such patients conform to the usual hospital routine, be sure that such conformity is *really necessary*.

## Listening and Observing

The patient who has fears and anxieties can benefit from talking out these feelings. Most patients, however, do not readily "open up." Be sensitive to subtle indications that something is bothering the patient. Linger in the patient's unit to chat casually and respond to any hint of anxiety by showing interest in how the patient feels. Be available as an interested listener. A patient's readiness to express feelings to you is, in a sense, a test of the effectiveness of your relationship with that patient. Usually acceptance, demonstrated interest, and concern pave the way for a patient to express fears, anxieties, and uncertainties.

## Recognizing Significant Behavior

Nonverbal behavior often provides a clue to the patient's feelings. Nervous movements, restlessness, unwillingness to participate in conversation, and many other behaviors signal that a patient needs extra attention (Figure 16-2).

The patient who states, "My doctor says I should have surgery," is probably signaling a need to talk about it. You can shut off conversation, or you can encourage it by your response.

**FIGURE 16-2** Observation of behavior can help you recognize a patient's needs. *Delmar/Cengage Learning*

Saying, "I know that. I took your preoperative orders from the doctor," may be interpreted by the patient to mean, "This health care provider doesn't care how scared I am." On the other hand, if you respond, "How do you feel about having surgery?" the patient is more likely to verbalize feelings about the impending surgery.

When you encourage patients to express feelings, you are providing a valuable service. A patient may gain more from verbalizing anxieties than from taking a tranquilizer.

## Using Appropriate Responses

When patients make "loaded statements," it is usually effective to repeat what the patient has said, using essentially the same words but with a questioning inflection. This type of response, known as *echoing*, is a safe response; it does not give information, and it does not show your reaction to what the patient said. It merely says to the patient that you heard; the rising inflection in your voice implies, "Please continue. I am listening." Some patients will not understand the meaning of the rising inflection and simply be annoyed by your use of echoing.

It is good to have a range of communication techniques so you can use the most appropriate one for a particular situation. Some other useful techniques are: reflecting, clarifying, validating, questioning, and confronting. *Reflecting* is similar to echoing, but requires that you restate what the patient said, indicating that you have heard the message and are aware of the patient's feelings. Your response may begin with a phrase such as, "It sounds like. . ." or "It seems like you. . ."; this type of response is also called *mirroring*. When you use reflecting, you are essentially providing a mirror for the patient to view what he or she just said. The patient then has an opportunity to confirm, deny, or modify the meaning of the comment.

*Clarifying* is a technique used to test your interpretation of what has been said. After stating something like, "Let me see if I understand what you mean," you state the message, as you understand it, in your own words. The speaker can then confirm or deny that you understand the intended meaning. This may require several repetitions before the speaker will agree that you understand the message.

*Validating* is a technique used to check the meaning of certain nonverbal behaviors of the speaker. Often, the spoken message conveys one meaning, but certain nonverbal clues indicate a different meaning or indicate that the speaker's emotional state is different from what the verbal message implies. The technique for validating involves such statements as, "I sense that. . ." followed by a description of a feeling or "I notice that. . ." followed by an observation of some behavior, posture, or facial expression. This technique invites the patient to express feelings, doubts, anxieties, worries, annoyances, and frustrations.

*Questioning* is often required in the performance of patient care, usually to obtain specific information. Questioning can also be used as a therapeutic tool and as a means of avoiding a misunderstanding. Questioning should be done with a caring attitude. It is better to ask only one question, allow time for the patient to answer, then converse briefly before asking another question. It is especially important that you *listen* while the patient responds and allow the patient to finish before you speak again.

*Confronting* is a technique that challenges the patient's statement. It must be done in a calm and friendly manner, not in the adversary manner associated with the word "confrontation." Confronting can be used to clarify a message discrepancy (verbal/nonverbal), challenge a belief, or examine an attitude that may block effective therapy. A summary of these five communication techniques is shown in Table 16-1.

**TABLE 16-1**

**Techniques of Helpful Communication**

| TECHNIQUE | EXPLANATION | EXAMPLE |
|---|---|---|
| Validation | A statement that attempts to verify the nurse's perception of the client's message in both content and feeling areas | "You really look distressed, like something is wrong." |
| Clarification | A statement used to clear up possible misunderstandings to seek information necessary to understanding | "If I understand you correctly, you are upset because your daughter has just told you she is getting married." |
| Reflection | Stating the nurse's perception of the client's message in both content and feeling areas | "You are afraid you will not be needed after your daughter marries." |
| Broad questions | Questions used to encourage the client to talk | "What would you like to talk about?" |

*Source:* From Waughfield, Claire G. (2002). *Mental health concepts* (5th ed.). Clifton Park, NY: Delmar, Cengage Learning.

## Maintaining Confidentiality

Legally and ethically, health care providers are required to protect patients' privacy and to hold patients' health information in confidence (Figure 16-3). In 2003, the Health Insurance and Portability and Accountability Act (HIPAA) Privacy Rule took effect. This federal legislation protects the privacy of individuals' medical information. Clients are generally given information about their privacy rights on their first visit to a particular health care office or facility. HIPAA stipulates that consumers have the right to request copies of and to correct any errors in their medical records. Consumers also have the right to decide who can receive their medical information and for what purposes. Violations of the HIPAA Privacy Rule may be reported to the Office of Civil Rights.

An exception to confidentiality is information *relevant to the patient's well-being*. For this reason, it is unwise to commit yourself to promises. If a patient offers to tell you something that requires a promise "not to tell," do not be flattered that the patient wants to share a secret. Even more important, do not make such a promise. Simply state, "Whatever I learn about a patient is kept in confidence, unless the patient's well-being requires that I share the information with the health care team." Then indicate that you are listening if the patient wishes to talk.

Suppose you made such a promise to Mr. Zel, a very personable young man who has been admitted to the hospital with a possible bleeding ulcer. After extracting a promise of secrecy from you, he confides that his brother is bringing clothes tonight, and they are going to slip out of the hospital and "hit the bars." What should you do, once you know that his "secret" involves a plan that would be harmful to Mr. Zel? Should you break your word and report his plan to your supervisor? Should you keep your word and not tell his secret? Suppose he really does slip out of the hospital? Suppose you report his plan; when your supervisor confronts

FIGURE 16-3 Patient information is always confidential and must never be discussed casually. *Delmar/Cengage Learning*

him, he denies everything. Avoiding any promise of secrecy can prevent getting caught in such a trap.

### Being Sensitive to Feelings

Unpleasant behavior is usually due to a negative emotional state, ignorance, or an unfavorable attitude. Few people are "mean" in the sense of gaining satisfaction from being unpleasant.

When patients behave in undesirable ways, it is almost always the result of inner feelings. These feelings affect the patient's well-being. *Whenever you encourage a patient to adopt a positive, realistic outlook, you contribute to that patient's well-being.* Negative feelings indicate a need. Try to identify the need and respond appropriately.

### Identifying Patient Needs

Any behavior that may indicate a negative emotional state should signal to the health team that the patient needs additional attention. All too often, such behavior results in the patient being labeled "difficult," and the patient is avoided as much as possible. The health care provider who labels a patient with an unflattering term (e.g., "impossible") demonstrates ignorance of needs and lack of caring about that patient.

For experienced health care providers who have mastered the routine procedures and techniques, the real challenge of patient care lies in identifying needs of patients and establishing a therapeutic caregiver/patient relationship. The patient's behavior provides the clues for identifying a need. Once identified, a need may require medical intervention, but many patient needs can be met through nursing interventions.

Mrs. K. was in a room at the end of the hall, many steps away from the nurses' station. She turned on her call light every few minutes. Sometimes, the person who answered her call could not return to the desk before Mrs. K. had her light on again. The staff was irritated about the extra mileage being walked to take care of trivial requests. Sunday morning, Jennifer had a few minutes before giving out medications, so she went—unsummoned—to Mrs. K.'s room. She found little things to do for Mrs. K., rearranged her flowers, and showed interest and concern. It was about an hour before Mrs. K. turned on her call light again. As other members of the nursing team spent more time with her, Mrs. K. volunteered the information that a neighbor, who had recently been discharged from the hospital, told her, "It is impossible to get any attention in the hospital." Mrs. K. feared she would not be able to get a nurse if she needed one. When the staff demonstrated interest and showed that they were available, Mrs. K.'s fear was relieved and she no longer made excessive demands.

### Being Willing to Serve Patients

Lilia was a student in the dietary aide program. She noticed that one patient always asked her to do several things each time she carried a tray in. Lilia was increasingly irritated because it was not her responsibility to "wait on" the patient. She decided to get in and out of the room before the patient could ask her to do something. She was still asked to do things, in spite of her great haste. When she mentioned this to the head nurse, she was told, "Never appear to be in a hurry. Never talk about how busy the staff is. This makes some patients think they must ask for things while someone is in the room, for fear help will not be available later."

Lilia then tried walking into the patient's room in a leisurely way, putting the tray in position and then asking, "Is there anything I can do for you?" The surprised patient answered, "No, I can't think of anything."

Lilia's haste in getting out of the room had contributed to the patient's anxiety and distress. Lilia found that she could complete her assignment just as quickly by appearing calm and unrushed as by dashing in and out of patients' units.

## COMMON BEHAVIOR PATTERNS OF PATIENTS

### Egocentrism

Most people become egocentric during illness. This means that the patient becomes self-centered—the primary concern is with self. Much of the demanding behavior that health care providers (and families) resent in patients is actually a manifestation of the egocentric reaction to illness. In the extreme, this type of behavior can test your acceptance of the patient, yet egocentrism is just as much a reaction to illness as physical symptoms. If you accept egocentrism as a reaction to illness, you will find it easier to tolerate a patient's self-centered behavior.

### Regression

Regression, another common reaction to illness, involves reverting to behaviors that are appropriate to an earlier level of development. The most extreme form of regression is lying in the fetal position and not responding to one's surroundings. This is often seen in elderly patients who have been bedfast for a long period of time.

In the home, a young child may regress when a new baby arrives. For example, a toddler who has mastered drinking from a cup may ask for a bottle. Regression can be seen with patients of all ages. Dependence on others for personal care, when one is capable of self-care, is an example of regression. Understanding regression as a common reaction to illness can help you avoid impatience and a judgmental attitude toward a patient who exhibits regressive behavior.

## Unfriendly Behavior

Place yourself in the following situation. Today you are assigned to Mr. A., who is totally indifferent to all your efforts to be pleasant. You feel annoyed and wonder why you are wasting good cheer on this cold, unfriendly person.

Then you tell yourself that there may be reasons for Mr. A.'s behavior. Your thoughts run through some of the possible reasons. "Maybe Mr. A. fears his illness, but he does not want me to know he is frightened. Perhaps he does not admit to himself that he is frightened. He may have had unfavorable experiences with health care providers and is transferring hostility from his previous experiences to me. Perhaps his unfriendliness is a form of passive aggression. On the other hand, he may perceive health care providers as cold, indifferent, unsympathetic, or incapable of understanding how he feels."

If you are really trying to understand Mr. A.'s behavior, your thoughts might be: "My behavior may have annoyed Mr. A. Was I too cheerful when he felt there was nothing to be cheerful about? Maybe he just wants to be left alone! I should accept him and acknowledge his right to behave according to his present feelings. I will not perceive his lack of responsiveness as a personal affront."

*There is no one way to cope with an unfriendly patient.* Every person reacts as an individual and may or may not be aware of the reaction or its effects on other people. Do not allow unfriendliness to affect your own mood. Accept it for what it is, namely, a manifestation of how the patient feels at the moment. Maintain your own pleasant manner. Continue to show interest and concern. Visit the patient's room at intervals, but not so frequently that you are an annoyance. Sometimes your efforts will pay off without your knowing. The patient will be aware of your interest and this, in itself, will contribute to a sense of well-being. Sometimes your persistence pays off—your sincerity and interest lead to trust and the patient begins to respond to you.

## Aggressive Behavior

Aggression, a form of behavior that usually indicates hostility, may be physical or verbal. Physical aggression is most likely to occur if the patient is a child, is emotionally or mentally disturbed, is inebriated, or is in an irresponsible state. A simple aggressive act such as pushing your hand away may indicate fear, anger, or other negative emotional reactions to you or to what you are planning to do (Figure 16-4). It may be an effort at self-defense. If the aggression is more serious—an actual attack on you, for example—you must handle the situation as best you can to avoid being hurt and then summon help from a professional worker. *Because there are legal and ethical implications in handling aggression, avoid any action that could result in your being accused of assault on the patient.* Protect yourself from injury, but secure the assistance of your supervisor as quickly as possible.

**FIGURE 16-4** Patients may demonstrate feelings of frustration and anger. *Delmar/Cengage Learning*

A child is likely to use physical aggression defensively, due to the expectation of pain. The child's age, condition, and other factors determine the best way to handle aggressive behavior. If you are in doubt about how to work with a particular child, discuss the problem with the pediatric supervisor and obtain specific instructions. Your general approach, however, must include an accepting attitude. Never say to a child, "You are bad." Instead, tell the child you cannot accept kicking, biting, or whatever form the aggression is taking (Figure 16-5). Set limits to the behaviors you will accept. Even if the child does not respect these limits (e.g., no more kicking), he or she will understand why you are using restraints during a procedure.

**FIGURE 16-5** A patient who understands a procedure is more likely to cooperate. *Delmar/Cengage Learning*

When you have finished working with the child, demonstrate acceptance with friendly behavior. Keep in mind that the child who fights you is manifesting an intense emotional state.

With adults, aggressive behavior is usually in the form of verbal attack or resistance. Verbal aggression may involve criticism, loud talking, profanity, or arguing. If the patient is critical, listen to the complaint and how it is described. If there is a valid complaint, corrective steps should be taken immediately. If the complaint does not seem to be valid, consider the complaint to be an expression of feelings. Arguing may be a disguised request for an explanation: the patient is challenging you to justify some aspect of the therapeutic plan, some policy of the health agency, or some procedure.

**Passive aggression,** on the other hand, is likely to consist of overt or covert noncooperation. In **overt** noncooperation, the patient balks—refuses to take medicine, accept a treatment, undergo a diagnostic procedure, or carry out some self-help routine. **Covert** noncooperation involves deceit. The patient wants the health team to think he or she is cooperating, but actually is not. Patients who ask that their medication be left on the bedside table ("I'll take it later") may intend to flush it down the commode. If you discover that a patient has been covertly noncooperative, you will probably feel anger. It is hard to accept that someone has deceived you. But consider for a moment: why would a patient not cooperate with the therapeutic plan?

Perhaps the patient fears drug reactions and believes that quietly disposing of the drug is easier than trying to explain to health care providers "who do not understand how I feel about drugs." Perhaps the patient's religion discourages the use of drugs. Perhaps the patient knows (or thinks) that this is a terminal illness and does not want to prolong life, if the cost is pain and helplessness or depleting the family's financial resources. Whatever the reason for this noncooperation, you may be sure it makes sense to the patient. It is your responsibility to (1) refer this problem to the professional staff, (2) remain nonjudgmental toward this patient, (3) accept that you may never understand the reasons for the patient's behavior, and (4) remember that noncooperation serves a purpose for the patient.

## Hostility

Dealing with verbal or passive aggression is largely a problem of dealing with hostility. Team planning is more likely to be effective than isolated efforts by one or two members of the team. In general, each health care provider should give undivided attention to the hostile patient, listen without defensiveness or argument, indicate respect for the patient's feelings, show concern, and encourage expression of thoughts and feelings (Figure 16-6). Sometimes, it is effective to reflect what the patient has just said: "You think the food is terrible." At other times it may be more appropriate to question, using the patient's ideas but adding your own interpretation followed by "Is that what you mean?" It may be more appropriate to test your guess about the feelings behind the patient's comments: "Are you unhappy about this?" Or, "You seem to be quite angry about this." Use a pleasant tone and phrases that help the patient feel free to express feelings. Your responses should convey acceptance, caring, and willingness to listen. Sometimes such an approach has unexpectedly good results. The patient, after airing feelings, may say something such as, "I guess that's a pretty small thing to be fussing about."

The worst thing you can do with a hostile patient is to return hostility. This simply confirms the patient's belief that you do not care or understand—your hostility has justified the patient's hostility. To avoid hostile behavior toward the patient, you *must* avoid

**FIGURE 16-6** Listening to the patient's concerns provides emotional support and relieves anxiety. *Delmar/Cengage Learning*

hostile feelings. Accept the patient's hostility as indicative of a need, perhaps a need to develop trust in the health care team. If you develop negative feelings toward a patient, avoid defensiveness, criticism, arguing, short answers, or otherwise showing your negative feelings. If the patient detects your negative feelings, someone else should be assigned to care for that patient.

## Crying

Crying can result from any degree of anger, fear, or grief. Some people cry whenever they experience sentimental feelings. Crying is an emotional release and should not be stifled. Women tend to cry more readily than men. This is a result of cultural influence: little boys are taught that it is unmanly to cry. Do not make the mistake of thinking that men do not have emotional reactions just because they do not cry readily. Any male patient may be experiencing just as much fear, anger, or grief as the woman crying in the next room.

When you find a patient crying, avoid such comments as, "Let's stop crying now," or "You are much better, so there is nothing to cry about." These remarks may make you feel better, but they indicate to the patient that you are not trying to understand the patient's feelings.

Sometimes it is appropriate to ask the reason for the crying. At other times, it is better just to show acceptance, encourage freedom to express feelings through crying, and wait for the patient to volunteer information. It is not difficult to find out if the patient is crying because of pain and discomfort, fear, or sadness. If the crying seems to be due to personal problems, avoid prying questions, which could be an invasion of the patient's privacy.

With the crying patient, always indicate that you approve of crying as a means of relieving feelings. Sometimes holding the patient's hand or placing your hand over the patient's hand provides reassurance and conveys your interest and concern. Offer to stay, but if the patient shows a preference for being left alone, then say you are available if anything is needed, and leave. But return after 15 to 20 minutes and use appropriate behavior to respond to the patient's status at that time.

Each situation with a crying patient must be handled according to your best judgment and knowledge about the patient. Exactly what to say and do is dependent on the patient's situation. In every case, however:

- Do not offer false hope.
- Do not make promises you cannot keep.
- Do not minimize the patient's cause for crying.
- Do not express disapproval of crying.

Crying is sometimes exhibited by patients suffering from mental/emotional disturbances. These patients need your reassurance, caring, and concern, in addition to specific approaches that are part of the therapeutic plan. If your course includes care of the psychiatric patient, you will learn additional techniques for dealing with crying.

## Noncooperation

When an adult patient is uncooperative, there is usually a reason. Most adults recognize that cooperation with the health team is in their interest. Some possible reasons for noncooperation are lack of understanding, misinformation, suspicion or distrust, preference for one's own way of doing things, or negative feelings.

To understand a patient's failure to cooperate, inquire in an interested but uncritical manner about the reason for the patient's behavior. You may find that an explanation is needed, the patient needs to be taught a health principle, a false belief needs to be corrected, a misunderstanding needs to be cleared up, or feelings of fear or distrust need to be relieved.

Suppose your patient refuses a medication. Perhaps the patient believes the physician intends to discontinue that medication. The patient may have grown up with the belief that taking pills is a sign of weakness. Perhaps the patient has heard about health care providers giving patients the wrong medication. (Let's admit it: medication errors do occur and are inexcusable.) The patient may be convinced that the "little red pill" is causing nausea or some other discomfort. (And it may be.) Maybe the patient resents the health team's expectations that the patient adapt personal habits to their routines. The patient who is accustomed to going to bed at midnight may resent being told to take a pill and go to bed at 10 o'clock.

*Patients cannot be forced to cooperate.* Cooperation must be gained by eliminating the cause of noncooperation. If you are unable to learn why the patient is not cooperating, discuss the situation with your supervisor. Sometimes the problem must be referred to the patient's physician. If cooperation is essential to recovery, then it must be secured in some way. If the patient is objecting to a procedure that is not essential to recovery or well-being, then the physician may discontinue it rather than antagonize the patient. Table 16-2 discusses strategies for coping with difficult behaviors.

## The Overly Cheerful Patient

Convalescent patients usually are optimistic and happily anticipating full recovery from illness. Such cheerfulness is genuine and can be accepted at face value.

Any patient who is awaiting surgery or the results of diagnostic studies, however, probably has some anxiety. Some of these patients appear quite cheerful, in spite of great anxiety

## TABLE 16-2
## Coping with Problem Behaviors of Patients

| BEHAVIOR PATTERN | COPING STRATEGIES |
| --- | --- |
| Egocentrism | Accept egocentrism as a common reaction to illness; practice tolerance and patience. |
| Regression | Recognize regression as a common reaction to illness; encourage the patient to perform tasks he or she is capable of doing; avoid a judgmental attitude. |
| Unfriendly behavior | Do not perceive unfriendly behavior as a personal affront; maintain a calm and friendly approach; occasionally ask if there is anything you can do for the patient. |
| Aggressive behavior—child | Recognize that the child is probably frightened, may expect you to perform a painful procedure, be angry, or have had bad experiences with health care providers in the past. Maintain a friendly and caring attitude; explain procedures; express regrets if the procedure is painful; set limits on what behaviors you will tolerate (i.e., no kicking, no biting); obtain assistance or use restraints in accordance with policies of your agency. |
| Aggressive behavior—adult | If the patient is physically aggressive, protect yourself but avoid any behavior that could be construed as assault on the patient; call for assistance if needed; consult the supervisor. |
| Verbal assault | Firmly but pleasantly state that you do not wish to be spoken to in such a manner. Consult the supervisor if the behavior continues. |
| Criticism | Consider whether or not the criticism is valid. If so, take steps to correct the problem. Offer an apology if one is due. If the criticism is unreasonable or does not have a basis in fact, confrontation may result in the patient reconsidering the criticism. |
| Arguing | Does the patient need an explanation? Is the arguing really based on unexpressed fear or anger? Use various communication techniques, but avoid the attitude that you have to "win" an argument. |
| Hostility | Listen without defensiveness or argument; show respect for the patient's feelings; show acceptance, concern, caring; use various communication techniques to encourage expression of feelings. Avoid hostile feelings toward the patient. |
| Crying | Express concern; show acceptance of the patient's feelings; consider whether the crying may be due to pain or discomfort; ask if the patient would like to talk; indicate approval of crying as an expression of feelings; offer to stay or, if the patient prefers, leave; if you leave the patient, return in 15–20 minutes to express concern and caring. |

(Continued)

**TABLE 16-2**

**Coping with Problem Behaviors of Patients (Continued)**

| BEHAVIOR PATTERN | COPING STRATEGIES |
|---|---|
| Uncooperative | Use various communication techniques to determine the reason for noncooperation. (Remember that a patient's right to refuse a medication or procedure is protected by federal law.) Ask if the patient has any questions; offer to explain. Consider: Does this patient resent not being included in decisions about his or her care? |
| Overly cheerful | Is the patient using cheerfulness to cover up fear about an impending surgery or the outcome of diagnostic tests? Use various communication techniques to encourage expression of feelings. |
| Overly friendly | Is the patient merely showing interest with questions about your personal life? Does the patient's touch indicate a need for reassurance? Or is the patient being "too familiar"? If needed, calmly state limits on what is acceptable behavior between a patient and caregiver. Show caring and concern, and provide reassurance. Discuss the behavior with your supervisor. |

*Source:* Delmar/Cengage Learning.

(Figure 16-7). Do not allow apparent cheerfulness to make you indifferent to the needs of such patients. Some may handle their anxiety quite effectively without help. Others may need to talk about their feelings. Your observation skills and awareness of subtle signs of stress can help you know which patient is handling feelings effectively and which one is covering up with outward cheerfulness that is inconsistent with inner feelings. By being available and encouraging patients with anxiety to bring their fears into the open and talk about them, you can contribute to their well-being. Secret fears loom very large. When brought out into the open and discussed, they often become less frightening.

## The Overly Friendly Patient

Occasionally, you may have a patient who is overly friendly. Such behavior may consist of personal questions or physical contact. The person who begins to ask personal questions may be trying innocently to make conversation or may be attempting to establish an overly familiar relationship. It is better to avoid discussing your personal life and your own experiences with patients. Instead, direct the conversation to the patient or to impersonal topics.

Unnecessary physical contact may indicate a need for reassurance or it may be an attempt at familiarity. If you are sure the behavior is an attempt to be familiar, calmly state that you prefer that the patient discontinue the behavior. Whenever behavior exceeds desirable limits, make the limits clear. Do not, however, be so expectant of familiarity that you misinterpret a patient's plea for reassurance. To many patients, touch provides a source of strength and comfort.

Situations involving familiarity should be discussed with your supervisor. *Be sure to report facts—what actually happened.* Do not color your report with what you would have liked

FIGURE 16-7 Some behaviors are a cover for fear. *Delmar/Cengage Learning*

the situation to be, with judgmental statements, or with opinions. The supervisor can best assess the situation if you give an accurate account of what the patient said or did and what you said or did. The supervisor's professional judgment can provide guidelines for members of the health team who are caring for the patient.

## REFERENCES AND SUGGESTED READINGS

Duchek, David. (2008, October). Staying calm when a patient's behavior is out of line: A good day at the practice can be maintained if difficult patients are dealt with the right way. *Ophthalmology Times, 33*(19), 62–64.

Elliot, Rachel, et al. (2008, July–August). Understanding medication compliance and persistence from an economics perspective. *Value in Health, 11*(4), 600–610.

Munoz, Cora, & Luckman, Joan. (2005). *Transcultural communication in health care* (2nd ed.). Clifton Park, NY: Delmar, Cengage Learning.

Tamparo, Carol D., & Lindh, Wilburta Q. (2008). *Therapeutic communication for health professionals* (3rd ed.). Clifton Park, NY: Delmar, Cengage Learning.

U.S. Dept. of Health and Human Services. (2009). Understanding health information privacy. Retrieved from http://www.hhs.gov/ocr/privacy/hipaa/understanding/index.html

Waughfield, Claire G. (2002). Relieving anxiety. In *Mental health concepts* (5th ed., pp. 112–132). Clifton Park, NY: Delmar, Cengage Learning.

## REVIEW AND SELF-CHECK

1. List eight guidelines for improving health care provider relations with patients.

2. List nine behaviors commonly manifested by patients; beside each behavior, describe an appropriate response or behavior for the health care provider.

3. List five behaviors that may indicate a patient's emotional reaction to illness.

4. Explain the following terms and name a behavior that would be an example of each:
   Egocentrism
   Regression

Aggressive behavior

Hostility

5. List five communication techniques that can be used to respond to patients; write a brief explanation of each.

___

## ASSIGNMENTS

1. List four examples of *nonverbal* behavior that may indicate a patient is worried or upset.
2. List four examples of verbal behavior that may indicate hostility.
3. List four examples of "loaded" statements that appear to be "small talk" but could indicate underlying anxiety.
4. For each statement in Assignment 3, list two or more "safe" responses that a health care provider could make to the patient's statement.
5. In a whining tone, Mrs. Z. often asks a member of the health team to do things she could do for herself. List four other behaviors that would be a manifestation of regression.
6. Mrs. H. is crying. She tells you her husband is not paying any attention to her while she is sick. You have noticed that he visits each day for about 30 minutes. Mrs. H. told you when she entered the hospital that her husband would be trying to work and manage their home while she is hospitalized. There are two school-age children. Is Mrs. H. being unreasonable? Be prepared to justify your answer.
7. Mr. R. is scheduled for a lobectomy because of lung cancer. He tells you he has smoked two packs of cigarettes a day for 20 years. He is very cheerful, joking with all members of the health team. You have been caring for him for several days and notice that he paces back and forth in his room when he is alone. Discuss this patient in terms of his probable emotional state, his needs as a patient, and the health team's responsibilities to him.
8. Write a brief description of a situation in which a patient exhibited a pattern of behavior discussed in this unit. Indicate the response or behavior you think would be most appropriate for a health care provider.

# UNIT 17

# Human Relations and the Health Care Provider

## OBJECTIVES

Upon completion of this unit, you should be able to:

- List three guidelines for improving one's interpersonal skills.
- List seven ways a health care provider can help patients adjust to illness.
- Explain the health care provider's role in identifying a patient's needs.
- List three ways a health care provider can provide emotional support for a patient.
- State five guidelines for becoming an effective member of the health care team.
- List three beliefs that contribute to a favorable work attitude.
- State three ways in which a health care provider can maintain up-to-date knowledge and skills.

## KEY TERMS

Compensation
Counterpart
Dynamic

Horizontal
   communication

Vertical
   communication

You are now more aware of human behavior than you were at the beginning of this course. You can use your knowledge about human behavior to understand yourself and others. You can consciously evaluate the outcomes of your life experiences in an effort to understand how your behavior influences such outcomes. You can strive to eliminate ineffective behaviors and develop behavior patterns that produce favorable results. If you are making such efforts, then you have gained from this study of human behavior.

Skill in interpersonal relations does not develop overnight, nor does it suddenly appear as a result of wishful thinking. It develops through continuous striving. Slow and steady progress in developing human relations skills is your goal, rather than sudden and complete achievement. The approaches described can help you apply your present knowledge to various areas of living.

## HELPING PATIENTS ADJUST TO ILLNESS

Your patients come to the health agency with the effects of illness added to their usual problems. There are some—perhaps many—stressors in their life situations; illness is an additional stressor. To some people, the health agency is a strange place. For some, it is so threatening that the patient enters only as a desperate effort to get help. In a stressful situation such as the hospital, the patient uses patterns of behavior that have proven useful in past threatening situations. Then, the patient meets you.

You are at home in this environment. The instruments and equipment are useful and meaningful items that make up a large part of your daily routine. You may or may not like your work. You may or may not like your coworkers. You may feel good, or you may feel terrible today. You may have problems at home. You have your own frustrations and conflicts.

### Rising above Your Own Problems

Do you have the right to inflict your personal problems on this troubled patient? Your role is to provide health care. To do so effectively, you must handle your own problems of living well enough to give your full attention to your patients. When you report for work each day, the problems of your personal life must be set aside until you have completed that day's work. *You cannot deal with job problems and home problems at the same time.* Put personal matters aside while you are on the job, so you can give your full attention to your patients (Figure 17-1).

**FIGURE 17-1** Do not carry your personal problems to work with you.
*Delmar/Cengage Learning*

## Identifying a Patient's Needs

You have learned about some influences on patient behavior. Use this knowledge to understand and accept each patient as a person. You do not serve Mrs. Jones's needs when you tell your coworkers "she just acts like that because she has a conflict." You may or may not be right about the cause of her behavior. Your role is to be aware of *possible* meanings of behavior in terms of patient needs. Recognizing some of the possible influences on behavior is the key to identifying patient needs, not the source of conversational topics.

If you think a patient's behavior indicates unmet needs, discuss the patient's behavior with your supervisor. Sometimes, the health team needs to study a patient situation in an effort to identify needs. Striving to understand the behavior of your patients should be approached *in a thoroughly ethical and responsible way* (Figure 17-2).

## Introducing a Patient to the Health Agency

Each new patient should have health agency procedures explained so the patient knows what to expect. Explain a procedure before doing it. Answer the patient's questions or refer the question to the appropriate person (Figure 17-3). Through careful orientation of a patient to the health agency, its policies and procedures, and the plan of care, misunderstandings can be minimized. These measures can relieve a patient's fear of the unknown. Your interested, sincere, and pleasant manner can build the patient's confidence in members of the health care team.

## Adapting Your Behavior

Accept each patient as a worthy person. Remember that the patient's behavior is an effort to deal with the present situation. If it becomes apparent that you are having an adverse effect on the patient, change your behavior. Some patients enjoy a cheerful, talkative health

**FIGURE 17-2** There are ethical and unethical ways to use knowledge of human behavior.
Delmar/Cengage Learning

**FIGURE 17-3** Report to the proper person. *Delmar/Cengage Learning*

care provider; others find cheerfulness annoying. As you become more sensitive to the feelings of others, you will be able to adapt your behavior to each patient. If you insist on being the same with all patients, you will be accepted by some but not others.

### Providing Emotional Support

Some patients need emotional support; others draw on their own resources. With increasing sensitivity, you will be able to detect a patient's need for emotional support. Give extra time and attention to such patients, be available to listen, and accept their feelings and behavior. *True emotional support comes more from your availability and acceptance of the patient than anything you actually say.*

### Using Good Judgment

With increasing experience, you will learn which observations should be reported to the appropriate person and which provide clues regarding your appropriate behavior. It is better to report an observation the supervisor considers unimportant than to fail to report something significant. Good judgment in this respect comes from applying learnings from all your courses and from having experience with many different patients.

## BECOMING A MEMBER OF THE HEALTH TEAM

As a health care provider, your interpersonal skills will be a major factor in determining how effective you are.

## Understanding Your Role

The primary requirement for getting along with your coworkers is to know your role and stay within it. Your preparatory course is helping you understand your role as a health care provider. When you accept a position with a specific health agency, you should clearly understand your role within that agency. Most health agencies and hospitals have job descriptions for each position.

If you accept a position in a solo practice office, or even in a small clinic, you may find that roles and responsibilities have not been specified in writing. If there is no job description, discuss your role with the person who employs you and with your supervisor. Take notes, and write out a list of your responsibilities as you understand them. Then ask your supervisor to sign it. Several revisions may be required. Your goal is to have a *written* list of responsibilities. Role confusion can be the cause of misunderstandings, so a written list is your best protection.

It is possible that policies of the employing agency will not permit you to perform some procedures you learned during your course. Many new health care providers are appearing in the health field; responsibilities have not been clearly defined for some of them. In agencies that use several levels of care providers, the division of responsibilities is often based on the availability of prepared workers at each level. If there is an adequate supply of professional workers, those at the technical level are not given as much responsibility as when there is a shortage of professional personnel.

Your exact role in the agency, then, is influenced by the functions of that agency within the community, by the policies and practices of that agency, and by the availability of personnel. If you accept employment with a clear understanding of your role, do not complain later about that role. If an agency offers you a position that does not allow you to use your educational preparation fully, consider whether or not you should accept that position. Being overqualified for a position usually leads either to frustration and job dissatisfaction or to violating existing policies and job descriptions by performing beyond the prescribed role. Both are undesirable situations. It is usually preferable to obtain employment where your role will be consistent with your educational preparation.

Do not assume responsibilities that are beyond the scope of your educational preparation. If the employing agency expands your role, then educational preparation for your expanded duties must be provided; do not assume your expanded duties until after your additional training.

## Maintaining Good Relationships

Satisfactory job relationships include working cooperatively with members of other services in the agency (Figure 17-4). *All* services have responsibilities for serving patients. Respect the role of each service. Recognize that staff members of a service are responsible to the supervisor of that service. Do not give orders to people from another service. Give information if it is needed, but not orders. If there is a problem, your supervisor should discuss it with the supervisor of the other service. This may appear to be a roundabout way to solve a problem, but observing lines of authority prevents confusion and interdepartmental conflict.

## Understanding Organizational Structure

Communication channels in an organization are referred to as vertical or horizontal. When the supervisor communicates with you, that is **vertical communication.** If someone works

**FIGURE 17-4** The health care team functions best when each member understands channels of authority and lines of communication. *Delmar/Cengage Learning*

under your direction, then your communication with that person is vertical. Your supervisor's communications with the top administrative level are vertical.

When your supervisor communicates with the supervisor in another department, that is **horizontal communication.** Usually horizontal communication does not occur below the supervisory level. This does not mean that you cannot talk to people from other departments. It means that problems, policy changes, and other matters affecting two or more departments are handled through horizontal communication at the supervisory level or above. Therefore, if you are aware of a problem involving your **counterpart** from another department, do not approach that person directly. Instead, inform your supervisor who can then use either vertical or horizontal channels of communication to correct the problem.

Interdepartmental conflict can result if appropriate lines of communication are not observed. As a member of the health team, you occupy a position on the vertical organization of your own department and a horizontal position in relation to health care providers of your same level in other departments. *Your communication lines for assignments, problems, reports, and complaints are limited to vertical relationships.*

Be aware of where your specific job fits within the organizational chart. Be clear about who is in a vertical relationship to you and who has a horizontal relationship. It is possible to learn from experienced workers whose relationship to you is horizontal. But you receive your orders from the person who has a vertical relationship to you—your supervisor or team leader—and you report to that person.

The principles of effective human relations and effective communication also apply to your interactions with coworkers, friends, and relatives. As you strive to improve your human relations skills, practice interacting and communicating effectively with everyone, not just patients. Over time, your communication skills will improve and you will find it easier to form satisfying relationships with others.

## Job Satisfaction, Standards, and Self-Respect

It is each health care provider's responsibility to know the extent and limitations of a role, to know how to carry out the responsibilities of that role, and to maintain high performance standards. You will see health care providers who use flawless technique in all that they do. You may see others who take every shortcut they can. If you set high standards for yourself and live up to them throughout your career, you will be able to take pride in your work.

If you set high standards for your performance, you may be told occasionally that you are being too particular. Some people not only make minimal effort themselves, they also try to get others to do as they do. It requires determination to hold high standards. In the health field, high standards protect patients from errors or the results of poor technique. Through practice, high standards of performance become part of one's value system. By upholding high standards at all times, a person can become incapable of violating good technique. On the other hand, if one uses sloppy technique most of the time, any attempt to use good technique seems to require much effort. Actually, good technique requires no more effort than sloppy technique, and it enables one to take pride in a job well done. Such pride contributes to self-respect and job satisfaction.

## Attitudes

Attitudes consist of a mixture of feelings, beliefs, and behaviors. Many attitudes are learned early in life by imitating adults. Some attitudes are formed unconsciously on the basis of experience. A boy who was often severely punished by his red-haired first-grade teacher may go through life with a bad attitude toward redheaded people, but he may not associate his attitude with those early painful experiences.

Your attitudes affect your adjustment as a health care provider. If you have a strong prejudice, you may find it difficult to work with some of your coworkers or care for some patients. Each of us has an attitude toward work. It may be a favorable attitude, such as "one can find much satisfaction in work." It may be unfavorable, such as "work is what you have to do to get some money."

If you have the attitude that work is worthwhile, that it is satisfying to serve others, that it is desirable to do every task to the best of your ability, then your attitudes will help you find much satisfaction from day to day. Dissatisfaction among workers is often the result of poor attitudes toward work and/or persons in authority.

Attitudes affect various aspects of one's performance, but they are especially relevant to teamwork. Consider the differences in attitude in the following examples. JoBeth often finishes her morning assignment before anyone else, then goes on an extended break because, "I've done my assignment." Anna approaches her work in a conscientious manner, often doing something extra for patients and encouraging them to talk. Sometimes she skips break, especially if she is scheduled for an early lunch. When Anna notices that Sarah's morning assignment includes several patients with extensive needs, she says to Sarah, "When I'm finished, I'll help you with Mr. Z." JoBeth overhears that offer and says, "Why do you take on extra work? Mr. Z is her problem."

## Compensation

Salary is sometimes a cause of dissatisfaction in a job. Salaries of health care providers are not as high as those in some types of industries. The choice to work in a health occupation should have been made on the basis of complete information, including knowledge that health agencies usually do not pay salaries comparable to those offered by profit-making organizations. Much progress has been made in recent years, however, and today's health care providers are receiving better salaries than ever before.

**Compensation** other than money can be found in serving others, especially the sick. Only you can decide whether or not the degree of job satisfaction you experience is sufficient to make up for a smaller salary than you might be able to make in some other type of work. Job satisfaction is a highly personal matter. If you know someone who is making a high salary but hates the job, then you are already aware of the importance of job satisfaction to one's happiness. Salary alone is not enough to provide job satisfaction.

## PRACTICING EFFECTIVE PATIENT RELATIONS

Becoming an effective health care provider includes knowing your job, performing well all tasks within the scope of your responsibilities, understanding and applying the concepts and facts relevant to each task, and observing safety precautions (including asepsis as appropriate). Most of the courses you are now studying prepare you to fulfill these requirements. But to be *truly effective*, you must also focus on developing human relations skills—a never-ending challenge. In this section, you have studied several topics that will help you be sensitive to the needs of a patient and understand common behaviors of patients:

- Physical and emotional effects of illness
- General effects of serious illness
- Influences on a patient's reaction to illness (age, life role, usual state of adjustment, dependency, cultural background, past experience)
- Common behavior patterns
- Strategies for coping with certain problem behaviors

You have also studied several topics that are relevant to you as a health care provider—*the beliefs and attitudes that you personally bring to the role*—important aspects of your personal effectiveness:

- Acceptance of each patient as a worthwhile human being (including tolerance for those who are different from you)
- Interest in and concern for each patient
- Willingness to listen
- Accuracy in observing
- Ability to recognize significant behaviors
- Respect for confidentiality
- Being sensitive to a patient's feelings and providing emotional support as needed

- Willingness to try to identify needs and serve each patient in accordance with those needs
- Ability to put your personal problems aside while caring for patients
- Willingness to adapt your behavior as needed to interact effectively with a variety of patients exhibiting many different behavior patterns

These topics deal with how you relate to your patients. Another major aspect of good human relations is how you communicate, verbally and nonverbally. In Unit 15, you learned how to convey caring, some reasons for ineffective communication, and responses that tend to block further communication. In Unit 16, you learned several specific communication techniques: echoing and reflecting, clarifying, validating, questioning, and confronting. Becoming a skillful communicator requires conscious effort and practice.

In Section V, you will have the opportunity to practice improving your communication skills. In Unit 18, you will practice interpreting nonverbal behavior and in Unit 19 you will learn additional aspects of effective verbal communication. In each of these units, you will have the opportunity to participate in role-play situations as a means of polishing your communication skills and increasing your sensitivity to the *real messages* sent to you by another person.

## THE CHALLENGE

One exciting aspect of the health field is that it is **dynamic**—ever-changing. Research produces new knowledge every day. No one knows for sure what the treatment for certain diseases will be in the future.

If you wish to be an alert and informed member of the health team, you will need to read your professional journals, be active in your professional association, attend staff development programs, and become active in community health programs. It is highly satisfying to be well informed, but remaining well informed in the health field requires continual effort. If you sit back and admire your diploma for 20 years, you will not remain up to date in your field.

Look around you at the health workers you see every day. Some are interested in their work and are up to date on information and techniques. Others come to work each day, but do not make an effort to continue learning. Which type of worker do you want to be in 15 years? Your attitudes toward work and your efforts to be informed will determine which type of health care provider you become.

## REFERENCES AND SUGGESTED READING

Breggin, Peter R. (2006). *The heart of being helpful: Empathy and the creation of a healing presence.* New York: Springer Publishing Company.

Munoz, Cora, & Luckmann, Joan. (2005). *Transcultural communication in nursing* (2nd ed.). Clifton Park, NY: Delmar, Cengage Learning.

Sanow, Arnold, & Strauss, Sandra. (2007). *Get along with anyone anytime anywhere! 8 keys to creating enduring connections with customers, co-workers, even kids!* Vienna, VA: Nautilus Communications.

Tamparo, Carol, & Lindh, Wilburta. (2008). *Therapeutic communications for health care* (3rd ed.). Clifton Park, NY: Delmar, Cengage Learning.

## REVIEW AND SELF-CHECK

1. List three guidelines you could use to improve your interpersonal skills.

2. List seven ways you, as a health care provider, can help a patient adjust to illness.

3. Explain why a health care provider should be concerned about identifying a patient's needs.

4. List three ways you can offer emotional support to a patient.

5. List five guidelines that could help you become an effective member of the health care team.

6. List three beliefs that contribute to a favorable attitude toward work.

7. List three ways to keep one's knowledge and skills up to date.

## ASSIGNMENTS

1. List five benefits of improving your interpersonal skills.
2. Participate in a class discussion about ways you can minimize a new patient's fears.
3. Explain vertical lines of communication (and authority) in relation to your role on the health care team within the health agency affiliated with your educational program.
4. Identify the job title of your counterpart (horizontal relationship) in another service within the affiliated health agency.
5. Explain why you should discuss patient problems with your supervisor rather than with coworkers.
6. List five guidelines for continued growth as a health care provider after you have become employed in a health agency.
7. One of your coworkers has been employed at a health care agency for 15 years when you arrive as a new employee. In spite of having seniority, this person has a horizontal relationship to you and others with your job title. Two or three times a week, this coworker tells you to do some task. Because she speaks with an authoritative tone, you tend to comply with her instructions. Yesterday, your supervisor said, "You are not assigned to Mrs. X. Why are you doing her treatments?" When you explain, the supervisor says, "You get your assignments from me."

    Today, this coworker says, "You walk Mr. Z this afternoon." Mr. Z is not assigned to you. How will you respond?

**Note:** Your instructor may allow class time for role-playing this situation or a full class discussion.

8. Develop a chart to show how your job title relates to other job titles in the agency where you are getting your clinical experience.

   a. Insert job titles to show vertical relationships:

   The person to whom your supervisor reports

   Your supervisor

   Your job title

   Any persons who report to you

   b. List three job titles that are not in your department but have a horizontal (equal) relationship to your job title.

SECTION V

# Practicing Effective Communication

You have learned a number of things about human behavior: ways people are alike and different; the basic needs of people and how they attempt to meet these needs; how people try to protect themselves against real or imagined threats to security, happiness, peace of mind, or general well-being; and ways people react to physical illness and the problems that accompany it.

Applying knowledge about human behavior to relationships with others is easily talked about, but difficult to practice. There must be a beginning, however, and that beginning can lead to a high level of skill for those who continuously strive for improvement. This section will provide opportunities for practicing three skills that are basic to understanding human behavior: observing the behavior of others, observing your own behavior, and adapting your behavior according to how you "read" another person's behavior.

# UNIT 18

# Observing Nonverbal Behavior

## OBJECTIVES

Upon completion of this unit, you should be able to:

- Explain the meaning of "skill in interpersonal relations."
- Describe selective observing.
- List five examples of nonverbal behavior that may convey a message.
- State five steps for improving your use of nonverbal communication.
- Observe nonverbal behavior.
- Interpret the message of nonverbal behavior.
- Recognize your own patterns of nonverbal behavior.
- Use nonverbal communication purposefully to improve interpersonal relations.

## KEY TERMS

Selective observing          Stance

You have heard much about "good human relations" since you began your preparation for a career in the health field. Have you thought about the *real meaning* of that expression? Does it mean that knowing about influences on human behavior makes it easy to develop good human relations? Perhaps you already recognize that such is not the case, because good human relations require far more than just *knowing about* human behavior. Actually, good human relations involve a conscious effort to *select your behavior* for a given situation, rather than allowing habit or emotions to determine what you say and do.

Skill in interpersonal relations may be thought of as *controlled* interaction with others. It means control over what happens by *consciously deciding* what to say or do to bring about the response you desire from another person. It is seldom possible to control what happens completely, but you can have an influence. When your behavior arouses positive feelings in others, then it is likely that the behavior of the other person toward you will be favorable. On the other hand, your behavior can arouse negative feelings in others: anxiety, anger, a sense of threat, self-pity, feelings of being "put down," or just plain irritation. When your behavior arouses negative feelings, then the behavior of the other person toward you may be unpleasant: noncooperation, complaints, withdrawal, or disagreement with whatever you say.

To learn how to select appropriate behavior, you must first learn to use any available evidence to determine the other person's feelings. Some of the evidence lies in *what* is said and *how* it is said. Some consists of the other person's behavior. Much of the evidence, especially in a stressful situation, lies in nonverbal communication. And so, your learning to influence the outcome of a given situation must start by learning to observe nonverbal behavior—a form of communication that is often more meaningful than spoken communication.

## OBSERVING AND INTERPRETING NONVERBAL BEHAVIOR

Most of us think we are observant and that our observations are reasonably accurate. **Selective observing** means that we notice some details of a situation, while completely missing many other details. Left to chance, observations are likely to be made according to one's interests or curiosity. To become skillful in observing nonverbal behavior, your selective observing must include nonverbal behavior.

Most people communicate feelings through nonverbal behavior, often unconsciously. But regardless of whether or not the nonverbal behavior is conscious, it signals that the person is responding to something—perhaps to you as a person, something you said or did, your tone of voice, the expression on your face, and the other person's interpretation of what it means. It is also possible that the behavior indicates the individual's response to the total situation: the stress of a job interview, anger at being ill, fear of surgery, or the expectation of an unfavorable diagnosis. Nonverbal communication, then, provides a clue to a person's inner feelings (Figure 18-1). In some cases, it is also a signal that more specific behavior, such as an angry outburst, is about to occur.

The message of nonverbal behavior is lost unless you note it and interpret the meaning correctly. To improve your use of nonverbal communication, consciously practice observing the nonverbal behavior of others. Next, practice interpreting that behavior and check your interpretation against further evidence. When you interact with another person, note any

**FIGURE 18-1** A patient's body language may reveal feelings of anxiety.
*Delmar/Cengage Learning*

changes in facial expression, slight movements of facial muscles, position of the lips, direction of gaze, position of the eyelids, body movements, **stance** (how a person stands), general posture, and the hands—position and movements. Experts use the ability to read people to help them select members for a jury or screen job applicants. Jury consultant and author Jo-Ellan Dimitrius suggests that physical traits, dress, and body language all provide clues to people's personalities and emotional states.

After noting the nonverbal clues, try to interpret that behavior. Does a twitching facial muscle indicate stress? Or repressed anger? If stress, why does the individual feel stressed in this situation? Do the restless movements of the hands indicate nervousness? If so, why does the person feel nervous in this situation? What is the person's emotional state? What expectations does the person have? Are you sending nonverbal messages to which that individual is responding? By associating the nonverbal behavior of a specific person with additional evidence as it becomes available, you can learn to "read" that person with a reasonable degree of accuracy.

Interpretation of nonverbal behavior carries the risk of misinterpretation. This is a serious risk, for *misinterpretation can lead to more misunderstanding than simply ignoring the nonverbal communication*. The risk of misinterpretation can be decreased by following six steps:

1. Note the nonverbal behavior.
2. Make a *tentative* interpretation.
3. Continue to observe for more evidence, especially evidence that is easily interpreted—a display of anger, statements of disapproval, objections, or complaints.
4. Revise your interpretation if there is evidence that the first interpretation was not accurate.
5. Watch for *consistency*, that is, occurrence of a specific nonverbal behavior every time that individual is in a particular situation, such as making a decision, doing something new, speaking before a group, or coping with conflict.
6. Use verbal communication to clarify the meaning of the nonverbal behavior. For example, if it is appropriate in a given situation, you could say, "Pat, you seem upset. What's going on?"

Once you have detected the pattern and determined that certain nonverbal behaviors consistently indicate a specific feeling state of that person, you have learned "to read" that person's nonverbal behavior (Figure 18-2).

With friends and coworkers, you may become quite accurate at reading their feelings without any words being exchanged. Accuracy in interpretation is achieved only over a period of time and through frequent opportunities to observe an individual in a variety of situations. Even then you may find it difficult to interpret some nonverbal behavior. You may practice trying to read one of your coworkers over a long period of time, and finally say, "Look, I have noticed that you often pick up a pencil and roll it between your fingers. At first I thought you do this when you feel irritated; then it seemed that you do this when you are bored; but just now you did it after laughing at Joe's story. Tell me, just why do you pick up a pencil and twirl it?" Your friend may give you an answer that indicates one of your interpretations was correct, may indicate a lack of awareness of the behavior, or may admit not knowing the reason for it. Your friend may say that all of your attempts at explaining the behavior are wrong: "I formed that habit when I quit smoking. Now, every time I see someone light up, I pick up a pencil and twirl it. I suppose it serves the purpose my smoking used to serve." Note that in this case you still do not have an interpretation of the *feeling state* when this behavior occurs. So continue to watch your friend's use of this particular behavior in different situations.

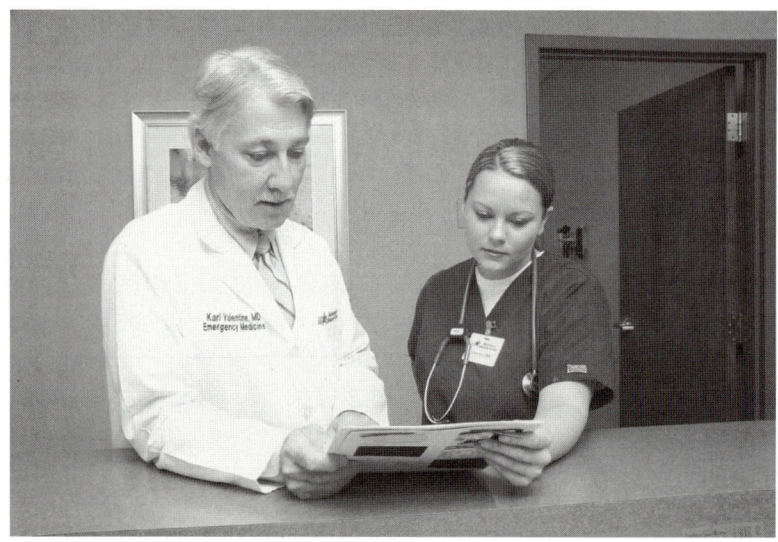

**FIGURE 18-2** Without observing nonverbal behavior, how can you be sure someone understands what you have explained? *Delmar/Cengage Learning*

With people you see less frequently, you will not be able to learn the meaning of their nonverbal clues as readily. And, with people you see only occasionally or for brief periods of time, you must make your best judgment of the probable meaning of nonverbal behavior and try to confirm that interpretation as the relationship proceeds.

In relating to patients and their families, look for nonverbal behavior that may mean a buildup of feelings, especially fear, anxiety, confusion, and anger. When you detect such signals, it is likely that the patient would benefit from extra attention in the form of sincere interest, concern, consideration, and emotional support while adapting to strange surroundings and illness.

The special attention you provide may encourage the patient to talk. You might invite questions with, "Is there something you would like me to explain? I will try to answer any questions you have." You may be able to answer some questions but find it necessary to refer others to appropriate persons—the patient's physician, the supervisor, or another department of the health facility. You will be safe in giving information about routines and the facility itself. Questions about the patient's condition should be handled by others, usually the physician. Your role is to provide emotional support for the patient when you listen to questions, show sincere concern, and state that you will pass any questions you cannot answer on to the person who can provide answers.

As you gain experience in reading nonverbal behavior, you will detect many different indicators of patients' negative feelings. With increased skill in relating to others, you will be ready for the next challenge: encouraging others to express their feelings. You can do this while performing a procedure or otherwise serving a patient's needs by physical actions. You may lead off with a casual statement such as, "I suppose this visit to us is something of a nuisance to you," or "Most people find our agency a little frightening on their first visit." You might ask a direct question, but select your words carefully to avoid the appearance of prying. "Were you surprised that the doctor wanted you to have these studies done?" Or, "Have you had this type of test before?"

A *full exploration of feelings* is best left to professionals with counseling skills. However, you can encourage *expression of feelings* and still remain within your role as a health care provider. Be aware that your patient is a human being going through a stressful experience, indicate your willingness to listen, and give your full attention to the patient. But, in order to recognize those who need an understanding listener, you must receive the message. A *message of need is most likely to be sent nonverbally.*

The purpose of observing nonverbal communication, then, is to become sensitive to—or aware of—the feelings of others as conveyed by small bits of behavior, rather than words. This sensitivity enables you to adapt your behavior to these feelings and select your response consciously. The favorable effect may consist of providing emotional support, conveying that you care, defusing the other's fear or anger, or providing an invitation to release pent-up feelings by talking about the situation that aroused the feelings.

## SETTING THE STAGE FOR PRACTICING INTERPERSONAL SKILLS

It is difficult to develop human relations skills without assistance from others. You need guidance from someone who has already developed a high level of skill: your teachers, other health professionals, a member of the school staff who has specialized in interpersonal relations, or possibly someone from the community who is a specialist in human relations.

### Early Practice

Your beginning efforts to develop skill are best conducted in association with your classmates. You are all striving for improved interpersonal skills. Through the common knowledge you have all gained from your course, you should now be able to accept one another's efforts without criticism, accept suggestions from one another about how to improve, and explore your own feelings in a situation in which others are also exploring their feelings. Ideally, your class will have a regular time for practicing interpersonal skills throughout the remainder of your course.

### Continuing Practice

When you leave the school setting, opportunities for group practice may not be readily available. If you wish to continue practicing in a group situation, find a course or workshop that will provide opportunities for continued practice of your communication skills.

When you are employed as a health care provider, you will have to rely primarily on your own assessment of outcomes. As you improve your observation skills, you will be more aware of the effect of your behavior on other people. As you interact over a period of time with coworkers and patients, you can test your interpretations of their behavior. You will never reach the point of always interpreting behavior correctly. There is the ever-present risk of being wrong. Keep an open mind and be ready to revise your interpretation as you make new observations.

Striving to improve communication skills begins with practice in noting behaviors that signal the inner feelings or thoughts of a person. An observer who is fairly accurate in noting and interpreting these signals can anticipate the type of behavior about to occur and encourage it, or possibly change it, by careful selection of words or actions (Figure 18-3). The following exercises are designed to help you practice recognizing and interpreting nonverbal communication.

**FIGURE 18-3** Feedback from an observer helps us to be aware of our own nonverbal behavior. *Delmar/Cengage Learning*

## EXERCISE 18–1: OBSERVING NONVERBAL BEHAVIOR

### PURPOSE

In this exercise, you will discuss the messages conveyed by a series of nonverbal behaviors.

### INSTRUCTIONS

1. Work in groups of two. One partner will be the actor and the other the observer. In round 2, you will reverse roles.
2. Without speaking, the actor will demonstrate each of the nonverbal behaviors listed. After each behavior, the observer will comment briefly on the message he believes the behavior is sending. (There are a number of possible explanations for each behavior.)

### NONVERBAL BEHAVIORS: ROUND 1

1. Cross your arms.
2. Roll your eyes.
3. Look at the floor.
4. Jiggle your leg for several seconds.
5. Fiddle with your pencil or pen.
6. Sit up very straight in your chair.

## NONVERBAL BEHAVIOR: ROUND 2

1. Clench your fists.
2. Sigh loudly.
3. Smile.
4. Tap your fingers on the table repeatedly.
5. Look at your watch.
6. Make direct eye contact with your partner.

## EXERCISE 18–2: OBSERVING AND INTERPRETING NONVERBAL BEHAVIOR

### PURPOSE

In this exercise you will observe and interpret nonverbal communication and test your interpretation against the person's explanation of the thoughts and feelings that accompanied the nonverbal behavior.

### INSTRUCTIONS

1. Divide into groups of four. Two people will be actors and two will be observers. In round 2, you will reverse roles.
2. Select one of the situations below to role-play. The actors may take a few minutes to plan their performance while the observers review the information in Unit 18.
3. Actors role-play the situation for five minutes. During this time, observers list the nonverbal behaviors they see and note what was happening in the role-play when the behavior occurred. One of the observers should call time after five minutes.
4. Observers describe the nonverbal behaviors they witnessed and offer a possible interpretation for each behavior. Actors confirm whether each interpretation matches what they were thinking or feeling at the time.
5. Reverse roles so that the actors are now observers and the observers are now actors. Repeat the exercise using a different situation.

### ROLE-PLAYS FOR EXERCISE 18–2

1. Jane often arrives late to work and asks to leave early. Her supervisor decides to discuss the matter with her.
2. Rob, an experienced lab technician, notices a new technician using sloppy procedures and taking shortcuts. Concerned about accuracy and a reprimand from the supervisor, he confronts his coworker.
3. Arturo has recently immigrated to the United States and must get a physical for his new job. He has never been examined by a doctor before, and his English is limited. A nurse sits down to help him fill out paperwork and to get a medical history.

4. Mrs. Jones, an elderly patient, is hard of hearing. She takes several prescription medications. She asks a staff person to explain how much of each medication she should take and when.

5. Fifteen-year-old Lisa has come to the clinic for a pregnancy test, which is positive. A clinic worker gives her the test results and discusses her options with her.

## REFERENCES AND SUGGESTED READINGS

Munoz, Cora, & Luckmann, Joan. (2005). *Transcultural communication in health care* (2nd ed.) Clifton Park, NY: Delmar, Cengage Learning.

Pease, Barbara, & Pease, Allen. (2006). *The definitive book of body language.* New York: Bantam.

Tamparo, Carol T., & Lindh, Wilburta Q. (2008). *Therapeutic communications for health professionals* (3rd ed.). Clifton Park, NY: Delmar, Cengage Learning.

## REVIEW AND SELF-CHECK

1. Explain the meaning of "skill in interpersonal relations."

2. Explain the meaning of "selective observing."

3. List five examples of nonverbal behavior that may convey a message about the sender's thoughts or feelings.

4. List five steps for improving one's own patterns of nonverbal communication.

5. Explain why a health care provider should develop skills in observing and interpreting nonverbal behavior.

___

## ASSIGNMENTS

1. The next time you watch a situation comedy on TV, concentrate your attention on one of the lead actors and note examples of nonverbal communication. Did the other characters react to or ignore the nonverbal communication? Did any specific example lead to a misunderstanding or conflict between two of the characters?

2. The next time you watch a comedian who does imitations, note the various mannerisms and facial expressions the comedian portrays. Comedians are keen observers of human behavior, and imitators are especially observant of small bits of behavior that characterize an individual. Note the specific mannerisms portrayed in the actor's imitation of a certain person.

3. Use your next movie or TV evening to study the communication styles of the actors. Especially note examples of the following:

    a. An actor who has a frozen countenance (facial expression does not change) most of the time. What nonverbal behaviors does this actor use to communicate?

    b. An actor who uses subtle changes in facial expression. What "body language" does this actor use to supplement facial expression?

    c. An actor who conveys feelings primarily through facial expression. Does this actor also make use of body language to communicate feelings and/or reactions to the action occurring?

    d. Turn down the volume for at least five minutes during a television show and observe the characters' facial expressions and body language without sound. Can you follow the plot, based on the actors' nonverbal communication?

# UNIT 19

# Verbal Communication

## OBJECTIVES

Upon completion of this unit, you should be able to:

- List three sources of communication breakdown.
- List three reasons why it is difficult to avoid ambiguity in verbal communication.
- List three ways to minimize ambiguity.
- List four sender-related causes of message discrepancy.
- List four receiver-related causes of message discrepancy.
- List two reasons why assumptions are a source of communication breakdown.
- Explain why expectations may cause a communication breakdown.
- List five ways to send a clear message.
- List four ways to "hear" a message correctly.

## KEY TERMS

| | | |
|---|---|---|
| Ambiguity | Clarification | Inconsistency |
| Assume | Enunciation | Paraphrase |
| Assumptions | Expectation | Reprimand |

Workers in the health field spend much time communicating with others: patients and their families, visitors to the health agency, other members of the health team, and supervisors. As a health care provider, you need a high level of communication skill. Whenever and wherever people talk to one another, communication problems may occur.

It is tempting to assume that whatever you say to another person is understood—that your listener gets the meaning you intend to convey. In reality, there are numerous sources of communication breakdown: our language permits different meanings for many words, speech and hearing factors may distort what is heard, and nonverbal messages may differ from the spoken message. Many examples of misunderstanding, noncooperation, criticism, and other forms of conflict between people can be traced to a communication problem. Your preparation for working in the health field includes practice in improving your communication skills so you will have a minimum of communication problems (Figure 19-1).

**FIGURE 19-1** Successful communication is a two-way exchange.
*Delmar/Cengage Learning*

## AMBIGUITY

**Ambiguity** means vague, unclear. The opposite of ambiguity is clarity. The word *unambiguous* is sometimes used to mean completely clear or free of ambiguity.

It is difficult to avoid ambiguity in verbal communication for a number of reasons:

- A word may have several different meanings.
- The word used by the speaker may not be the best word for expressing the desired meaning.
- A pronoun may not clearly indicate whom or what it represents.

For example, the word *smart* is used by some people to mean very intelligent; another person uses *smart* to mean sassy or disrespectful. Can you think of other meanings for this one word?

Some words or phrases have double meanings. They can be interpreted literally, or they may be used to mean something entirely different. The following illustrates this type of ambiguity:

*A: "This cat is really good for mice."*

*B: "How can you say that? He is afraid of mice. He even runs from them."*

*C: "That's just what I mean. He is very good for the mice."*

A pronoun that may refer to more than one noun is another source of ambiguity. Suppose a patient tells the nurse, "Dr. Brown and Dr. White (both males) both came by to see me last night. They think I'm doing fine. He even said I may go home today." Does "he" refer to Dr. Brown or to Dr. White?

In attempting to avoid ambiguous statements, you should:

- Use words that have a single, precise meaning whenever possible.
- Use the best word for what you want to say.
- Use a noun to indicate who or what; if you use a pronoun (he, she, it, they), it should clearly refer to *one specific noun* used in the same sentence.

## DISCREPANCIES IN A MESSAGE

Most of us are careless about verbal communication, especially when we are trying to attend to many things at once. In haste, we say *approximately* what we mean, then **assume** that the message received by the listener is the same as the message we intended to send. (To assume is to suppose that something is true, without having any proof.) Also, we sometimes send one message nonverbally and state a different message verbally. Which message is the listener to believe?

Message discrepancy means that the message sent and the message received differ in meaning. The difficulty may be with the sender of the message or the receiver. When the problem is with the sender, it may be caused by:

- Ambiguity in the message.
- **Inconsistency** in the verbal and nonverbal messages.
- Poor **enunciation,** causing some words to sound like other words with a different meaning.
- Use of language the listener does not understand. (This is likely to occur if the listener is a child, a person from a different culture, or an elderly person who may not be familiar with newer meanings of a word.)

If the problem of message discrepancy lies with the receiver, it may be caused by:

- Poor hearing.
- Selective listening (the individual listens only to certain parts of a statement).
- Inability to understand the words used by the speaker, such as medical terminology.
- Acceptance of the wrong message when there is inconsistency in the sender's verbal and nonverbal communication.

An example of inconsistency in verbal and nonverbal messages is the crying patient who says, "I'm all right. I feel fine." Sometimes the health care provider who is alert to nonverbal messages can pick up the true situation, as when a patient says, "There is nothing really wrong with me. The doctor says these are just routine tests." At the same time, the patient's countenance reflects a high level of anxiety. Whenever there is inconsistency in verbal and nonverbal messages, the listener must decide which message to believe.

In your endeavors to convey messages that are received (interpreted) as you intend:

- Avoid ambiguous statements.
- Select words and phrases the listener will understand.
- Speak clearly.
- Control your nonverbal signals to avoid sending a message that is different from your verbal message.
- Face the person to whom you are speaking.

## TONE

You have probably heard a parent or teacher scold a child, "Don't take that tone with me!" Tone of voice can be as important as the choice of words in conveying a message to a listener. Responding to someone who is angry in a calm tone of voice often helps diffuse the person's

**FIGURE 19-2** Telephone communication is almost entirely verbal, without the benefit of observing nonverbal behavior. *Delmar/Cengage Learning*

anger. On the other hand, an impatient or harsh tone of voice may hurt or anger the listener. Becoming conscious of your tone of voice helps your listener take your words in the spirit you intend them. Tone is particularly important when talking on the telephone, because the listener does not have the benefit of seeing your facial expressions and other nonverbal behavior (Figure 19-2).

## EFFECTIVE LISTENING

In addition to expressing ideas clearly, a good communicator takes care to "hear" others accurately (Figure 19-3). The following techniques will help you become an effective listener:

- Give your full attention to anyone who is speaking to you.
- Listen to the words and observe nonverbal behavior in an effort to get the "real message."
- **Paraphrase** or restate what the person says to make sure you have understood correctly.
- Use questions to clarify the speaker's intended meaning, especially (1) if the speaker uses ambiguous or unfamiliar words and (2) if the verbal and nonverbal messages are inconsistent.

## ASSUMPTIONS AND EXPECTATIONS

Underlying many communication problems are **assumptions** and expectations held by the speaker or by the listener. An assumption is *acceptance of something as fact without any evidence or proof.* Sometimes we assume that another person "knows" how we feel or what

FIGURE 19-3 Listen with empathy. Try to understand how the patient feels. *Delmar/Cengage Learning*

we are thinking, even though we did not verbally express our thoughts or feelings. Actually, the person to whom we are speaking may be completely unaware of how we feel or what we are thinking. Or the other person may make assumptions about how we think or feel and the assumptions are completely wrong! Making assumptions is certain to create misunderstandings and communication breakdowns.

Another frequent cause of communication problems is the expectation of a person, either the sender or receiver of the message. An **expectation** means thinking that something will occur. An expectation can cause the receiver to "read into" a message something that the sender did not intend. For example, suppose your supervisor walks in while you are taking a shortcut on a task, then later the supervisor sends for you. Having been "caught" taking an unauthorized shortcut, your expectation is that the supervisor is going to **reprimand** you. You are probably set to defend yourself or to accept blame and say you will not do it again. But perhaps, instead of reprimanding you, the supervisor says, "I noticed you were not following procedure. Let's take a close look at the method you were using. It may be more efficient than our present procedure." Let us hope you did not misinterpret the supervisor's opening statement before you found out that your expectation was wrong! Sometimes an expectation can even lead the listener to "hear" a message that is quite different from the words spoken. This takes the speaker by surprise, because the speaker is unaware of the other person's expectations.

## IMPROVING COMMUNICATION SKILLS

Improving your communication skills requires that you test your habits as a sender-of-messages and as a receiver-of-messages. Fortunately, the same practice that helps you become more precise in your sending can also contribute to your skill in listening. As you become sensitive to ambiguities, inconsistencies, assumptions, and expectations, you will ask for **clarification** rather than risk a misunderstanding.

The following exercises are structured to provide practice in speaking, listening, and interpreting messages. In Exercise 19-1, you will increase your awareness of how the tone of a message can alter the meaning you convey to your listener. In Exercise 19-2, you will practice expressing your ideas clearly and listening effectively to the ideas of others.

When you have made progress on each of these skills, the probability of your having a communication breakdown is less. As an effective communicator, you will also be more effective in establishing good relationships.

## EXERCISE 19-1: USING TONE TO ALTER THE MEANING OF A STATEMENT

### PURPOSE

In this exercise, you will practice using and listening to different tones of voice.

### INSTRUCTIONS

1. Work in groups of two. One partner will be the speaker and the other the listener. In round 2, you will reverse roles. Note that although the statements are the same in both rounds, the tones of voice used are not.
2. Role-play the following situations, using the tone of voice indicated. After the speaker has made the statement, the listener comments on how the tone affects the message he or she "hears."

### ROLE-PLAYS: ROUND 1

In this exercise, you will practice making statements that convey your intended meaning to another person, with minimal chance of misinterpretation by the listener.

1. A nurse says to a patient, "Are you ready for your treatment, Mr. Jones?"
   Tone: impatient
2. A supervisor says to an employee, "I expected you at work an hour ago. What happened?"
   Tone: concerned
3. A patient says to a health care provider, "There was a mistake on the last bill I received from your office."
   Tone: hesitant
4. A lab supervisor asks a lab technician, "Are those test results ready yet?"
   Tone: curious
5. A health care provider comments to a co-worker, "Here we are, working the late shift again."
   Tone: resentful

### ROLE-PLAYS: ROUND 2

1. A nurse says to a patient, "Are you ready for your treatment, Mr. Jones?"
   Tone: kind
2. A supervisor says to an employee, "I expected you at work an hour ago. What happened?"
   Tone: irritated
3. A patient says to a health care provider, "There was a mistake on the last bill I received from your office."
   Tone: demanding

4. A lab supervisor asks a lab technician, "Are those test results ready yet?"
   Tone: hurried
5. A health care provider comments to a co-worker, "Here we are, working the late shift again."
   Tone: joking

## EXERCISE 19-2: EXPRESSING IDEAS AND LISTENING EFFECTIVELY

### PURPOSE

In this exercise, you will express your opinion on a topic as clearly as possible. You will also use the listening techniques described earlier to check your understanding and to gain more information about another person's opinion.

### INSTRUCTIONS

1. Organize into groups of three. Each person should get a turn to play the role of the speaker, the observer, and the listener. The roles are described below.
2. The opinion statements that follow will serve as the basis for your discussion. Select a different opinion statement for each of the three rounds.
3. The speaker will discuss an opinion about one of the statements. The listener will use the listening skills described in this unit to check for understanding and to gain more information. After five minutes, the observer will call time and will provide feedback about the communication skills and listening skills observed.

**Speaker** Your objective is to communicate your opinion clearly to the listener. Select for discussion one of the opinion statements listed following this exercise. Explain why you agree or disagree with the statement. Feel free to use your personal knowledge and experiences to support your opinion.

**Listener** Your objective is to use effective listening techniques to gain a full understanding of the speaker's opinion. You are not to express your own opinion while playing the role of listener.

**Observer** Your objective is to provide feedback for the speaker and listener according to these guidelines:

- How clear was the speaker's first statement of opinion?
- How did the listener show that he or she was listening?
- Which listening skills did you observe?
- What additional information did the speaker share as a result of the listener's responses?

## OPINION STATEMENTS TO SERVE AS A BASIS FOR DISCUSSION

1. Health care providers should be allowed to go to classes during duty hours if they want to work on a higher certificate.
2. A health care provider should prepare for one role and remain in it throughout his or her career.
3. Advanced courses should be open to all health care providers who want to become professional practitioners.
4. Most people entering a health career want to help the sick.
5. Women make better health care providers than men.
6. Every health care provider wants to stay up to date.
7. People should be required to carry health insurance; then, when they need health care, they will be able to afford it.
8. Patients should not expect health care providers to listen to their problems.
9. The government should take over the costs of health care.
10. Women are more suited to the role of an auxiliary worker than to the role of a professional.
11. Health maintenance organizations are preferable to the fee-for-service system for the delivery of health services.
12. A woman who is pregnant has the right to decide whether or not she will continue the pregnancy.
13. Everyone who has AIDS should be quarantined.
14. Sex education should not be allowed in the public schools. Sex education is for adults, not children.
15. Managed care is the best system for providing health services.

## CLASS CHALLENGE

Some of the opinion statements just listed are related to one or more trends or issues in the health field. Are you informed about these trends and issues? Do you know what changes are being proposed? What are the pros and cons for each issue?

You may wish to continue your work on communication skills by studying an issue, then preparing an oral report, one side of a debate, or a written report. Thus, you will learn about important trends that may affect your work situation in the future and, at the same time, improve your ability to communicate ideas clearly.

## REFERENCES AND SUGGESTED READINGS

Donoghue, Paul, & Siegel, Mary. (2005). *Are you really listening? Key to successful communication.* Notre Dame, IN: Ave Maria Press.

McKay, Matthew, et al. (2009). *Messages: The communication skills handbook.* Oakland, CA: New Harbinger.

Munoz, Cora, & Luckmann, Joan. (2005). *Transcultural communication in health care* (2nd ed.). Clifton Park, NY: Delmar, Cengage Learning.

Tamparo, Carol T., & Lindh, Wilburta Q. (2008). *Therapeutic communications for health professionals* (3rd ed.). Clifton Park, NY: Delmar, Cengage Learning.

Unit 19: Verbal Communication   **289**

## REVIEW AND SELF-CHECK

1. List three common sources of communication breakdown.
   - different meanings for many words
   - speech & hearing _____
   - nonverbal _____

2. State three reasons it is difficult to avoid ambiguity in verbal communication.
   - word may have several meanings
   - speakers use word that is not best
   - pronoun used (use name instead)

3. List three ways to minimize ambiguity.
   - use single, precise words
   - use the best word
   - use noun to indicate who or what

4. List four causes of message discrepancy:

   a. By the sender.
   - ambiguity in the message
   - inconsistencies verbal & nonverbal message
   - poor enunciation

   b. By the receiver.
   - use of language listener does not understand
   - the listener may contribute to message discrepancy
   - by poor hearing, selective hearing, inability to understand,
   - acceptance of wrong message

5. Explain why a communication breakdown may be due to:

   a. Assumptions of the sender or receiver.
   - To assume means accept something as fact w/out proof; an expectation
   - is thinking that something will happen

   b. Expectations of the sender or receiver.
   - As sender, you can minimize message discrepancy by:
   - avoid vague words, select words that patient will understand,
   - speak clearly, avoid nonverbal signal

6. List five guidelines for sending a clear message.

   avoid vague words

7. List four guidelines for "hearing" a message correctly.

## ASSIGNMENTS

Complete the following exercises during the next month.

1. As you watch television or a movie, note examples of:

   a. Communication breakdown.

   b. Poor listening skills on the part of one or more characters.

   c. Message discrepancy.

   d. Nonverbal communication unnoticed by other characters.

2. In a class discussion:

   a. List movies or TV programs in which a communication breakdown is a major basis for the plot.

   b. Share examples noted in Assignment 1. Discuss the apparent cause(s) (e.g., faulty assumptions, message discrepancy, poor listening skills, etc.) of the communication problems in each example that was observed.

# Section VI

# Coping with Loss

You have now learned about human behavior, ways people react to threat, and how to communicate effectively. These learnings will be especially valuable as you work with people who are struggling to cope with loss. The ultimate losses are death (loss of one's own life) and bereavement (loss of a loved one).

In order to provide effective care to a terminally ill patient or to help those who are facing the loss of a loved one, the health care provider must have arrived at full acceptance of his or her own mortality and must have resolved any "unfinished business" related to past losses.

The purpose of Section VI is to help you acknowledge your own mortality, clarify your beliefs about death, and become sensitive to the needs of terminally ill patients and their families.

# UNIT 20

# Gains and Losses throughout the Life Span

## OBJECTIVES

Upon completion of this unit, you should be able to:

- State one reason that a happy life event may be accompanied by sadness or depression.
- State three reasons that it is important to consciously grieve for the small losses of life.
- List four steps for learning to cope with loss.
- Explain the significance of a loss.
- List three examples of loss that occur during each period of the life span: infancy, early childhood, the school-age years, adolescence, the young adult years, middle and late adult years, and senescence.
- Explain suicide in terms of six possible causes.
- Name five possible effects of suicide on the survivors.
- List five possible effects of suicide by a child or adolescent.
- State seven guidelines for using loss and grief as a growth experience.

## KEY TERMS

| | | | |
|---|---|---|---|
| Detachment | Invulnerable | Omnipotent | Transference |
| Displacement | Mortality | Survivor guilt | |

## LIFE CHANGES AS GAINS AND LOSSES

Life involves a continuous succession of changes that require us to adjust and readjust. Some of these changes represent a gain of some type—new home, new member of the family, graduation, new job, or a promotion. Some changes represent a loss—being fired, losing an important object, losing a spouse through divorce, losing a loved one through death.

Many events involve both gains and losses. Moving to a new home is exciting, but it involves losing the familiarity of the old home and relationships in the old neighborhood. Graduation is usually a happy event—it symbolizes moving on to bigger and better things. But graduation also means giving up a favorite teacher, no longer spending much of the school day with your classmates, and giving up a familiar role for a new role and new responsibilities. You expect the big events of life to have a happy effect, so it is confusing to find that, instead of being happy, you are sad or even depressed. These negative feelings are due to awareness (perhaps at the unconscious level) of losses that will result from an otherwise happy event.

Most people do not need to learn how to be happy about a gain, but many people do not know how to cope with loss. Loss definitely is one of life's most important lessons, because unexpressed grief is a powerful influence on behavior and on emotional/mental health. There is a relationship between significant loss and the occurrence of a serious illness or accident, usually within 18 months following the loss.

## LEARNING TO COPE WITH LOSS

If we learn early in life to deal effectively with "small deaths" (the losses that are part of living), then we are better prepared to deal with those losses that cause a radical change in our life situation. If we do not learn to "let go" (of whatever was lost) and to grieve appropriately for each loss, then there is an accumulation of suppressed emotions—grief, anger, guilt, and fear. Suppressed emotions are eventually expressed in some form, such as uncontrolled outbursts, depression, or inability to cope with daily life problems. Failure to express such feelings is characteristic of people who develop phobias, commit suicide, or develop alcohol/drug dependency.

Actually, we have a choice. We can learn to accept the inevitable losses of life and express our grief appropriately, thereby maintaining control and emotional well-being. Or we can go through life without learning how to deal with loss—reacting with anger about the "unfairness" of life or suppressing our grief, thereby risking loss of control when these feelings eventually erupt.

Dr. Elisabeth Kübler-Ross was a psychiatrist who worked with dying patients for many years. According to Dr. Ross, the dying process extends throughout life, and each of us goes through the stages of this process repeatedly as we experience specific life changes, especially those that involve some type of loss. The best preparation for dealing with death, according to Dr. Ross, is to learn to grieve appropriately for the "small deaths" (i.e., losses) that accompany any major life change. Once we have learned to grieve, we are able to cope better with the "big" losses that will, inevitably, occur in each of our lives. Learning to cope with loss involves several specific steps:

1. Recognize the losses involved in a life event.
2. Grant yourself the right to grieve for each loss—no matter how small.
3. Recognize and accept the various emotions involved in your reaction to a specific loss.
4. Allow yourself time to grieve.
5. Accept that grief is a *process* that extends over a period of time.

## SIGNIFICANCE OF LOSS

Losses are of many types: objects, people, relationships, jobs, money, body image (e.g., amputation, radical mastectomy), or intangibles such as beliefs, faith, one's sense of security, self-esteem. The significance of a loss is very personal (Figure 20-1). A person's reaction to a loss *reflects its meaning to that person*, rather than its value as perceived by others.

Some types of loss may be experienced at any time throughout life: moving, personal relationships, death of a loved one, personal property, health. Reactions to such losses are

**FIGURE 20-1** The significance of a loss is very personal.
*Delmar/Cengage Learning*

influenced by the period of life in which they occur. Children often do not understand the reasons for a loss, and adults may fail to note or accept the child's emotional reaction. Adults have the advantage of being involved in some decisions that result in a loss, such as moving, so their emotional reaction is tempered by an understanding of the reasons for the decision. For elderly people, a great loss is losing control over decisions that affect the remainder of their lives. Moving into a child's home or into a nursing home results in partial loss of control over one's daily activities. The reaction to such a change often includes hopelessness and resignation. The most devastating loss is the loss of life—one's own or that of a loved one.

## LOSSES DUE TO DEATH

The impact of a death on each survivor is influenced by numerous factors, including age of the survivor, relationship to the deceased, the survivor's past experience in coping with significant losses, age of the deceased, and circumstances surrounding the death (Figure 20-2). For example:

- Was the death expected? Did it follow a lengthy terminal illness?
- Does the death represent a release from pain and suffering?
- Was the death sudden and unexpected? In this situation, the survivors must cope with shock initially, then with loss.
- What was the age of the deceased? If the deceased was elderly and the survivors believe that he or she had "lived a good life," the loss is easier to accept. If the deceased was young, grief is likely to be accompanied by anger and a sense of injustice.

FIGURE 20-2 The impact of loss through death is influenced by factors surrounding the death. *Delmar/Cengage Learning*

Certain circumstances surrounding a death have an especially powerful impact on survivors:

- **The death was accidental.** Was the accident due to someone's negligence or carelessness? If so, anger and blaming may delay the beginning of a healthful grieving process. If a survivor was involved in the accident, that person may feel that he or she was responsible for the death. Or, that person may experience **survivor guilt,** wondering "What right did I have to survive?" or believing "I should have been the one who died." Anyone who is experiencing survivor guilt needs professional counseling.

- **The death was related to violence or criminal activity (mugging, burglary, or drive-by shooting).** Survivors of this type of death must deal with anger and perhaps a desire for revenge, as well as grief.

- **The death was a murder or homicide.** Survivors must deal with shock initially, then questions of "Why?" and "Who?" If the killer was a member of the family, survivors may divide into two groups. Some will refuse to believe the perpetrator's guilt and will loyally support his or her defense. Others will direct anger at the accused and seek "justice" for the deceased. In both cases, these emotions interfere with the grief process.

- **The deceased was on life support.** Who made the decision to discontinue it? Even when a living will and advance directives exist, the decision to discontinue life support is difficult for family members. If some family members disagree with the decision, then the decision maker has to cope with their criticism in addition to personal feelings about making that fateful decision. Unfortunately, there are still some physicians who do not respect advance directives, believing they must use all available measures to sustain life, in spite of the dying person's expressed wishes and hopeless condition. In those situations, the decision maker must be assertive about having the provisions of the advance directive carried out. The emotional impact of the loss may be delayed by the activities required for allowing the person to die and by the emotions aroused by that difficult situation—anger, perhaps guilt, loyalty and love for the dying person, and a sense of mission to ensure that his or her wishes are respected.

- **The death was due to self-inflicted injury—suicide.** This type of death is especially difficult for survivors. Because suicide is widely misunderstood, it is important that health care providers have a broad view of this type of death.

## SUICIDE

Any suicide attempt is a medical emergency. Although suicide is viewed as a mental health problem, it can be understood only within the context of the person's life situation: social isolation, abuse, pain, disfigurement, disability, loss of a body part, severe mood swings, the "voices" heard by a schizophrenic, or any life circumstance that has become intolerable. For a desperate individual, death may seem to be the only way to escape. Members of certain groups are at high risk for suicide: teenagers, the elderly (especially divorced or widowed men), and anyone who is seriously depressed.

Any death by suicide places family members and associates of the deceased in a soul-searching position:

*Why did I not recognize the signs that he or she was in such distress?*

*Why was I not more sensitive to his or her unhappiness?*

*What did I do that caused this terrible act?*

*Why did I not express my love?*

*Why was I so critical?*

*Why did I not insist that he or she seek help?*

*What could I have done to prevent this act?*

For parents there may be many questions, most pertaining to "how could I have been a better parent?" For siblings, the entire range of emotions is possible, depending upon the relationship with the deceased. For surviving spouses, the emotional impact may range from relief to a devastating sense of loss, depending upon the quality of the marital relationship. Friends and associates may be affected differently by suicide than by a death due to accident or illness. Some of the questions just listed may haunt those who associated with the deceased on a daily basis, especially the question, "What could I have done to help?"

Following a suicide, survivors have to deal not only with their loss, but also with psychological trauma: guilt, anger, remorse, confusion, helplessness, or feelings of failure for not having been a better parent, sibling, or friend. Suicide by a child or teenager may affect an entire school, setting off an epidemic of suicides or suicide attempts within the school population.

Suicide is considered an honorable death in some cultures. In certain Asian societies, someone who has lost honor, for whatever reason, is *expected* to commit suicide. Japanese pilots were trained during World War II for suicide missions, to sacrifice their lives for the honor of their country. Today there is a resurgence of belief in *honorable suicide* among fundamentalist groups throughout the world. The role of suicide bomber is willingly assumed, usually by an adolescent or young adult, in order to destroy members of a group perceived as the enemy. This activity occurs with disturbing frequency in the Middle East. The mother of a young male suicide bomber was quoted in the news media as declaring proudly that her son had died an honorable death. If the suicide bomber acted on instructions of a terrorist organization, that organization may pay the surviving family a large sum of money for this sacrifice of a family member. But in America, suicide is regarded by many people as a dishonorable act. Some insurance companies do not pay if a death is due to suicide; most life insurance policies exclude suicide for a specific period of time, usually two years.

Some suicides are accidental. It is well known among adolescent males that constriction of the throat can increase orgasm when masturbating. When a male is found hanging with a rope or belt around the throat, it is sometimes because his effort to enhance a sexual experience did not go as planned. Perhaps a chair or stool turned over or his foot slipped, and an accidental hanging occurred. Though a coroner's report may indicate whether or not this was the case, such information would not be made public. If this type of accident occurred but the victim was still found alive, he may be admitted to the hospital in an unconscious condition.

A more common hospital admission is the person who has ingested a poison, taken an overdose of some drug, shot himself, or attempted to cut a blood vessel. These are "incomplete suicides."

> **Note:** Do not describe a suicide as "successful" or "unsuccessful." A suicide is either "complete" or "incomplete."

One who completes a suicide by any means is found dead, and therefore will not come under your care. Most people who complete a suicide have a history of suicide attempts. Who is to know when a person who survived one suicide attempt will make another attempt that becomes a completed suicide? As a health care provider, avoid thinking that any suicide attempt is "just trying to get attention." The attempt may be a call for help, but "attention" is not the motive.

Why would anyone ingest a poison or take a lethal dose of a drug? Why do some people cut themselves? Why put a bullet through one's head? (Guns are used more often by males than females.) The only logical answer is that the individual is desperately trying to escape an intolerable life situation, a painful or debilitating physical condition, or the hopelessness that accompanies deep depression. Dr. Kay Redfield Jamison is the author of several books on depression and manic-depressive illness and coauthor of a comprehensive review of research and clinical findings related to mood disorders. She has found that persons with *bipolar disorder* (previously called manic depressive illness) or *unipolar disorder* (formerly called clinical depression) have an overwhelming need to escape the hopelessness of the depressive state. Some people use drugs, alcohol, or both as a means of escape for months or years. Some people cut themselves because the pain of cutting provides escape from "feeling nothing."

These victims of a biological illness (disruption of one or more neurotransmitters in the brain) are considered mental patients, but most are highly intelligent and capable of productive work when not depressed. In fact, many creative people—composers, musicians, writers, poets, actors—are bipolar and do their best work when in the hypomanic state, but are incapable of productive activity when depressed.

*The greatest danger of suicide is when the person is coming out of a depressed state.* Many depressed persons do not have the energy to carry out a suicide. As they recover from depression, they not only have the energy but also know that sooner or later they will again experience the hopelessness of depression. One journalist spoke of her depressed periods as a "bottomless hole" or a "black abyss" of hopelessness and despair. After two attempts, she completed a suicide just when her physician and family believed she was recovering from her latest bout of depression.

According to Dr. Jamison, the suicide of a person who is depressed *is not an act of will*; it is a desperate effort to escape the effects of depression. Approximately 45% of bipolar persons commit suicide by the age of 40. Dr. Jamison also estimates that only two out of five persons with bipolar disorder have been diagnosed and are under treatment. That leaves three out of five who may be using alcohol and drugs to escape their severe mood swings and who may eventually commit suicide, never having been diagnosed or given the opportunity for treatment.

It is likely that you will encounter a hospitalized patient who has attempted suicide. It is especially important for caregivers to keep in mind that they do not know the circumstances of that patient's life situation. Any one of us may at some time in our lives experience emotionally overwhelming circumstances. Without having experienced such conditions, we do not know how we would react. Only those who have experienced hopelessness, depression, or mood swings over a period of time can understand the distress of a person who attempts suicide. Two months stand out as the time of year when suicide rates peak: May and October.

The implications for you as a health care provider are clear. Do not judge the patient who has attempted suicide. Know that this person needs emotional support and respect. Keep in mind your philosophy of individual worth, be a compassionate caregiver, demonstrate caring, and *listen*. Anyone who has attempted suicide should be evaluated by a psychiatrist and, according to the diagnosis, given appropriate treatment. Long-term counseling is needed by most survivors of a suicide attempt, to learn effective ways of coping with depression, mood swings, and life problems.

## DEATH OF A PARENT

The death of one's parent is a unique type of loss, regardless of one's age and the age of the parent. For each of us, parents provide a link to our ancestry, our own life history, and most of what we learned as children. For a child, the immediate reaction may be anger: "How could Mommy (or Daddy) leave me?" There may also be feelings of guilt:

> *When she (he) sent me to my room I wished she (he) was dead. It's all my fault.*
>
> *If I had been a better daughter (son), Mommy (Daddy) would not have died.*
>
> *If only I had said, 'I love you' more often.*

A young child is likely to perceive the parent's death as abandonment. Loss of a parent during childhood also means the loss of parental guidance through current and future developmental tasks. The deceased parent will be missing from important life events: graduations, recitals, athletic performances, the wedding, the birth of one's own children.

The death of a same-gender parent means the loss of a parental role model. This loss is especially significant during adolescence, a time of struggling to establish one's own identity. Although adolescence is characterized by some degree of rebellion, this period of life involves developmental tasks that are best accomplished under parental guidance. Sometimes the death of a parent forces a child into an adult role. The oldest girl may assume maternal responsibilities for care of younger siblings and for managing the household. An adolescent boy may become "the man of the house" and seek work to help support the family.

Regardless of the ages of surviving children, the age of the parent at the time of death may become the age at which the child expects to die. Thus, a man whose father died of a heart attack at age 52 may develop high levels of anxiety when he approaches that age. Reaching the age of the deceased parent is known as the "parental trigger," a time when one becomes especially aware of one's own **mortality**—the fact that death is inevitable.

There is special significance to the loss of one's mother, because "mother" represents nurturing, caring, comfort, a sense of security, trust. The need to be mothered extends into adulthood. There are certain special times when mothering, or the help of one's mother, is needed, such as preparations for a wedding or the birth of one's first baby. Becoming motherless can lead to a longing that continues for years.

The loss of a father also has special significance, especially during childhood. "Father" to most people means protection and security. If the mother has been a homemaker, death of her husband may mean a financial crisis. If it becomes necessary that she seek employment, then the children experience two losses: Daddy abandoned us, now Mommy leaves us every day to go to work. The family's standard of living may be lower without the father's income.

Regardless of which parent died, surviving children may be profoundly affected psychologically, especially if they do not grieve appropriately for their loss. **Displacement** may occur if feelings were not fully expressed during the mourning period; they may emerge, greatly magnified, later in life when some other loss occurs. **Transference** is manifested by seeking fulfillment from others, placing them in the position of parental substitute. It is also possible to become "stuck" emotionally. While maturing in other respects, the individual remains emotionally immature in relation to death, authority figures, abandonment, or any other aspect associated with the parent's death. For example, Harry died of a sudden heart attack when his son was 12 years old. Numerous relatives pointed out to the 12-year-old son that he was now the man of the house. In his new role, Harry, Jr., did not feel free to cry or express his grief, but in fact he was emotionally devastated. Many years later, any talk about sickness or dying would result in an angry outburst or he would leave the room. The son was emotionally "stuck." As an adult, he still could not express the grief he felt at the loss of his father.

## LOSSES IN SPECIFIC PERIODS OF THE LIFE SPAN

Preparation for coping with a significant loss comes from experiencing a variety of losses throughout life. The individual who learns during childhood to grieve for "small losses" is better prepared to cope with a major loss than someone who has not learned to recognize and grieve for a loss. Learning to cope with loss begins in infancy; the types of loss and their significance vary according to the period of life.

### Losses of Infancy and Early Childhood

The prenatal period is a very special time for both mother and fetus. If there are no complications or difficult circumstances, the pregnant woman experiences positive feelings during most of the pregnancy. For the fetus, life in the womb is the ultimate in security and safety. At the time of delivery, the family gains a new member—one of life's happiest events. But birth is the end of pregnancy—the loss of a once-only relationship between mother and infant. If the baby is breast-fed, the mother and infant establish another very special relationship. Weaning is a "small death" because it requires both mother and infant to "let go" of this special relationship forever.

During infancy and early childhood, any separation from the parents (or other caregivers) is perceived as loss. The child, not knowing that the parents will return, feels deserted. Sadness is a natural reaction to separation; but separation from those who represent security can also arouse fear, anger, and even guilt. When a young child is hospitalized and no member of the family remains with the child, the child's emotional reaction may be manifested as withdrawal. Early separation experiences may be the source of fears and anxieties in later life about the loss of a relationship.

Separation anxiety manifests in three stages: protest, when the child cries and screams; despair; then, **detachment,** when the child greets the returning parent with coldness. *Detachment,* a shutdown of loving feelings, deals with loss by punishing the mother, by masking the rage that is felt, and by putting up a defense against the pain of being abandoned. The effects of detachment may last for a day or a lifetime, seriously interfering with the ability to love and trust others.

The importance of parental attachments, especially during infancy and childhood, should be understood by parents who must leave their children at frequent intervals. Special efforts should be made to establish a loving relationship and minimize the child's distress at being left in daycare or with a baby-sitter. A good daycare center offers a loving and supportive atmosphere for the child, in recognition of the distress felt by an infant/child as a normal reaction to separation from mother.

Health care providers need to understand separation anxiety, spend as much time as possible with a child whose parents have left, and provide emotional support as needed. Honest, age-appropriate explanations will help the child understand what has happened (Figure 20-3). Above all, do not subscribe to the value judgment that a crying child is "just spoiled." Be aware that the crying child may believe that he has been abandoned.

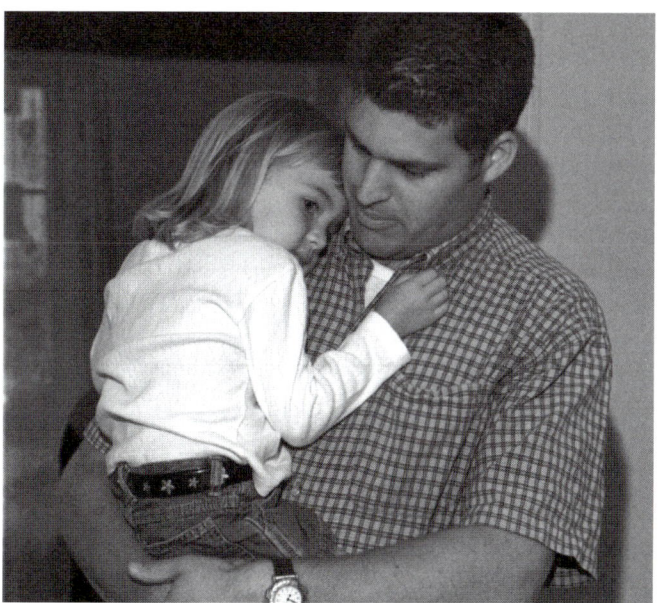

**FIGURE 20-3** A child needs honest explanations, but only enough detail to help the child understand the situation. *Delmar/Cengage Learning*

Many changes in relationships occur during early childhood. The child achieves more independence (and less dependence) as growth and development occur. Dependency is another type of special relationship, so the child's achievements also involve changes in relationships. Entering kindergarten or school is an exciting, sometimes frightening, experience. The child loses the comfort, safety, and security of home, but gains new experiences, a peer group, and new adult contacts. The mother loses her dependent "knee baby" and gains a school child who is increasingly independent.

## Losses of Middle Childhood

Throughout the school-age years a child repeatedly experiences losses and gains. Each promotion means leaving a familiar teacher and gaining a new one. There may be a loss of some classmates, although new children may come into the class at intervals. Friendships may break up, with any grief over the loss obscured by anger or guilt about the cause of the break-up. A change of school during this period includes numerous losses, which may or may not be offset by gains available in the new school. Completion of the elementary grades includes loss of some relationships and also loss of a familiar role. Promotion to middle school or high school usually means giving up childhood activities and entering the world of adolescence.

## Losses during Adolescence

Gains and losses related to growth and development, dependence versus independence, and promotion from one grade to another continue through adolescence. For the most part, emotional effects of these types of losses or gains are manageable. A person with adequate adjustment copes with these changes reasonably well. But some events of adolescence have the potential for arousing very strong emotional reactions: establishing a boy/girl relationship, becoming sexually active, experiencing peer pressure (to smoke, to use drugs, to consume alcoholic beverages), getting a job, and graduating. During this period social relationships are established with members of the opposite sex. When such a relationship ends, one or both parties may experience intense emotional reactions to the loss, regardless of whether or not the couple became sexually active and even if the break-up was agreed on by both. If the break-up resulted from parental interference, then the grief is complicated by anger and resentment that may have long-term effects on family relationships.

Adolescence is also the time when many young people obtain their first job, which requires learning a new role and includes a significant gain—one's own income. If the job is terminated, both role and income are lost; the circumstances may include loss of self-esteem.

Graduation from high school is perceived by students and their families as a happy event. The losses involved are seldom talked about. A high school graduation results in the breaking up of many relationships. It also represents the beginning of passage into adulthood and many new responsibilities. Although some students maintain their dependence on parents through additional years of education, for many the relatively carefree life of childhood and adolescence ends forever with graduation from high school.

## Losses of the Young Adult Years

The adult period of life is characterized by vocational choices, the struggle for financial independence, establishing adult coping strategies, affirming one's sexuality through marriage or a relationship, starting a family, setting up a home, and developing a satisfying lifestyle. Each of these activities may provide much satisfaction and happiness. Each is also fraught with the possibility of loss: getting fired from a job; ending a marriage through divorce; losing property through theft, fire, or natural disaster; losing friends or family members through death; moving, which often includes loss of a support network of friends, family, or both.

The adult period of life involves a continuous sequence of gains and losses, both large and small. Accepting the joy that life may bring and also learning to cope with the pain of loss leads to continued growth and a full life. Trying to escape pain by avoiding life experiences that include the risk of loss, such as marriage or a loving relationship, does not lead to growth and precludes living a full life. *Part of the adult life experience is accepting the risk of losing some of what we have gained.*

## Losses of Middle Age

Ideally, middle adulthood is a period for enjoying the rewards of one's labors during the early adult years. For many, however, this is a period of continued struggle for financial survival. The expenses of a family peak as children reach high school and college. If the family's income has increased through the years, these expenses are manageable. Otherwise, adolescent members of the family may have to become wage-earners.

The struggle for financial security involves relatively frequent gains and losses. For example, a promotion may mean additional salary and prestige, but result in the loss of free time if new responsibilities require longer hours or taking work home at night. Any unexpected expense may result in loss. For example, a long-awaited vacation at the beach may be lost because the car needs a new transmission.

Parents usually welcome the growing independence of their children. There may also be some sadness at the loss of the child/parent dependent relationship. As children leave home to attend school, set up their own apartments, or marry, parents experience a sense of loss. A woman who has been a homemaker for many years is prone to experience a loss of life purpose as the children leave home. Departure of the youngest child is especially difficult. "Empty nest syndrome" is a well-known depressive reaction to this event.

A loss of purpose is not limited to the middle-aged homemaker. Most young adults have goals—for achievement, recognition, making the world a better place, proving themselves in one way or another. During the middle adult years, these goals may still inspire a worker to strive harder. At some point, however, many people begin to realize that they will not be able to achieve some of their goals. As this realization reaches full consciousness, the individual may experience a profound sense of loss. Attitudes toward the job may change, the quality of work may be lower, and there may be expressions of hopelessness.

Recognition of a significant loss—namely, the loss of one's youth—occurs sometime during the middle years. This may occur on a 40th or 50th birthday, or it may develop gradually as physical stamina diminishes, physical proportions change, baldness develops, wrinkles appear, or once-firm tissues become flabby. Many people accept the effects of time and adapt their lifestyles to accommodate physical changes. Some people, however, experience a "midlife crisis" and set out to prove to the world (and to themselves) that they are still young. A long-term marriage may break up during this period, as one partner seeks younger companions to bolster the belief, "I am still young and attractive." Loss of youth is very painful to those who subscribe to the current emphasis on youth and sex appeal in the mass media. Menopause represents a very significant change for a woman—namely, loss of the ability to reproduce. For a man, occasional periods of impotence threaten self-esteem.

Middle age is a period when some loss of sensory capacity begins. This period of life is sometimes spoken of as the time of the five Bs: baldness, bifocals, bridges, bulges, and bunions. But this is also the time of life when potentially serious health problems may develop. As life span has increased during the past 50 years, the incidence of chronic diseases has risen markedly. Loss of health is so unacceptable that many people, upon being told that they have a particular disease, react with, "I don't believe it."

Denying a newly diagnosed disorder is not limited to serious illness. An adult who is told that recurrent sore throats are due to allergy may refuse to have allergy studies performed. This person's self-concept may not include "I am a person with an intolerance for certain foods and other substances in my life situation." A person who is diagnosed as having early arthritis may think immediately of people with deformed hands or those who complain constantly of their joint pain. The initial reaction is, "I will not become deformed, and I will not accept continuous pain in my life." Denial eventually gives way to acceptance of the diagnosis, after the individual has had time to adjust to symptoms and changes in body function.

## Losses during Senescence

The senescent period of life—old age—is now considered to consist of three periods: the young-old period, ages 65 to 74; the middle-old period, ages 75 to 84; and the old-old period, age 85 and above. The fastest-growing population segment in the United States is the 85 and older group. Because of this increased life span, we are seeing a relatively new phenomenon—elderly persons caring for their even more elderly parents. For these caregivers, death of a parent is a loss that is experienced during old age.

The senescent period of life includes more losses than gains. Physical losses eventually include diminished vision, hearing, taste, mobility, and memory. These losses usually develop gradually, but may be accelerated by any serious illness. Any chronic condition, such as arthritis, increases awareness of losses. When buttoning a shirt or tying a shoe becomes difficult, the individual is reminded daily of lost mobility and dexterity.

Psychological losses are also numerous during senescence. Retirement is a serious threat to mental health. For people who have not developed interests and activities outside of their work, there is no longer a daily routine of meaningful activity. One's work-related identity is lost. Daily interaction with co-workers is lost. Because retirement benefits seldom equal work-related income, financial loss may be significant. All of these losses are a serious threat to self-esteem, so serious that a period of depression following retirement is relatively common. In fact, some retirees develop a life-threatening illness within two years following retirement. This emphasizes the importance of having a purpose in life and being actively involved in meaningful activities other than work.

Social losses affect the elderly more than other age groups. Friends and close family members move or die. The loss of a specific friend may also mean the loss of a social activity shared with that person. The loss of a spouse may mean being left out of social activities in which the couple has participated for years. A son or daughter moving to another town means the loss of daily contact with immediate family, especially grandchildren. For many elderly persons, social life gradually diminishes. Loneliness and aloneness may characterize the daily life of an elderly person.

The loss that is feared by most elderly people is loss of independence. When an elderly person is deemed unable to live alone, the result is loss of one's home, loss of a familiar bed, loss of choices in what to eat and when. Loss of independence is accompanied by loss of self-esteem. Moving to a retirement home or confinement in a nursing home involves so many losses for the individual that there is often an immediate decline in health. All too often the emotional reactions of elderly people to these radical changes in lifestyle are not recognized or acknowledged by caregivers or by family members.

## STRIVING FOR READJUSTMENT FOLLOWING SIGNIFICANT LOSS

Loss involves pain. The intensity of the pain depends upon the degree of commitment to what was lost. *Coping with the pain of loss is a life skill that is essential to mental and emotional health.*

Loss, although painful, can be an opportunity for growth. In order to grow, we must acknowledge that we are not **invulnerable** (immune to harm), nor are we **omnipotent** (all-powerful). Growth includes learning what we can and cannot control. Once we accept that there are limits on what we can control, it is easier to deal with the fears, guilt, and anger related to losses over which we had no control.

Loss requires saying "good-bye" to someone or something that has been an important part of our life. Letting go of the past does not mean forgetting, nor does it diminish the value of what was lost. Letting go is necessary for closing the door on what has been and opening the door to a new chapter of life—a life without that which has been lost.

A loss, then, is more than just a loss. It is a threat to our belief system, and therefore to our reality. And because we tend to cling to our beliefs and what we perceive as reality, the first reaction to loss is disbelief, or denial. So, in addition to adjusting to a void created by the loss, we must also restructure our reality and our belief system. It is not uncommon to hear one who is grieving state, "I just don't know what I can believe in anymore."

Throughout life, each significant loss requires that we restructure our belief system and also work through the feelings involved in our reaction to the loss. Until the belief system has been restructured, a person may be disorganized and unable to function effectively in personal life or on the job. *It is essential that each of us learn about losses, reactions to loss, and the grief process.* Such learnings enable us to provide emotional support to others who are grieving, prepare us for coping with the loss of loved ones through death, and help us accept the ultimate loss of our own being. It is especially important that health care providers understand the significance of loss, recognize reactions to loss, and encourage those who have experienced loss to grieve. There are many opportunities in health care agencies for a sensitive caregiver to recognize someone's need for emotional support when dealing with significant loss.

## GUIDELINES FOR USING LOSS AND GRIEF AS A GROWTH EXPERIENCE

The following guidelines may appear simple. They are relatively easy to accept—intellectually. Accepting them at the *emotional level*, however, requires dealing honestly with one's feelings and beliefs. The result should be an increase in readiness to cope with the reality of loss and to help others who have experienced a significant loss.

1. Learn to recognize the small losses that occur in your life.
2. Accept anger, fear, and guilt feelings as part of many grief reactions.
3. Allow time for grieving.
4. Acknowledge your own vulnerability to losses and pain.

5. Acknowledge your lack of total control. You may control some aspects of your life, but some events are beyond your control.

6. Acknowledge your own mortality—the fact that your life will end at some time.

7. Accept that life involves change, including losses. Some changes require that we modify our belief systems to fit the new reality.

8. Following a loss, work through the feelings. When you are ready, "let go" of the past (which includes the loss).

9. Believe that you can cope with whatever loss you may experience.

10. Be supportive of those who have suffered a loss.

## REFERENCES AND SUGGESTED READINGS

*Indicates a classic reference that introduced new ideas.

*Jamison, Kay Redfield. (1999). *Night falls fast: Understanding suicide.* New York: Vintage.
*Kübler-Ross, Elisabeth. (1969). *On death and dying.* New York: MacMillan.
*Kübler-Ross, Elisabeth. (1975). *Death: The final stage of growth.* Englewood Cliffs, NJ: Prentice-Hall.
*Kübler-Ross, Elisabeth. (1978). *To live until we say goodbye.* Englewood Cliffs, NJ: Prentice-Hall.
Ross, Catherine, & Mirowsky, John. (2008, June 15). Age and the balance of emotions. *Social Science & Medicine, 66*(12), 2391–2400.
Tamparo, Carol D., & Lindh, Wilburta Q. (2008). *Therapeutic communications for allied health professionals* (3rd ed.). Clifton Park, NY: Delmar, Cengage Learning.

## SOURCES OF ADDITIONAL INFORMATION

http://www.suicidology.org

**American Geriatrics Society,** http://www.healthinaging.org (1-800-563-4916)

**Alzheimer's Association,** http://www.alz.org (1-800-272-3900)

## REVIEW AND SELF-CHECK

1. Explain why a happy life event, such as graduation, may be accompanied by feelings of sadness.

   *When a person is sad or depressed at the time of a "happy" event, it is because it can be accompanied by losses*

2. List three reasons it is important to recognize and grieve for the small losses we experience in life.

   *Coping w/ small losses prepares for big ones; if we don't grieve for small losses, they will accumulate; repressed emotions will be expressed as a loss of control*

3. List four steps for learning how to cope with losses.

   recognize loss; grant right to grieve for loss; recognize feelings about loss; allow time to grieve

4. Explain the significance of loss to physical and mental health.

   is repressed grief influencing behavior, accident or illness w/in 18 months, repressed grief — repressed in subconscious and these feelings might appear or not in the future

5. List three losses that occur in each of the following periods of life:

   a. Infancy

      Loss of infancy & early childhood in birth

   b. Early childhood

   c. The school years

      promotions from grade, change of schools, graduation from grade school

   d. Adolescence

      childhood toys, dependence on others, grad from middle or high school, relationships, loss of leisure time, job.

   e. Young adulthood

      leaving home, displaced worker, divorce, loss of property, moving

f. Middle adulthood

   _dependent parent/child relationship; leisure time w/ family or friends; purpose or goals, stamina, youth + vitality; sexual function, vision, hearing, taste, health_

g. Late adulthood

   _friends + family members; income, purpose, associate due to retirement; independence, choices,_

h. Senescence  _personal belongings_

6. Write out seven guidelines for using loss as a growth experience.

   _Loss + grief can lead to personal growth if the individual grieves small losses; accept feelings associated w/ losses; allows time for grieving; accept one's vulnerability to loss; accepts limits on control of event; acknowledge one's own mortality; accepts life is series of changes; works through feelings of losses; supportive of others who have suffered a loss._

7. Find out if your community has a support group for survivors of:
   a. Death of a child.
   b. Death by suicide.
   c. An incomplete suicide.

## ASSIGNMENTS

1. List significant changes that have occurred in your life, starting with your earliest memories and continuing to the present.

2. Set up a worksheet with three columns with the following headings: EVENTS, GAINS, LOSSES. In Column I, list significant events in the past two years of your life. Beside each

event, list in Column II what you gained and in Column III what you lost as a result of that event.

3. List three of your possessions that are important to you. How do you think you would react if you learned that these items had been destroyed in a fire?

4. What would be your behavior following the death of your best close friend? Write a description of your feelings, how you would express these feelings, and the people with whom you would share your feelings.

5. Prepare a set of guidelines to help you improve your ways of coping with loss. Be prepared to share these guidelines during a class discussion.

6. Participate in a small-group activity:

    a. Describe reactions to a significant loss that you have experienced or observed.

    b. Which of these examples are healthy reactions to loss?

    c. Which represent an unhealthy reaction to loss?

7. Compare the items below with your list of significant life changes (developed in Assignment 1). Add any of these events that have occurred in your life, so that your list is relatively complete.

    a. Death of a grandparent, parent, brother, or sister

    b. Death of a spouse, son, or daughter

    c. Death of any other relative who was important to you

    d. Death of a friend or classmate when you were a child

    e. Separation, divorce, or end of a long-term sexual relationship

    f. Marriage or establishment of a sexual relationship

    g. Any move—from one neighborhood to another, one city to another, or one state to another

    h. Change of school

    i. Major purchase—house, car, other

    j. Loss of personal possession—theft, foreclosure, fire, other

    k. New family member

    l. Pregnancy

    m. Serious illness of a family member

    n. Diagnosis of a serious or chronic illness (yours)

    o. Obtaining a new job; being fired from a job

    p. Change in job responsibilities or work schedule

    q. Radical change in financial situation

    r. Moving out of parents' home

s. Your child moves out of your home

t. Loss of freedom—confined to your room, not allowed to date or use the car, jail time

u. Radical change in lifestyle

v. Entered military service, college, other educational program

> **Note:** Continue to add to your list as you think of other changes that have occurred in your life.

8. Review your list of changes. Place a checkmark beside each change that involved a significant loss.

9. Review your list of significant losses in Assignment 8. Is there any loss in that list for which you have not grieved? If so, plan how you will grieve for that loss and begin the process. If there is more than one loss for which you have not grieved, decide now that you will grieve for each of these losses, but *only one at a time.* When you believe you have completed the grief process for one loss, then you may begin to grieve for another loss on your list.

10. Participate in a class discussion about a health care provider's responsibilities when caring for a patient who attempted suicide.

# UNIT 21

# Death: Changing Attitudes and Practices

## OBJECTIVES

Upon completion of this unit, you should be able to:

- List three contrasts between past and current practices related to death and dying.
- List five examples of beliefs about death.
- List three reasons death education can allay fears about death.
- State five conditions that contribute to "death with dignity."
- Name five issues related to end-of-life care.
- Name four reasons the courts are sometimes involved in end-of-life decisions.
- Compare euthanasia, suicide, and assisted suicide.
- State one purpose of the living will.
- State one purpose of the medical durable power of attorney.
- Name the two legal documents included in an advance medical directive.
- List four provisions of the Patient Self-Determination Act.
- Develop a personal philosophy about death and end-of-life care.

## KEY TERMS

| | | |
|---|---|---|
| Advance medical directive (AMD) | Durable power of attorney (DPA) | Patient Self-Determination Act (PSDA) |
| Bereavement | Euthanasia | Proxy |
| Conservator | Immortal | Thanatology |
| Do not resuscitate (DNR) order | Mortality | |
| | Near-death experience (NDE) | |

Many people view death as the absolute end of life. Thus death is an enemy to be feared and avoided at all costs. A totally different view is reflected in the writings of Dr. Elisabeth Kübler-Ross, who titled one of her books *Death: The Final Stage of Growth*. As a result of her many years of attending dying patients, Dr. Kübler-Ross proposed that the dying process involves a series of emotional/spiritual changes that, ideally, terminate with feelings of peace and tranquility prior to death. The dying process, then, can be an opportunity for spiritual growth. Some dying people need help to move through this process. Others seem to undergo this growth through their own beliefs, values, and inner resources.

Between these two opposite views of death, there is a wide range of beliefs. These differences are due in part to cultural attitudes and practices in care of the dying, which have undergone a marked change during the past half-century. This unit reviews those historical changes, examines some influences on beliefs about death, discusses current and emerging attitudes and practices related to death and dying, and reflects on a variety of issues pertaining to health care decisions.

## PAST ATTITUDES AND PRACTICES

In 1789, Benjamin Franklin wrote, "In this world nothing is certain except death and taxes." His comment reflects an awareness and acceptance of death that was common until the era of modern medicine. Prior to the last century, the leading cause of death was infection. Infant and child mortality rates were high; few families escaped the loss of a child. Death was familiar—a common experience that was highly visible to people of all ages. Illness and death were most likely to occur in the home, with family members and friends gathered around. It was the custom for each member of the family to bid the dying person farewell. In return, the dying person gave his or her blessing to favored relatives. The deathbed scene often included advice and charges to the survivors—to develop certain virtues, care for other survivors, gain honor for the family name.

Death was viewed as a reunion with deceased loved ones. The joyful anticipation of this reunion overshadowed any sadness at leaving the survivors. In some cultures, death was (or still is) celebrated as a release from the troubles of this life and a welcome passage to a happy and trouble-free existence in "the hereafter."

Mourning was public, as well as private. A widow was expected to wear black for at least a year following the death of her husband. Men wore a black band on the left sleeve as a public display of mourning for the deceased. The survivors did not participate in social events for many months. Women, in particular, were expected to remain in seclusion during the mourning period. There were frequent visits to the cemetery. The gravemarker and subsequent care of the grave symbolized respect for the deceased and the devotion of the survivors. In many other ways survivors demonstrated to relatives and the community their love and respect for the deceased. Until recently, both illness and death were a family affair.

## CHANGING ATTITUDES AND PRACTICES

Beginning in the early 1900s, infection was brought under control through improved sanitation and immunization. During the late 1930s and 1940s, the sulfa drugs and penicillin were discovered. These changes in the treatment of infection resulted in a dramatic decrease in deaths due to infection, especially among infants and children. As the life span increased, the primary causes of death became cancer, heart disease, degenerative disorders, and accidents. Care of the sick and injured shifted from the home to the hospital. Responsibility for care of the sick was delegated to health care personnel, with family members in the role of bystanders. This trend resulted in isolation of the patient from family members, who were "protected" from personal experience with serious illness and death. Children, especially, were excluded from contact with the hospitalized patient. Illness and death ceased to be a family affair.

As a result of this trend, many people today have never been personally involved with serious illness or the dying process. They have been deprived of involvement in the dying process—the opportunity to learn to accept death as a part of the cycle of life. Death is now perceived by many people as a terrible tragedy that "ought not to happen, especially to me and my family."

These changes of the past 50 years have great significance for emotional and mental health. Due to the invisibility of the dying process and the abandonment of many mourning rituals, there is a growing tendency to deny death. In American society, it is almost as though there is a conspiracy of silence. One just does not talk, or even think, about death until it strikes within one's circle of relatives or friends.

When death does touch a family, there may be a tendency to deny the grief process. Today, the community generally does not provide for bereaved people the kind of long-term support that can facilitate the grief process. Instead, survivors are expected to "pick up the pieces and get on with their lives" soon after the funeral.

In the work setting, life may go on as usual the day after a colleague's funeral, with no one willing to introduce the subject of death into the informal communication channels. The formal communication channel may acknowledge this loss of a member of the organization with a memorandum or floral offering. Otherwise, the work routine continues with minimal recognition that a member is missing, unless the deceased held an important position. Thus, death is kept out of sight and out of consciousness as much as possible.

## CURRENT ATTITUDES AND PRACTICES

Changes in infant and child mortality have had a particular effect on societal attitudes toward death as it relates to age. Whereas death is acceptable for older people (generally age 60 and above), it is viewed as inappropriate for someone under the age of 30 to die. Yet less than a hundred years ago, parents felt blessed if half of their children survived to age 12. Today, we find it especially tragic—unacceptable and terribly unfair—when a child dies. This attitude is especially prevalent among teenagers and young adults, who tend to think of themselves as **immortal** because "death is for old people." This attitude tends to modify with the passing years and accumulated life experiences. By middle age, most people begin to accept the reality of death, even if they are not yet able to acknowledge their own **mortality.**

Changes in the health care system have contributed to changes in societal attitudes toward death. In fact, a highly significant change in attitudes toward death has occurred *within* the health care system. Instead of accepting death as an inevitable outcome of some diseases, death is perceived as an enemy to be conquered with whatever resources the system can offer: new and better drugs, life-support systems, surgical replacement of body parts, heroic measures to restore vital functions. Some physicians believe they have a responsibility to maintain life in the physical body as long as possible, regardless of the patient's potential for recovery or a meaningful existence. Concern for the *quantity of life* has replaced concern for the *quality of life*. When all measures available prove inadequate to keep a patient alive, some personnel view the death as a personal failure ("If only I had made rounds 30 minutes sooner!") or as a failure of the system ("If we had been able to use such-and-such, we could have saved that patient.").

Recently, however, there is increasing awareness of a need to examine societal attitudes toward death and care of the dying. Some hospitals have modified their policies regarding visitors, some even permitting small children to visit a dying grandparent, parent, or sibling. Hospice and home care of a dying person are increasingly recognized as alternatives to hospitalization. More families now participate in the dying process, thereby permitting the dying person to retain a sense of family membership until the end. These recent trends recognize and respect the *human needs* of the dying person.

## THE EMERGENCE OF THANATOLOGY

During the 1950s a new interest and concern about death and dying emerged, largely due to the work of Dr. Elisabeth Kübler-Ross, sociologists, social workers, and pastoral counselors. Many professionals who were working with dying patients recognized that their educational programs had not prepared them for this role. The concern of these professional workers to meet the needs of patients with terminal illness led to the emergence of **thanatology,** the study of death and dying, and to death education for health care providers and for the public.

Thanatology involves people from a variety of disciplines: sociology, theology, psychology, counseling, social work, nursing, and medicine. Their work has led to increased awareness of the needs of dying persons, the importance of the grief process, techniques for helping patients and their families cope with death and **bereavement,** and the need for death education.

## THE MEANING OF DEATH

An important aspect of death education is learning to accept one's own mortality. In the past, this important lesson was learned early in life through direct experience with serious illness and death itself, usually in the home. Current practices that isolate dying patients prevent this direct involvement. But death education can help people think through the meaning of death, resolve their fears, reach some level of personal acceptance, and come to terms with their own mortality. In addition, death education can prepare people to accept their feelings as legitimate reactions when they do have to cope with a death crisis. It is especially important that health care providers who care for dying patients resolve their own fears about dying, because subconscious fears about death influence how one interacts with a person who is dying.

The meaning of death for each person is influenced by cultural background, religious beliefs, and life experiences. Following are examples of beliefs about death:

- Death is the end of existence.
- Death is only the end of physical existence.
- Death is a natural, biological event that concludes life.
- Death is the loss of everything—life itself, the future, loved ones, possessions.
- Death means separation from loved ones.
- Death means a reunion with loved ones who have already died.
- Death is the enemy. It should be fought with all available resources up to the end.
- What follows death is unknown; therefore, it is a fearsome event.
- Death is a test of one's faith; therefore, it must be faced with courage and a willingness to accept pain and suffering.
- Death is a change to another form of existence.
- Death is a transition; the soul moves to another plane of existence.
- Death is the beginning of a new life—perpetual existence in heaven or hell, depending upon Divine judgment of one's deeds on earth.

Some of these beliefs perpetuate fear of death. Others reflect acceptance of death as natural or as a transition to another dimension of existence.

Fear of death is, in part, the result of medicalizing and institutionalizing death. The result is that most people today have not had the opportunity to participate in the dying process. According to Dr. Kübler-Ross, "Any child who has experienced the death of a brother or sister, mother or father, grandfather or grandmother in his own home, surrounded by peace and love, will not be afraid of death or dying anymore..." (Kübler-Ross, 1969).

Death education can help people deal with their fears and clarify their own beliefs about death. It can help them understand that preparing oneself for dying includes grieving for what must be given up: relationships with family members and friends; ambitions, goals, purposes, and dreams for the future; material possessions; and, finally, one's own physical body. Thinking through these losses while in a state of good health usually results in a new perspective on what is important in life. The survivors of **near death experiences (NDEs)** report a peaceful interlude that left them with no fear of death and with new attitudes toward the value of each life experience.

## DEATH WITH DIGNITY

Increased attention to death and dying has resulted in several trends: the hospice movement, preparation of personnel to provide counseling for dying patients, and advance directives for end-of-life care. The right to die with dignity is inherent in the philosophy of hospice. Death with dignity embodies at least the following:

- The dying person is permitted to retain some control.
- The dying person has the freedom to choose his or her style of dying.
- The dying person is allowed to discuss death openly.
- The dying person is allowed to prepare for dying in his or her own way.
- Human mortality is a biological fact.
- The dying patient's care focuses on maintaining *quality of life*, rather than *quantity of life*.
- Intervention in the dying process, when the prognosis is hopeless, is inappropriate if such intervention violates the patient's wishes.
- Some interventions prolong the dying process.

Death with dignity, then, implies that the highest possible quality of life is maintained and that the dying person's rights and wishes are respected by caregivers. By participating in decisions and being allowed to make choices, the dying person maintains self-esteem and a sense of integrity as a human being. Familiar surroundings help the patient maintain a sense of identity. Those who die at home have the advantage of familiar surroundings and the presence of family members, friends, and even pets. Arrangements that permit the person to die at home can also benefit survivors, though some families are not able to cope with full-time care of a dying person. In any case, dying at home is now recognized as an alternative to dying in the institutional setting.

## EUTHANASIA

The word **euthanasia** is derived from two Greek words: *eu* (good) and *thanatos* (death). Euthanasia is a complex and controversial subject that involves philosophical views of life and death, ethical considerations, religious beliefs, and legal questions. Before taking a position for or against euthanasia, become informed about each of these aspects. With increasing knowledge and exposure to a variety of viewpoints, you will be prepared to formulate an opinion based on information, rather than value judgments alone.

The following discussion is limited to basic information that you, as a health care provider, should know and understand. For that reason, the definition that forms the basis of this discussion is more restricted than that used by authors who present a comprehensive discussion. As used here, *euthanasia is any action, requested by the patient but performed by someone else, that accelerates the dying process.* The request may be made because of intractable pain, loss of bodily control, or a deteriorating condition that will inevitably result in helplessness. Modern writers differentiate active and passive euthanasia, based on how the death occurs. *Active euthanasia* involves an *intentional intervention* (usually, administration of medication) for the purpose of causing death. *Passive euthanasia* consists of *withholding* and/or *withdrawing treatment*, with the intention of allowing the person to die of the underlying disease process. This definition of passive euthanasia includes withholding or discontinuing life support procedures, such as artificial ventilation, cardiopulmonary resuscitation, and tube feedings.

The primary argument in favor of euthanasia is that present end-of-life care does not provide adequately for relief of suffering. Derek Humphrey, founder of the Euthanasia Research & Guidance Organization (ERGO), defines *euthanasia* as any form of hastened death, *voluntary euthanasia* as a requested death by a doctor's lethal injection, and *physician-assisted suicide* as a doctor-prescribed lethal overdose that the patient takes orally (i.e., self-administered). Humphrey considers that euthanasia is a *rational planned deliverance from a painful and hopeless disease.*

Humphrey (2003) specifies three reasons that justify a patient's request for euthanasia: (1) terminal illness that is causing extreme suffering despite good medical care, (2) greatly diminished quality of life due to an incurable medical condition, (3) a physical condition so handicapping that the patient chooses to die rather than live under such conditions. Consideration of a patient's request requires that the patient be a mature adult, the patient has been given full information and can make an informed choice, the condition has existed for some time, and the attending physician has been involved in full discussion of the patient's condition and the patient's request.

The danger of euthanasia is *misuse*—someone other than the patient may benefit from the death. Obviously, beneficiaries from the patient's estate should not be allowed to influence the decision, although this is difficult to control when family members are involved in the patient's care. Every effort should be made to ensure that the patient truly desires relief from suffering and has reached that decision independently. Supporters of the right-to-die concept believe that euthanasia should be considered only under clearly defined conditions and with the expressed wish of the patient. The decision should not be left to one doctor and one patient, but should be reviewed by a panel of experts that includes at least two members who have conducted a face-to-face interview with the patient.

## EVOLUTION OF THE RIGHT-TO-DIE MOVEMENT

In Switzerland euthanasia has been legal since 1941; in Belgium since 2002; and in the Netherlands since 2002, although it has been permitted since 1984. In Holland doctors must follow a 28-step checklist, and all euthanasia incidents must be reported to the government.

In all other situations, at least two doctors must certify that the patient is dying and has requested accelerated death. If there is any question about the patient's competence for making such a decision, or any possibility of coercion, a psychologist must certify the validity of the patient's request. With the exception of Switzerland, all have a "residents only" rule, but Switzerland does require that a foreigner entering the country to seek euthanasia must be terminally ill.

Choices regarding one's mode of dying have been slow to develop in the United States. Initial efforts were spearheaded by Derek Humphrey, founder of the Hemlock Society as well as ERGO. Other organizations evolved from these early efforts: End of Life Choices, Compassion and Choices, Death with Dignity, Final Exit, First Freedom First, and other right-to-die groups. The World Federation of Right to Die Societies includes 44 member organizations in 29 countries. The various efforts of these organizations led to the first U.S. state law to legalize a patient's right to seek aid in escaping an intolerable health situation.

In 1997, following a state referendum, the Oregon state legislature passed the Death with Dignity Act, which permits a doctor to prescribe a lethal dose to a terminally ill patient, provided the patient is of sound mind and requests it verbally and in writing, with at least two witnesses. In addition, a consulting physician must confirm that the patient has a life expectancy of less than six months and *the drug must be self-administered*—it cannot be administered by the physician.

In 2008 the Washington state legislature enacted the Washington Death with Dignity Act, which took effect in March 2009. Thus Washington became the second U.S. state to legalize physician aid-in-dying. In January 2009, California's Right to Know End of Life Options Act went into effect. This law requires doctors to inform a dying patient of *any and all options* (legal and medical) *if* the patient asks. These options would include not only those related to pain management and hospice care but also those that hasten death, such as discontinuing treatment and withholding nutrition and hydration.

In December 2008, a Montana district court judge ruled that "the Montana constitutional rights of individual privacy and human dignity" include the right to "die with dignity." The Montana Attorney General then announced that he planned to appeal the judge's ruling. So, during 2009, Montana became the site of the next legal battle over a patient's right to choose physician-assisted dying.

The Oregon Department of Human Services (ODHS) now uses value-neutral language in discussing assistance with dying, avoiding the use of "suicide," "assisted suicide," and "physician-assisted suicide," all of which are inflammatory and misleading. Those who place their own beliefs and/or religious doctrine ahead of individual rights continue to oppose the right to aid-in-dying. These opponents and members of the press generally use value-laden and inflammatory terms.

Suicide involves a choice: to live or to die. For terminally ill patients and those who have a debilitating illness with no potential for recovery, the choice is between continued suffering and loss of function versus having control over the time and place of dying. Health care providers should be aware that a more accurate term for describing such a choice is "aid-in-dying."

Meanwhile, public interest in the right-to-die movement is spreading, and various health organizations are addressing the issue. For example, the American Public Health Association has adopted a policy of supporting the right-to-die concept. With increased public awareness, involvement of more health care organizations, and new challenges to existing laws, end-of-life practices will continue to evolve during the next decade.

## SOCIETAL ISSUES RELATED TO CARE OF THE DYING

The availability of life-support technology has given rise to ethical, moral, and legal questions previously unknown to any society. New types of decisions face the physician, the patient, and next-of-kin—decisions that can contribute to guilt feelings, inappropriate procedures, and medical practices based on fear of litigation. It is important for health care providers to be aware of issues pertaining to the care of dying patients.

Issues that concern society as a whole are those that establish medical and legal precedent for future decisions. Issues that concern the patient and family are largely those that involve constitutional rights. Some of these issues are currently being argued in the courts; others are appearing in the medical literature and at conferences as ethical, moral, and legal questions. Issues of particular concern to everyone participating in care of the dying are (1) the definition of death, (2) quality of life versus quantity of life, and (3) rights of patients and their families.

### The Definition of Death

What indicates that a person is dead? This question is especially important now that donor organs are needed for transplants. Each state has a Determination of Death Act that specifies the legal definition of death for that state. The *medical definition* is based on cessation of respiratory or circulatory functions or irreversible coma. In some hospitals brain death is measured in terms of (1) cerebral functions (consciousness, responsiveness to stimuli) and (2) brain-stem functions (control of vital processes). Where both measurements are made, the patient is not declared brain dead unless at least two physicians agree that brain-stem function is absent. The definition of death is especially relevant to the care of young accident victims. It is indeed difficult to give up hope for a young person whose body appears normal, even when tests indicate that there is no brain activity.

Determination of the moment of death is a pressing decision when other patients are waiting for a donor organ. A surgeon waiting to perform an organ transplant is understandably impatient about any delay in pronouncing a potential donor dead. The Uniform Anatomical Gift Act specifies that the physician who declares a patient dead must not be involved with a patient who is awaiting a donor organ. The Uniform Determination of Death Act specifies that both cardiopulmonary and brain function criteria must be met before body organs may be removed. Any state that adopts these statutes, or develops its own statute with clearly stated criteria for determination of death, is providing legal protection for any dying person who is a potential organ donor.

### Quality of Life versus Quantity of Life

Which is more important, the *quality* of life or the *quantity* of life? When the current state of medical practice offers no hope for a patient's recovery, to what extent should life-extending procedures be used? Intravenous fluids, blood transfusion, and tube feedings are used to maintain life, rather than to cure disease. Often such procedures are continued even when a patient's condition is hopeless. Life can be maintained for days, or even weeks, until the body refuses to continue to function. Is the physician or family obligated to "do everything possible" to *extend* life? Or should life-maintenance procedures be discontinued when there is no hope of recovery and the quality of life is nil? Who should make such a decision—a mentally competent patient, the next-of-kin, or the physician? Who should make such a decision if the patient is *not* mentally competent or is comatose?

The right-to-die issue was brought to public attention by the Terri Schiavo case. In 1990, Terri suffered a cardiac arrest; heroic efforts restored heart function, but she remained comatose. Medical procedures indicated that she was brain dead, but she was kept alive by a gastric feeding tube. After Terri had been comatose for 10 years, her husband obtained court approval to discontinue the gastric feedings, but Terri's parents went to court to oppose this action. The following seven years of controversy in the courts led to interventions by Governor Jeb Bush and the Florida legislature, then by the U.S. Congress and President George Bush. Laws that were enacted to prevent the removal of Terri's gastric feeding tube were declared unconstitutional by the courts.

The publicity regarding the Schiavo case was inflammatory, including derogatory accusations against her husband. Eventually, in 2005, the feeding tube was removed and Terri was allowed to die. This case clearly reveals the zeal of opponents of the right to die. Should strangers and politicians make decisions about a patient's medical care, especially about dying? Is quality of life as important as being kept alive by artificial means? Terri Schiavo's case aroused a high level of public interest in patients' rights and end-of-life care.

## Rights of Patients and Their Families

When the recommended medical treatment of a condition has extreme side effects, causes more pain than the disease itself, or involves radical surgery that permanently alters body appearance, does the patient (or the parents, if the patient is a minor) have the right to refuse treatment? Medical opinion is that *any medically approved treatment should be used*. But some patients reject surgery or treatments such as chemotherapy, choosing instead to *let the disease run its natural course*. Although a physician cannot force surgery or chemotherapy on an adult, there have been court judgments that required a child's parents to allow physicians to administer chemotherapy to a child.

Does a patient who is mentally sound have the right to refuse extreme measures for maintaining life (Figure 21-1)? This issue, also, has been before the courts. Judges generally use brain death as the criterion for authorizing a physician to discontinue treatment of a comatose patient. The question is far more complex when a patient is conscious and mentally competent. If the patient has no hope of recovery and does not want to continue to suffer, does that person have the right to say "pull the plug"? Some people view the use of life-support procedures for dying patients as *prolonging death, rather than extending life*. The concept of death with dignity includes the patient's right to reject life-support and resuscitation procedures.

## Do Not Resuscitate Orders

After the technique for cardiopulmonary resuscitation (CPR) became an integral part of the curriculum for all health care personnel, it became common practice to "call a code" for any patient who stopped breathing, even if the person was terminally ill. This was especially true in teaching hospitals, where numerous medical students and interns were expected to learn resuscitation procedures, including open-heart massage. When it was recognized that resuscitation is inappropriate for some patients, a new type of physician's order came into being: **do not resuscitate (DNR).** This order is written by the attending physician for patients who are expected to die and for whom no further treatment is feasible.

**FIGURE 21-1** Patients have the right to refuse treatment, including life-support measures and resuscitation. *Delmar/Cengage Learning*

With the development of hospice and a growing trend toward care of a dying person in the home setting, there was need for end-of-life procedures for patients outside the hospital setting. If caregivers called emergency services after the patient died, the paramedics who responded were legally obligated to begin CPR, unless there was a written DNR. Forty-five states and the District of Columbia now authorize nonhospital DNRs.

## LEGAL ASPECTS OF THE RIGHT TO DIE

Numerous right-to-die issues have now been addressed by the U.S. Supreme Court, the U.S. Congress, and some state legislatures. In the Mary Beth Cruzan case the Supreme Court ruled that there is a constitutional right to die, but that it is up to the states to define that right. Later, Congress passed the **Patient Self-Determination Act (PSDA),** which mandates that patients be informed about the right to participate in medical decisions regarding their treatment. Living will laws have now been passed by forty-five states and the District of Columbia. As of 2003, Michigan, Massachusetts, and New York do not have a living will law but recognize the legality of a living will. All states and the District of Columbia have a medical **durable power of attorney (DPA)** law. The living will and medical DPA laws are the result of widespread consumer resistance to indiscriminate use of medical technology that can prolong life indefinitely. Both documents pertain to *self-determination*—the right of a patient to participate in medical decisions and, specifically, the right to refuse medical treatment. An **advance medical directive (AMD)** refers to both medical DPA and the living will.

## The Living Will

The living will permits individuals to indicate their wishes regarding medical care. It is especially valuable when an individual becomes incapable of conveying such wishes to the doctor and family. People who have the foresight to prepare a living will protect their families from having to make painful decisions regarding medical treatment if there appears to be no chance of recovery. Living wills also provide guidance for the physician regarding extreme measures such as life support and resuscitation.

The living will is especially useful in cases of coma or prolonged dying when there is no hope of recovery. Ideally, a living will should be prepared and signed *before* the onset of illness or accident. If a patient wants to sign a living will after being admitted to a health care facility, additional witnesses and safeguards are required. The living will presents the patient's wishes in writing. Some court cases (e.g., Mary Beth Cruzan, Karen Ann Quinlan) have been based on statements the patient made to family and friends indicating that he or she would not want to be kept alive in a vegetative state. In the absence of a living will or other written instructions, lengthy legal proceedings may be required before the patient is allowed to die a natural death by discontinuing life support and/or artificial nutrition.

Everyone who completes a living will and/or a medical DPA should discuss their advance directive(s) with the physician, their families, and especially the **proxy** (the person named as decision maker in the medical DPA) (Figure 21-2). The discussion should be specific about

**FIGURE 21-2** A patient should discuss AMDs with the physician, nursing staff, family, and especially the "proxy" named in a medical DPA. *Delmar/Cengage Learning*

one's beliefs and wishes regarding end-of-life care and about any medical interventions that are not wanted. Without such meaningful discussions at intervals, there is risk that one's wishes will be ignored, even if an advance directive has been completed.

It is not necessary to involve a lawyer in preparing a living will. Each state has a specific form. A living will form should be filled out according to the instructions, signed in the presence of witnesses who are not family members or beneficiaries, and then signed by the witnesses. The original should be filed in a safe place; copies should be provided to members of the family. Upon admission to a hospital, a copy should be added to the patient's chart; *a family member should obtain a receipt from a hospital representative, acknowledging that an AMD for that patient is on file.*

## The Durable Power of Attorney

The medical DPA is a document that designates a specific person to make medical decisions if the patient is unable to do so. The desires of the individual should be made clear to the decision maker at the time the document is prepared. When illness or accident occurs, the decision maker is responsible for seeing that the patient's wishes are carried out. Some DPA forms include statements pertaining to life support, resuscitation, and artificial feeding, so that specific instructions are included in the legal document.

## Advance Medical Directives

The living will and the DPA constitute an AMD. Arizona, California, Louisiana, North Carolina, Montana, and Vermont have established AMD registries. Several other states are considering such a registry. Even more important, a U.S. living will registry has been created. Once the use of AMDs, especially the living will, has become common practice, the right to die is less likely to involve legal actions.

## The Patient Self-Determination Act

Under the PSDA, any hospital, nursing home, hospice, or health maintenance organization (HMO) that receives federal funding (Medicare and Medicaid) must inform patients about their rights, specifically the right to refuse certain types of treatment. This federal law also prohibits health care providers from discriminating against a patient who elects to forgo life-sustaining procedures. The PSDA specifies that any patient who enters a hospital or nursing home must be informed about:

- The right to make decisions about medical treatments
- The right to refuse a treatment (medical or surgical)
- The right to prepare an AMD if the patient does not already have a living will or medical DPA
- The procedure in that institution for preparing an AMD
- The right to have an AMD made part of his or her medical record

This law resulted from the proliferation of court cases regarding the right to die. A number of families have experienced emotional trauma and incurred tremendous legal expense in the effort to allow their loved one, in a state of irreversible coma, to die. Health care providers, regardless of their own opinions, must respect the wishes of patients that have been stated in an AMD.

The PSDA will serve the needs of many patients, especially those with terminal illnesses and those who choose to forgo certain medical procedures. But it does not solve the problem of a comatose person who does not have an AMD. Who knows when an accident or sudden life-threatening illness will result in brain damage and a vegetative state? The only sure protection against the use of undesired measures, when there is no hope of recovery, is to have an AMD prepared *before* illness or accident occurs.

Box 21-1 shows some of the requirements of the Patient Self-Determination Act.

### Involvement of the Courts in Health Care Decisions

Increasingly, the legal system is becoming involved in health care decisions. This is most likely to occur when (1) relatives of a comatose person believe life support should be discontinued, but there is no advance directive, (2) an advance directive is ignored by health care personnel, or (3) the family wants to do "everything possible" for their loved one, even though the physician and hospital believe life support/nutrition should be discontinued.

---

**BOX 21-1**

### The Patient Self-Determination Act

Provisions of the PSDA apply to all health care agencies that receive federal funds (Medicare and Medicaid reimbursement).

Each health care institution will:

- Provide written information to each patient regarding:
  a. The right to make decisions concerning medical care, including the right to refuse medical or surgical treatment.
  b. The right to prepare AMDs.
  c. The institution's policies concerning the implementation of such rights.
- Document in the patient's medical record whether or not the individual has completed an advance directive.
- Provide care without discrimination against the patient who has completed an advance directive.
- Establish policies and procedures to ensure compliance with state law regarding advance directives.
- Provide educational activities for staff and the public on the matter of advance directives.

The Department of Health and Human Services will:

- Provide a national public education campaign.
- Develop written materials explaining patients' rights, to be distributed by health care facilities.

*Source: Delmar/Cengage Learning*

In the first type of situation, the courts use one of two standards for determining whether or not life support may be discontinued. The "substituted judgment" standard recognizes that many individuals have not prepared advance directives and that their loved ones can best decide that individual's preference for end-of-life care. The "clear and convincing evidence" standard requires that the patient's preferences have been clearly stated to relatives or friends prior to the patient becoming unable to make medical decisions personally.

The second type of situation is discussed under the topic "A Dilemma for Health Care Providers." The third situation is less common, in that most families of a comatose patient accept the recommendation of the physician. If a family does demand that treatment continue, even though there is no hope of improvement in the patient's condition, the hospital or physician may request that the court appoint a **conservator.** The responsibility of the conservator would be to evaluate the situation and recommend a course of action based on what the patient probably would choose, if able to express those preferences.

## A DILEMMA FOR HEALTH CARE PROVIDERS

Sometimes health care personnel choose to ignore an AMD, believing that they are obligated to do everything possible to keep a patient alive. This behavior involves conflict between the health care provider's philosophy of health care and the legal rights of patients. The conflict may extend beyond the staff, involving hospital policy and established procedures.

### Liability for Performing Unwanted Treatment

Performing heroic measures to restore breathing or a heartbeat can be enormously satisfying. As conveyed on television, it is an exciting part of being a health care provider. But keeping someone alive who has provided written instructions that prohibit life-support measures not only violates the patient's rights, but is also illegal. Ignoring a DNR can result in prolonged suffering, further medical expenses for the patient and family, and possibly litigation against health care providers and the hospital. Every health care provider should understand the legal aspects of AMDs; knowing which patients have advance directives is the responsibility of each caregiver.

### Preparation for Death-and-Dying Situations

You may or may not be preparing for a role in health care that includes the care of dying patients. Regardless of your expected role, you should be prepared for participation in a life-or-death situation, either in your career or in your personal life. Know the provisions of federal laws and the laws of your state pertaining to the rights of patients and their families, know the policies of your employing health care agency, and be aware of your own beliefs about death and dying. The concept of death with dignity, knowledge about AMDs, and awareness of the provisions of the PSDA should help you accept that patients have a right to participate in decisions about end-of-life care. You should also learn to accept the inevitability of death, the limitations of medical science, and the inappropriateness of heroic measures in some situations. *It is especially important that you develop your own philosophy about death, which includes facing your own fears about death and accepting your own mortality.*

Thoughtful consideration of the following questions will help you clarify your beliefs and develop your own philosophy of death:

- What do I believe about death?
- What do I believe about my own death?
- What fears do I have about dying?
- What would I have to give up if I were dying?
- What work do I want to complete before I die?
- What relationships do I want to mend before I die?
- What do I want to say to my loved ones before I die?
- What do I want to say to a loved one before he or she dies?
- Who should dispose of my possessions following my death? Who is to receive what?

By developing your own personal philosophy of death, you will have clearer beliefs about the care of a dying patient. If the health care provider role you expect to assume does not involve caring for dying patients, you may be tempted to ignore this exercise. But you cannot be sure what the future holds—in your career or in your personal life. So consider the following in terms of "What do I believe about the care of a patient who...":

- Does not want to be resuscitated if a cardiac arrest occurs?
- Refuses intravenous fluids or tube feedings during the final stages of an illness?
- Refuses dialysis, even though the kidneys are not functioning?
- Refuses chemotherapy, even though the oncologist insists there is a 20% chance it will help?
- Begs the doctor, "Just let me die."
- Begs the doctor, "Just put me out of my misery."

Inadequate management of pain is the reason some patients wish for death or consider suicide. The expression of a wish for death, then, may mean that the patient needs improved management of pain. However, many dying patients have accepted death and are ready—mentally, emotionally, and spiritually—even before the physical body ceases to function. Be sensitive to the needs of such patients, and especially to a patient's readiness for death.

## Ethics Committees

The Karen Ann Quinlan court decision included a recommendation that ethics committees, rather than the courts, should handle controversial patient care situations. In 1995, the Joint Commission on Accreditation of Health Care Organizations began requiring that health care facilities set up a code of ethical behavior. As a result, most hospitals are establishing ethics committees to review patient care conflicts. Some ethics committees involve patients' families in hearings, thereby ensuring that all viewpoints will be heard and increasing the probability that a decision will be acceptable to the hospital, the physician, and the family. In other hospitals, the ethics committees exclude families from the hearing, relying on reports of the medical staff for rendering a decision. The latter approach carries the risk of having the patient's end-of-life choices ignored in favor of aggressive medical treatment.

Ideally, ethics committees would always protect the patient's well-being and respect the expressed wishes of the patient and family for end-of-life care. Ethics committees can and should encourage staff training in the legal and ethical issues most often involved in patient care/institutional conflict.

Numerous issues are being addressed in the medical community, the mass media, and the courts: definition of death, when life support may be discontinued, when artificial feedings for persons in a persistent vegetative state may be discontinued, the right of a patient to choose accelerated death, culpability of a person who assists a patient to commit suicide, and the moral/ethical/legal aspects of euthanasia. Some legal issues may be resolved within the next several years. In the meantime, everyone involved in end-of-life care must resolve for themselves the ethical and moral issues related to the dying process.

## REFERENCES AND SUGGESTED READINGS

Buchwald, Art. (2007). *Too soon to say goodbye*. New York: Random House.
Compassion and Choices. (2009, Summer). *Compassion and Choices Magazine: Special resource issue, 8*(2).
Eisenberg, Daniel. (2006). *The right vs. the right to die: How to stop it from happening again*. San Francisco: Harper San Francisco.
Humphrey, Derek. (2007). *Good life, good death—A memoir*. Junction City, OR: Norris Lane Press.
Humphrey, Derek. (2008). *The good euthanasia guide: Where, what and who in choices in dying*. Junction City, OR: Norris Lane Press.
Kiernan, Stephen P. (2006). *Last rights: Rescuing the end of life from the medical system*. New York: St. Martin's Press.
Preston, Tom. (2006). *Patient-directed dying: A call for legalized aid in dying for the terminally ill*. Lincoln, NE: iUniverse.
Relman, Arnold S. (2007). *A second opinion: Rescuing America's health care*. Cambridge, MA: Perseus.
Terman, Stan, et al. (2007). *The best way to say goodbye: A legal, peaceful choice*. Carlsbad, CA: Life Transitions Publications.
Wanzer, Sidney, & Glenmullen, Joseph. (2007). *To die well: Your right to comfort, calm, and choice in the last days of life*. Cambridge, MA: De Capo Press.

## SOURCES OF ADDITIONAL INFORMATION

**AARP,** http://www.aarp.org/endoflife
**Aging with Dignity,** http://www.agingwithdignity.org
**Compassion and Choices,** http://compassionandchoices.org/cid/
**Critical Conditions,** http://critical-conditions.org
**Death with Dignity National Center,** http://www.deathwithdignity.org
**Euthanasia Research and Guidance Organization (ERGO),** http://www.finalexit.org
**Partnership for Caring,** http://www.partnershipforcaring.org
  Advance directive packages, including legal forms for each of the 50 states, can be ordered by phone—1 (800) 989-9455—or downloaded from the Web site.
**Physician's Order for Life Sustaining Treatment (POLST),** http://polst.org
  Source of a standardized form for converting a patient's treatment choices into doctor's orders.
**Right to Die Organization,** http://www.worldrtd.org and http://www.finalexit.org

## REVIEW AND SELF-CHECK

1. List three practices related to death and dying that have changed over the past hundred years.

   Death was accepted as part of life; Death was common experience; Death was visible; Illness/death would occur at home; Family/friends would say good-bye to dying person; Dying person gave blessing to survivors

2. List five examples of beliefs about death that fit your current beliefs.

   Death is acceptable for the aged persons; Death of children is viewed as tragic; Within health care system — death is enemy to be conquered
   — goal is to maintain physical existence
   — death is seen as person's failure in dying process
   — patient is isolated from loved ones

3. How can death education alleviate one's fears about death? State at least three reasons.

   awareness of needs of dying persons; importance of grief process; techniques for helping patient + families cope w/ death

4. Name five conditions that contribute to "death with dignity."

   modified hospital policies for terminal patients; homecare of dying; hospice care; more family participation; recognition of human needs

5. List five current issues related to end-of-life care.

   Dying person allowed some control
   Dying person allowed to prepare in their way
   Mortality is fact of life
   Dying person should focus on quality of life
   Intervention discuss w/ patient
   Dying person should be allowed to discussed dying openly

6. Name three reasons the courts are sometimes involved in end-of-life decisions.

   Living will, DPA, PSDA, Assisted Suicide

7. Compare euthanasia, suicide, and assisted suicide in terms of purpose, responsibility, and actions.

   Euthanasia is any action, requested by the patient, but carried out by someone else that accelerates the dying.

8. State the purpose of:

   a. The living will

   allows individuals to indicate their wishes regarding the med. care before they are unable to do so

   b. The medical durable power of attorney

   is that specific person can make medical decisions if patient can't do

9. List four provisions of the PSDA.

   Be more accepting of limitations of science
   Accept man's mortality
   Accept that heroic measures might be inappropriate

10. List your beliefs about:  student's own belief

    a. Death

    b. End-of-life care

## ASSIGNMENTS

1. Draw a line that represents your life span. It can be any shape or length. The beginning represents birth; the end, death. Mark several significant losses at points along the line.

2. Study your life line. Does it make you uncomfortable? If so, consider possible reasons for this effect.

3. Think about death for 15 seconds, then write down 5 to 10 adjectives that immediately come to mind.

4. Think about your own death for five seconds. Write down two words that describe your feelings.

5. Consider your losses if you were to die in an accident tomorrow:

    a. List the relationships you would lose.

    b. List the possessions you would be giving up.

    c. List uncompleted tasks you would leave behind.

6. Refer to your list of relationships and your list of possessions. Decide how you would want your property distributed. Prepare instructions to guide your survivors in carrying out your wishes:

    a. Disposition of your body

    b. A funeral or memorial service

    c. Disposition of your property

    d. Care of your survivors, if you have dependents

7. Write your obituary, including age at time of death, the cause of death, the achievements or affiliations for which you will be remembered, your survivors, and the final arrangements.

8. Now that you have thought about your death, list tasks you will complete as soon as possible.

9. Participate in a class discussion about the following topics:

    - Withholding artificial feedings from a patient who is in an irreversible coma

    - Withholding artificial feedings from a patient who is conscious but approaching death

    - "Do not resuscitate" orders

    - A patient's right to refuse a treatment the doctor wants to administer

    - Discontinuing life support for a patient in a persistent vegetative state

    - Discontinuing life support for a conscious patient who requests that it be discontinued

    - Discontinuing dialysis for a patient who does not want to live as a quadriplegic

10. At the top of a blank sheet of paper, write "What I believe about death." List your present beliefs.

11. At the top of a blank sheet of paper, write "What I believe about care of a dying patient." List your present beliefs.

12. Obtain a copy of the legal document used in your state for AMDs. Read through the document. Is it a living will? Is it a medical DPA? What rights does it give the patient? What rights does it give the family?

13. Interview all members of your immediate family to find out what they know about AMDs. Provide information and encourage them to complete an AMD.

14. Using the appropriate form for your state, prepare your own AMD, sign it (with the necessary number of witnesses), and inform your family that you have an AMD.

15. Discuss the specific choices you have indicated in your AMD with your family, the proxy named in your medical DPA, and your physician.

16. Use the Internet to find sources of information/Web sites related to:

    a. The right to die

    b. Euthanasia

    c. Rights of dying persons

    d. Right to refuse life-prolonging treatments

    e. Choices related to dying

17. Use the library and/or the Internet to learn about one of the following cases: Terri Schiavo, Mary Beth Cruzan, Karen Ann Quinlan.

# UNIT 22

# Grief and Bereavement

## OBJECTIVES

Upon completion of this unit, you should be able to:

- List four influences on a person's reaction to loss.
- List five emotional components of grief.
- List physical effects of grief—five immediate effects and four delayed effects.
- List five mental/emotional effects of grief.
- List five effects of grief on behavior.
- List two needs of a bereaved person.
- List five conditions that facilitate the grief process.
- List six conditions that inhibit the grief process.
- Name the five stages of the grief process as described by Dr. Kübler-Ross.
- List five indications of unresolved grief.
- State five guidelines for assisting the family of a dying patient.

## KEY TERMS

Anticipatory grief
Bereavement
Condolences
Grief work

Grief is a normal and natural reaction to loss that ranges from mild disappointment through various degrees of sadness, up to the intense and painful state that we call grief. **Anticipatory grief** occurs prior to the actual loss, usually during a terminal illness. **Bereavement** is separation from or loss of someone who is significant in one's life. Grief is the predominant emotional response to bereavement, although anger and fear may also be experienced. **Grief work** is a process of working through the emotional reaction to loss, reorganizing one's life patterns, and achieving some degree of adjustment. Grief work is important to future emotional and mental health. Uncompleted grief work will eventually manifest as physical illness, poor adjustment, or tendencies to avoid or overreact to situations involving loss, dying, or bereavement.

## REACTIONS TO LOSS AND BEREAVEMENT

Each person reacts in his or her own way to each of life's losses. Some people react mildly for a short period of time to a specific loss. Another person may experience intense feelings for days, weeks, or months following a similar loss. Dr. Kübler-Ross has noted that many people experience a grief reaction similar to the five stages of dying, even if a loss is relatively small. For example, Mr. B. lost a set of keys that included the house key, several office keys, and the car keys. He went through the following stages during a period of 10 days:

- I just don't believe I would lose my keys. (Denial)
- I am furious that those keys haven't been found. (Anger)
- If those keys turn up, I will always put them on the refrigerator as soon as I get home. (Bargaining)
- I'm not worth very much if I can't even keep up with my keys. (Depression)
- The keys are definitely lost. I may as well have some additional keys made. (Acceptance)

The reaction to loss of an object may be relatively mild and of short duration, depending on the meaning of the object to its owner. Losses that are related to one's self-esteem, such as loss of a job or the end of a relationship, tend to produce intense emotional reactions of longer duration than losses that do not threaten self-esteem. A sudden or unexpected loss produces an intense reaction that begins with shock and disbelief.

Some grief reactions include not only sadness, but also some degree of anger, hate, guilt, anxiety, or even panic. *Anger* is usually a major component in grief when the age of the deceased is "inappropriate" for dying, such as infancy and childhood, adolescence, young adulthood, or "the prime of life." A survivor may actually feel anger toward the deceased for "going away and leaving me." This reaction is especially likely in a child whose parent has died. *Anxiety* is related to the future: "How can I live without . . . (that which was lost)?" or "How can I make certain this never happens to me again?" *Panic* is related to the recognition that one does not have the power to control the loss of a loved one. *Guilt* may be concerned with control: "Could I have prevented this from happening?" or blame: "If I had been more loving, this wouldn't have happened." Children who are not old enough to understand terminal illness or death are especially prone to guilt, because a child's anger toward a family member or playmate is sometimes expressed as an explosive "I hate you!" or possibly, "I wish you were dead!" A child may recall past actions, words, or thoughts and perceive that behavior and the death or illness as having a cause/effect relationship.

Grief is painful. Grief related to loss of a loved one through death usually results in a profound grief reaction. The remainder of this unit limits discussion of grief to this type of loss.

## EFFECTS OF GRIEF

The death of a loved one has both physical and psychological effects on the survivor (Figure 22-1). Shock is the immediate reaction. Profound shock is likely if a death is sudden or unexpected, the result of an accident or act of violence, or a suicide. In contrast to sudden bereavement, a lengthy illness provides time for anticipatory grieving prior to the actual death. Intensity of the immediate grief reaction, then, is determined by whether the death was expected or unexpected, a sudden or slow process, violent or nonviolent. If shock is severe, the survivor cannot begin grief work until the physical effects of shock have subsided.

**FIGURE 22-1** Grief has both physical and psychological effects.
*Delmar/Cengage Learning*

In the absence of severe shock, a grief reaction can range from little or no visible reaction to uncontrolled, destructive behavior. The immediate physical effects include tightness in the throat, a choking sensation, shortness of breath, weakness, a feeling of emptiness or a knot in the stomach, and nausea. These effects may subside within a few hours, to be replaced by loss of appetite and/or digestive problems, disturbed sleep patterns, restlessness, frequent sighing, and crying that may continue intermittently for days, weeks, or months.

The mental/emotional effects of bereavement include preoccupation with thoughts of the deceased, lack of interest in other people, irritability, difficulty in organizing thoughts or making decisions, difficulty in concentrating or remembering, feelings of hopelessness, feelings of guilt, and possibly a tendency toward blaming self or others for the loss. Some behavioral effects of grief are lack of interest in grooming, refusal to participate in previous activities or hobbies, poor performance at home or on the job, reminiscing about the deceased, idealizing the deceased (forgetting negative aspects of the deceased), and clinging to personal reminders.

These effects of grief vary in intensity and duration according to a survivor's relationship to the deceased, personal ways of dealing with strong emotion, and patterns of behavior learned in previous life crises. *How a survivor deals with grief influences future adjustment.*

## IMPORTANCE OF THE GRIEF PROCESS

Grief is a period of pain from which one recovers over time. It may also be a growth experience in which one learns to accept certain realities:

- We are vulnerable to certain life experiences, including losses.
- We are not all-powerful. We only have control over *some* aspects of our lives.
- We are mortal, not immortal.

- There will be a time for each of us when life comes to an end.
- Loss requires saying "good-bye" to some aspect of life, but loss can also mean a new beginning.
- "Letting go" does not diminish the importance of what was lost, but it does free the survivor to make the necessary adjustments for living without the deceased.

The bereaved should make his or her own decisions about involvement with other people and participation in activities. Some people need a period of time for withdrawal or denial before accepting the finality of the loss. If the grief process is delayed too long, however, the person's adjustment deteriorates, and a delayed grief reaction eventually occurs, possibly with destructive effects. Because grieving leads eventually to adjustment and denying grief leads to deterioration in adjustment, anyone who has suffered a loss should (1) be encouraged to grieve and (2) continue to have emotional support until grief work has been completed.

## INFLUENCES ON THE GRIEF PROCESS

Any person who has experienced a significant loss has the right to grieve. A person's grieving tends to be consistent with the personality and usual coping styles. The intensity and duration of grieving are influenced by the relationship to the deceased and past experiences with loss. Friends and family should grant each survivor the right to grieve in his or her own way.

Working through the stages of denial, anger, and bargaining prior to the actual death seems to facilitate grief work during the bereavement period. Spending quality time with the dying person—sharing memories, expressing feelings, touching and holding—facilitates anticipatory grieving and also eases the dying process.

### Emotional Support

Grieving is facilitated if family members share their feelings and if relatives and friends are supportive throughout the process (Figure 22-2). It is especially important that this emotional support comes from those with whom the bereaved must restructure his or her life—resume the daily routine of old responsibilities, assume new responsibilities, and restructure relationships

**FIGURE 22-2** A survivor may need encouragement to express the feelings that accompany loss. *Delmar/Cengage Learning*

that no longer include the deceased. This support network is especially important on significant dates—anniversaries, birthdays, and holidays—throughout the first year of bereavement.

## Acceptance of Loss

Grief work begins with acceptance of the loss—the finality of death. Sometimes there is intellectual acceptance without emotional acceptance. Only when the finality of the loss is accepted at the emotional level can grief work begin. The survivor needs encouragement to "be with" his or her feelings by expressing the sadness and pain, rather than denying the feelings or hiding them from others.

## Making Final Arrangements

Participating in the tasks related to death seems to facilitate acceptance. Before or immediately after the death, someone must notify relatives, friends, coworkers, the minister, and the family lawyer; prepare an obituary; care for and remove the body; plan for the disposal of the body (burial, cremation); plan a service (funeral, memorial); purchase a cemetery lot (or decide how to dispose of the ashes if cremation is chosen); complete paperwork (death certificate, notices to insurance and annuity companies, government agencies, banks). Insofar as possible, the tasks that involve decision making should be completed prior to the actual death, because one who is experiencing powerful emotions may not be able to make important decisions. The closest survivors should make certain decisions; however, some people are unable or unwilling to make funeral plans while the patient is still living.

Some people want to be involved in the final stages of the dying process, and some want to assist with final care of the body. Being present at the final moments of life is beneficial to survivors and also to the patient. Many dying patients state that dying alone is their greatest fear. For survivors, being with the patient in those last moments is preparation for emotional release. Bathing, dressing, and grooming the body provides an opportunity for saying "good-bye" in the most loving and caring way possible. This is especially appropriate if the deceased is a child. Sometimes the survivors participate in closing the grave with handfuls of dirt. This, too, is a way of saying "good-bye" and moving toward emotional acceptance of the loss.

The body of the deceased and the final service both play a role in acceptance of death. The body is a stimulus to the release of feelings. The funeral service and interment provide opportunities to express the intense feelings that immediately follow the death and help prepare the survivors for grief work. Alternatives to a traditional funeral, such as a memorial service, can also facilitate the grief process.

## Grief Inhibitors

In the belief that people need to be protected, someone may try to keep those closest to the deceased from participating in these tasks. Friends or relatives may encourage survivors-to-be to withdraw from the death scene and to delegate final tasks to others. The survivors may even be deprived of time with the loved one, either during the final moments or immediately after death, in the mistaken belief that witnessing the death or being with the body would be traumatic. No matter how good their intentions, people who influence the family to withdraw from the death scene deprive family members of an experience that facilitates "letting go" and beginning the grief process.

Children, especially, are likely to be excluded. As they observe atypical adult behavior and disruption of the family's normal routine, they may be confused, frightened, or angry. They need explanations about what is happening, much comforting, and a chance to say "good-bye" to the dying person *if they wish to do so.*

Numerous other conditions can inhibit the grief process: a sudden death, an untimely death, the mode of death (accident, suicide, violence), unresolved grief from past losses, past tendency to suppress anger and grief, ambivalent feelings toward the deceased, the use of drugs or alcohol to suppress feelings, resuming normal activities too early, isolation from a death (war in a foreign country), or uncertainty about a death (a plane crash or fire in which the remains are difficult or impossible to identify). The uncertainty created when the body cannot be viewed makes it especially difficult for survivors to accept the death. There is, instead, a tendency to cling to the belief that "(name of the victim) will come back home some day."

## Condolences

Most people find it difficult to express **condolences** to the bereaved. All too often, statements that are offered as words of comfort or as reassurance actually deny the importance of grief or imply that the person has no right to grieve. The following are examples of such statements:

- "You must be strong" implies that showing one's grief is a sign of weakness.
- "You must be a little man" denies a boy the right to grieve and also implies that, as a male, he is not allowed to cry.
- "It's time to get on with your life" is a way of saying, "I do not grant you any more time for grieving."

Often, the most effective form of condolence is simply silence, accompanied by a hug or kiss if appropriate. Friends and relatives who take time to "be there" for a bereaved person are helpful. Staying in touch, either in person or by phone or mail, keeps the bereaved person believing that you care. As time passes, having friends and family who are willing to listen facilitates the grieving process for a bereaved person.

If a year has passed, the person may need professional counseling to facilitate the completion of grief work. But a statement such as, "It's time to get on with your life" is totally inappropriate a month, or even several months, after the death of a loved one. An inappropriate statement may indicate that the speaker does not understand the grief process or its importance to a survivor's future adjustment.

## GRIEF WORK

The grief process does not flow smoothly, nor is it effortless. Management of grief requires time and energy and involves much psychological pain (Figure 22-3). The grief process requires at least a year for completion. A bereaved person experiences a sequence of emotional states over a period of time. The expression *grief work* is used to describe these experiences.

Ideally, grief work should begin within a few days of the death. Following the initial stage of shock and denial, there is a release of feelings, which may be followed by a period of confusion. There may be recurrent dreams about the deceased. Memories may crowd the mind, making it difficult to concentrate or even to sleep. This is a time when talking about

**FIGURE 22-3** The grief process requires time but should be completed.
*Delmar/Cengage Learning*

the deceased is therapeutic. There is a need to remember and to review the relationship with the loved one—the good memories and the bad memories. The survivor must work through not only the sadness, but also any anger, fear, and feelings of guilt. This "working through" is best accomplished through talking with others about one's loss and expressing the feelings of the moment. Some people need to talk *to* the deceased—say what was left unsaid during their time together, ask for forgiveness, or express regrets. Crying is effective for expressing both sadness and anger, but verbalizing is especially effective for diffusing sadness and anger and resolving guilt feelings. Those with creative talent may express their feelings through music, art, or writing. Each mourner must work through these feelings in his or her own way, sometimes in private and sometimes with the help and support of others.

Eventually, the sadness is replaced by loneliness—an intense loneliness that is not relieved by the presence of others (Figure 22-4). The bereaved is beginning to realize that the void left by the deceased cannot be filled by anyone else. The unique relationship with the deceased is lost forever. This is a period of freeing oneself from the deceased; with time, loneliness gives way to hopefulness. When talk begins to focus less on the loss and more on changes needed to adjust to life without the deceased, the grief process is nearing completion.

With additional time, the survivor resumes some former activities, establishes new relationships or modifies old relationships to exclude the deceased, and begins to find satisfaction in daily activities. At that point, the survivor is "getting on" with his or her life. Successful completion of grief work leads to a greater understanding of life, greater compassion for the suffering of others, and higher levels of sensitivity to the needs of others who have suffered loss.

## Uncompleted Grief Work

Some survivors fail to complete the grief process, either because feelings are suppressed or because certain conditions inhibit the grief process. Grief that is not resolved may be indicated by hyperactivity, inappropriate feelings, physical illness (possibly with the symptoms of the

**FIGURE 22-4** Grief often includes a profound sense of aloneness. *Delmar/Cengage Learning*

deceased, if he or she dies of an illness), changes in relationships with others, hostility, depression, or a lack of feeling. Sometimes the grief reaction becomes chronic; that is, the bereaved becomes locked into the early stages of the process and does not progress toward readjustment. Denial of grief at the time of the loss may result in a delayed grief reaction after weeks, months, or even years, usually at the time of another death or when a close friend is grieving.

Supportive friends and relatives can contribute greatly to successful grief work. Professional counseling is needed, however, when a survivor manifests denial or evidence of uncompleted grief work after one year.

## ROLES OF HEALTH CARE PROVIDERS

The health care provider is likely to be in contact with relatives of a dying patient when they are survivors-to-be, rather than throughout the bereavement period. Because the physician has primary responsibility for providing information about a patient's condition, health workers must know what the patient, as well as the family, has been told. This can be determined by carefully worded questions and by observation of nonverbal behavior. Active listening is effective for learning what the physician has told the patient and family and identifying where the other person is emotionally. Sometimes it is appropriate to use open and honest communication, such as "I feel sad that your husband is so sick."

The health care provider's goal is to help the family, not by giving information or expressing personal opinions, but by helping the other to express feelings and work toward acceptance of the loss at his or her own pace. Various professional workers are prepared to provide skilled counseling for patients and their families. Large hospitals have chaplains and social workers, some of whom have special preparation for helping others cope with a life crisis.

Smaller hospitals and most nursing homes rely on community resources to provide this specialized service.

Nurses have the advantage of providing care throughout the day and night. Other personnel visit the patient or stay with families for a relatively brief period of time. Each death/bereavement situation is unique, so there cannot be a single procedure to guide the health care provider. But there are guidelines that may help the caregiver adapt to each situation.

## GUIDELINES FOR ASSISTING THE FAMILY OF A DYING PATIENT

1. Be available to the family as much as possible. (Do *not* use the nurses' station as a refuge to avoid interacting with the family.)
2. Use active listening to encourage the expression of feelings.
3. Interact with the patient as you provide physical care. Model for family members the expression of caring, even if the patient is not responsive.
4. Be tolerant of what you see and hear. Various members of the family are at different stages of grieving, and each is reacting to a life crisis in his or her own way.
5. Encourage close family members to stay with the patient, to talk and touch as much as possible throughout the dying process. This is important, even if the patient is comatose.

**Note:** Be aware that the hospital has an intimidating effect on many people. To "stay out of the way," they may miss their final opportunity to be with the loved one who is dying, unless you encourage them to stay close by.

6. As appropriate, offer to call the family minister, priest, or rabbi. If you observe that a family seems to need assistance in dealing with their grief, contact the hospital chaplain or social worker.
7. Know the available sources of help in your community and share this information with a family as appropriate. For example, *Compassionate Friends* is a support group for parents who have lost a child.
8. Work on your own "unfinished business" related to past losses and on your own fears related to death. Until you have accepted your own mortality and completed your own grief work, you cannot be fully effective in helping others to cope with death and dying.

## REFERENCES AND SUGGESTED READINGS

Deits, Bob. (2009). *Life after loss.* Cambridge, MA: DeCapo Press.
Hollerand, Andrew. (2007). *Grief.* New York: Hyperion.
James, John W., & Friedman, Russell. (2009). *The grief recovery handbook, 20th anniversary edition: The action program for moving beyond death, divorce, and other losses, including health, career, and faith.* New York: HarperCollins. (Note: Some counselors give a copy of this book to each member of a bereavement group.)
Kübler-Ross, Elisabeth, & Kessler, David. (2005). *On grief and grieving: Finding the meaning of grief through the five stages of loss.* New York: Simon & Schuster.
Wright, H. Norman. (2004). *Experiencing grief.* Nashville, TN: Broadman & Holman.

## SOURCES OF ADDITIONAL INFORMATION

**AARP,** http://www.griefandloss.org

**GriefNet.org,** http://www.griefnet.org; http://kidsaid.com. E-mail support groups directed by a clinical psychologist who is also a death educator and traumatologist.

## REVIEW AND SELF-CHECK

1. List four influences on a person's reaction to loss.

    individuals pattern of reacting to loss
    type of loss (object, job, person)
    significance of loss
    whether or not loss is a threat to loss to self-esteem

2. List five emotional components of grief.

    sadness
    anger
    hate
    guilt
    anxiety & panic

3. List five immediate physical effects of grief.

    tightness in throat, choking sensation, shortness of breath, weakness, knot in stomach, nausea, feeling cold

4. List four delayed physical reactions to grief.

    lack of appetite, disturbed sleep habits, restlessness, frequent sighing, crying

5. List five mental and/or emotional effects of grief.

   Pre-occupation of the thoughts of the deceased
   Lack of interest in other people; irritability
   Difficulty in organizing thoughts, making decision
   Feeling of worthlessness
   Feelings of guilt

6. List five possible effects of grief on a person's behavior.

   Lack of interest in grooming → being depressed so a person has no interest in grooming himself
   Refusal to participate in previous activities
   Poor performance; Reminiscing about deceased
   Refusal to listen to criticism about deceased
   Forgetting negative aspects; clinging to personal reminders

7. State two needs of a bereaved person.

   encourage the to grieve & have emotional support

8. Name five conditions that can facilitate the grief process.

   right to grieve is granted ; Bereaved accepts finality of loss
   Anticipatory grief is experienced ; survivors expresses sadness & loss
   Family members share feelings ; Survivor participates in tasks
   Relatives and friends must be supportive   related to death
   Support is provided on all significant dates

9. List six conditions that may inhibit the grief process.

   Protecting the survivor from tasks related to death ; sedation through use of chemicals
   Denying family time during final moments of life ; Resuming normal activities too soon
   Not participating in final services ; Uncertainty about death
   Not being allowed to express feelings ; Inappropriate statement about
   Ambivalent feelings towards deceased         death

10. List five indications that a person has unresolved grief.

    *hyperactivity, inappropriate feelings, physical illness, changes in relationship w/ others, hostility, depression, lack of feeling*

11. Develop five guidelines for assisting the family of a dying patient.

    *Be available to family as much as possible*
    *Be tolerant of what you see and hear*
    *Encourage family members*
    *Ask for the chaplain assistant*
    *Know available resources*

## ASSIGNMENTS

1. If you have lost a member of your immediate family, write a brief description of your reaction—immediate and throughout the first year. Evaluate your grief work: Was it effective? Or do you have "unfinished business"?

2. If you have never experienced the loss of a loved one through death, prepare for the time when you will have such an experience by writing out a set of guidelines to help you complete the grief process.

3. Participate in a small-group discussion on:

    a. The stages of grief as described by Kübler-Ross.

    b. Your own experiences with grief compared to the Kübler-Ross model.

4. Participate in a class project to identify your community resources for assisting bereaved people. Which of these provide immediate but short-term assistance? Which ones provide long-term assistance?

5. Think about the following situations and be prepared to participate in a small-group discussion about the (1) reactions reflected in each situation and (2) conditions that could have changed the reaction:

    a. A family of four adult children and one adolescent experienced the sudden death of their father. Sarah, being a nurse, took charge of the situation. She delegated tasks to each of her brothers and sisters. One sister was so overcome with grief that she could not perform her assignments, so Sarah took care of those tasks in addition to her own. Sarah was described by relatives as a "tower of strength for all of us." From the time when news of the death was received until the estate was settled, Sarah stayed busy "doing what has to be done." Approximately 10 months following her father's death, Sarah was admitted to the hospital in critical condition. Although she recovered, her convalescence required almost a full year.

    b. Lissa was a college graduate who had worked for six years to help her husband finish law school and set up his law practice. As soon as she became pregnant, Lissa quit her job to be a full-time homemaker. When her two children were two and four years old, Bob went to a distant city on business. He decided to fly so he could be home in time to spend the weekend with his family. On Friday evening, a plane crashed as it was landing at the local airport. News of the crash was broadcast within minutes. Lissa heard the newscast and knew that Bob was supposed to be on that flight. Her parents heard the newscast and rushed over to be with their daughter. They found her cheerfully setting the table for dinner. When they told her about the crash, she responded, "I heard that newscast. But I know Bob didn't get on that plane." After several weeks, workers at the crash site still had found nothing that could provide positive identification of Bob. Two years later, Lissa is still saying, "I know Bob is alive. Someday he will walk through the front door."

6. Beside each of the following statements, write a more appropriate statement for conveying compassion and emotional support to someone who has just lost a loved one:

    a. You must be strong.

    b. Now you are the man of the house.

    c. He is no longer suffering.

    d. She is in heaven now.

    e. You know it was his own fault; he just loved to drive fast and wouldn't use a seat belt.

    f. Start putting your life together; it's been a month now.

7. In a class discussion, add other inappropriate statements that might be said to a bereaved person, then discuss how those statements could be reworded to provide emotional support and encouragement.

# UNIT 23

# Caring for the Dying Person

## OBJECTIVES

Upon completion of this unit, you should be able to:

- List five fears commonly expressed by a dying person.
- List the five stages of dying, as proposed by Dr. Kübler-Ross.
- Describe a "healthy" reaction to dying, as proposed by Lindemann.
- List seven conditions that contribute to the adjustment of a dying patient, according to Carey.
- Discuss three personal and family issues related to the care of a dying person.
- Name three medical issues related to the care of a dying person.
- List five issues related to the rights of a dying patient.
- State five guidelines for meeting the needs of a dying patient.
- List five advantages of dying at home.
- State the primary focus of "palliative care."

## KEY TERMS

Curative
Humane
Palliative
Transformation

## REACTIONS TO DIAGNOSIS OF A TERMINAL ILLNESS

As a result of current practices in the care of terminally ill patients, many middle-aged people today have had little or no personal contact with a dying person. Their experience with death is limited to occasional attendance at a funeral. There is a universal tendency to fear that which is unknown and foreign to one's own experience, so death and dying have been relegated to the closet. Death is taboo as a topic of conversation for most people. But diagnosis of an illness for which there is currently no cure brings a patient and family members face to face with the reality of death. The reaction to such news includes fear—fear of the unknown and fear of death.

Counselors who work with dying patients have identified a number of fears expressed by many patients:

- What happens after death? What lies beyond death?
- Will I be forgotten?
- Will my loved ones be cared for adequately without me? If they can get along without me, does that mean I was not important to them?
- What will become of my work, my lifelong efforts to accomplish something? Will my work be continued by someone else? Will someone else take credit for my work?
- What will happen to my property? Will my possessions be cared for? How will they be distributed?
- Will I become dependent on others?
- Will I be a burden? Who will pay my medical bills?
- Will I lose my mind?
- Will I lose control of my life? Who will make important decisions that affect me?
- Will I have more pain than I can bear?
- Will I be left to die alone?

A major responsibility of caregivers is to recognize manifestations of fear and encourage a patient to verbalize them. Expressing fears about death to an understanding listener facilitates the dying process.

## STAGES OF DYING

According to Dr. Elisabeth Kübler-Ross, a dying person goes through five stages, beginning with denial and ending with acceptance that death is approaching. At some point, the dying patient begins to grieve for all that must be given up: relationships with loved ones and friends, material possessions, ambitions, life goals and purposes, plans for the future, and, ultimately, one's body.

Hope is important throughout the five stages. Without hope, the patient would lapse into despair. Fear also may be part of a patient's emotional state in any or all of the stages.

Although some thanatologists disagree with Dr. Kübler-Ross about the stages of dying, her model does provide a framework for understanding the feelings a dying person may experience. Naming these stages undoubtedly has helped caregivers recognize the needs of dying patients and accept behaviors that represent a patient's progress in relation to the dying process.

### Denial

The first stage of dying involves denial—"No, I am not dying. It just isn't true." This reaction seems to occur regardless of whether or not a person is told directly that he or she has a terminal illness. Denial may be manifested in many ways: changing doctors several times, continuing one's daily routine as though nothing is wrong, refusing to talk about the illness, refusing treatment, or embarking on a search for any and all treatments.

Denial serves a useful purpose. As a defense mechanism, it gives the patient time to deal with the shock of knowing that life is coming to an end. Denial may recur at intervals throughout the dying process.

### Anger

The second stage of dying is characterized by anger. As the patient begins to face the reality of terminal illness, the reaction is, "Why me? Why not somebody else?" During this stage, the patient may direct anger at anyone and everyone. It is a difficult time for health care providers as well as the family. The caregivers, it seems, cannot do anything right during this period. The patient's behavior is easier to tolerate if one remembers that this patient is in the process of learning to face his or her death.

### Bargaining

In the third stage of dying, the patient begins to bargain—with God, fate, the doctor or nurses, or the family. This bargaining may be unknown to the caregivers, or it may be shared. Perhaps the patient prays to stay alive until some particular event—the birth of a grandchild, a wedding, a child's graduation. Perhaps the patient promises to change behavior or lifestyle, if he or she can have a second chance: "If only I can be well again, I'll never take another drink." Bargaining may take the form of being a "good" patient—cheerful and cooperative regardless of annoying treatments or pain.

### Depression

The fourth stage is marked by depression. With increased symptoms, especially pain or weakness, the patient can no longer maintain denial; bargaining seems pointless; anger gives way to sorrow over impending losses. Dr. Kübler-Ross believes that this period involves two different types of depression: (1) a *reactive depression* to the impending losses faced by the patient and (2) a *preparatory depression* related to the impending separation.

### Acceptance

The fifth stage is one of acceptance. *Provided the patient has enough time and is helped to work through the previous stages*, this stage represents several accomplishments:

- The patient is neither depressed nor angry.
- The patient has grieved for the many losses.
- The patient is tired and/or weak and dozes frequently for short periods.

The stage of acceptance is not a happy stage. It is more likely to be, according to Dr. Kübler-Ross, devoid of feeling. But the patient is at peace (Figure 23-1).

Health care providers should not expect a dying patient to move systematically through these five stages. One patient may appear to skip a stage; another may continue in denial up to the time of death; still another may appear to reach acceptance very quickly. The stages do, however, provide a useful framework for identifying a specific patient's needs. By responding appropriately according to a patient's current emotional state, each health care provider can contribute to a patient's progress toward acceptance.

FIGURE 23-1 As death approaches, the patient becomes less responsive and body functions slow. *Delmar/Cengage Learning*

## DYING AS A GROWTH PROCESS

When death is viewed in light of the many losses involved, it is difficult to think of dying as an opportunity for growth. Viewed in terms of the emotional changes and the **transformation** that may occur as the dying process is completed, both spiritual and emotional growth become evident. According to Dr. Mwalinu Imara, author of "Dying as the Last Stage of Growth" in Dr. Kübler-Ross's book *Death: The Final Stage of Growth*, ". . . the dying stage of our life can be experienced as the most profound growth event of our total life's experience . . . if we are fortunate enough to have time to live and experience our own process, our arrival at a plateau of creative acceptance will be worth it."

The dying person has a choice: to withdraw in despair, to suppress negative emotions, or to reach out to others (Figure 23-2). It is through the third option that growth occurs. Growth requires commitment to experiencing self, becoming aware of one's own identity, communicating one's experience to others, and accepting that one's life had purpose and meaning. These changes are facilitated by a support network of loving and caring people, who also have the opportunity for growth as they share in the dying experience.

Many people need the help of a skilled counselor to work through the negative aspects of life experiences. The goal of helping a person work through the dying process is to have the individual achieve emotional adjustment and live life to the fullest during whatever time remains. Arrival at the stage of acceptance with a sense of peace indicates successful resolution of the emotions of the dying process. Dr. Kübler-Ross states, "Anyone who has witnessed a patient in peace and not in resignation will never forget it. . . ."

Erich Lindemann suggests that a "healthy" reaction to dying requires free expression and sharing of feelings with loved ones and close friends. Once the dying person can deal with the notion of having an illness for which there is no cure, the person can enrich the time remaining through a series of activities:

- Review one's life—various experiences and relationships and the meanings of each.
- Visit places and people that are important.
- Review memories with friends and relatives.
- Make up for missed opportunities.

**FIGURE 23-2** The dying person can withdraw in despair, suppress feelings about approaching death, or reach out to others. *Delmar/Cengage Learning*

- Resolve old conflicts.
- Think through and talk over with loved ones such questions as "What will happen to my survivors?" and "How will my place be filled?"

Although these activities may be painful, there will also be joy as these experiences are shared with others who have been a part of one's life experience. Raymond G. Carey, author of "Living until Death: A Program of Service and Research for the Terminally Ill" in Dr. Kübler-Ross's *Death: The Final Stage of Growth*, reports a number of conditions that contribute to successful adjustment of dying patients:

- Interest and concern of relatives, family, and clergy
- Warm, supportive relationship with at least one person
- Relatively good adjustment and past patterns of successfully coping with problems
- Strong religious beliefs, especially if the person has truly tried to live according to these beliefs
- Belief that one's life has meaning
- Belief in life after death
- Willingness to talk about the illness and approaching death
- Previous contact with a dying person who achieved a state of inner peace
- Honesty combined with reassurance (not of cure, but of continued support and control of pain) from the physician
- Control of pain, because pain interferes with adjustment

In addition to striving for emotional adjustment, the patient must face a number of challenges. The illness and impending dependence on others necessitates changes in lifestyle and relationships. For those who have a high level of independence, certain changes in self-concept are difficult, but necessary:

- From "I am an independent person" to "I must let others do some things for me."
- From "I am self-directing, capable, and in control of my life" to "I must let others have control over some aspects of my life."

In addition to these changes in self-concept, there must be a change in planning. Instead of thinking "Some day I will . . .," a dying person must think, "Today I will . . ." It is also important that the dying person continue to feel that life has meaning.

## PERSONAL AND FAMILY ISSUES RELATED TO CARE OF THE DYING

When a person is diagnosed with an incurable illness, certain decisions must be made. What treatments should be used? Should drugs or treatments that are known to have serious side effects be used? Should experimental drugs or procedures whose effects are not fully known be used? Should the patient find another physician? Another clinic? Another medical center that may have "a new cure"?

If the patient's condition is deteriorating or the patient is in the terminal phase of illness, questions about care must be decided. Should the patient be in a hospital or nursing home? Should the patient be at home? Who will provide care? Can this responsibility be rotated among family members? Or will one person have to provide around-the-clock care? Is there a home health service that could provide skilled care as needed? Is there a hospice in the community? The most important questions are:

1. Where does the patient want to be during his or her final days?
2. If the patient wants to die at home, is the family willing and able to undertake the care of a dying person at home?

## HOME CARE

In *Coming Home: A Guide to Home Care for the Terminally Ill*, Deborah Duda states that dying at home is "the old, natural way which most of the world never questioned." She lists 18 advantages of dying at home and seven conditions under which this decision would not be appropriate. Among the advantages she lists are that the dying person feels wanted, can influence surroundings, has more freedom and control, maintains respect and dignity, can enjoy home-cooked food, has the opportunity to express feelings to various relatives and friends, and the familiar setting is conducive to family support as the patient does the inner preparation for death. Another advantage, not included in Duda's list, is privacy; the patient's last days are family-centered, with minimal intrusion by outsiders. Also, the monetary cost of dying at home is minuscule, compared to the costs of intensive care and life-maintenance procedures commonly used in hospitals during the final days of a patient's life (Figure 23-3).

Dying at home is *not appropriate*, according to Duda, when neither the patient nor the family does not willingly choose this alternative to institutional care. Some families are not able to provide care, either because of their own limitations or because the patient's needs cannot be met in the home setting. If family members cannot handle the emotional drain, the physical demands of caring for someone who is terminally ill, or the overall stress of such a situation,

**FIGURE 23-3** Home health care services instead of facility admission can reduce the cost of care. *Delmar/Cengage Learning*

then choosing to die at home would not be appropriate. If the patient has arranged to be an organ donor and the specific terminal illness does not preclude use of the organs, then the patient's death should occur in the hospital setting, with a surgical team on call to harvest any usable organs as soon as the patient is pronounced dead.

Arranging for someone to die at home requires careful planning. The family should contact hospice and home health services to arrange for assistance and consultation services as needed. Roles should be discussed and agreed upon; the primary caregiver should be selected, with others agreeing to assume care at specific times. This may draw family members closer together as they share the common goal of providing loving care for the person they will soon lose. Or the family may become divided by disagreements and unequal division of responsibilities, with one or two persons carrying most of the burden. Careful advance planning may prevent the latter situation and allow the patient to spend his or her final days in a harmonious family setting.

## HOSPICE CARE

Hospice care can be provided as home care or, if available, as residential care. Home care with the supportive assistance of hospice personnel is an appropriate choice if the patient does not need or want hospitalization. Hospice care is provided by a team: the patient's physician; nurses to assess the patient's needs, develop a care plan, and provide skilled nursing care as needed; home health aides to provide personal care and, in some cases, assist with household needs; a social worker to provide emotional support and direct the family to community resources as needed; a chaplain and/or the patient's religious advisor; trained volunteers to provide visitation, companionship, and emotional support. Other benefits of hospice care include providing periods of respite for the primary caregiver and, later, offering bereavement counseling for the survivors. Basically, compared to the hospital setting, hospice provides a more caring and comfortable way for a patient to live out the final days and also provides support and guidance for family members.

## PALLIATIVE CARE

**Palliative** care refers to the type of care that should be provided when a patient's illness is terminal (i.e., cure or significant improvement is no longer possible). The primary focus of palliative care is *comfort*, both physical and psychological, rather than *cure* (Figure 23-4). Effective palliative care provides relief from such physical symptoms as pain, shortness of breath, and nausea. Palliative care also includes emotional support to relieve anxiety, accept the dying process, grieve for impending losses, and to say "good-bye" to loved ones. The reason most often cited by patients who request euthanasia or assisted suicide is *intolerable pain*; palliative care is *not* being provided, nor is the patient's pain being managed effectively.

Family and close friends are an important part of palliative care. Their presence may relieve a patient's fear of abandonment—of dying alone. Frequent visits by the person designated as "agent" in an advance medical directive may provide reassurance that end-of-life decisions will be honored. Many patients who have prepared an advance medical directive do not want "high-tech" interventions, believing that *such measures prolong dying, rather than living*. Many physicians, with a strong commitment to prolonging life, recommend such measures

**FIGURE 23-4** Working with dying patients requires substituting palliative goals for curative goals. *Delmar/Cengage Learning*

as additional chemotherapy, mechanical ventilation, artificial feeding, or dialysis, even when the patient is in the final stages of dying. The patient, the family, and the "designated agent" should question the benefit of such recommendations and keep in mind the patient's right to refuse treatment.

Palliative care is most easily provided in the home or in a residential hospice. Most hospices in the United States are home-based, however, and the time hospice personnel can spend in each patient's home is limited. It is more difficult to provide palliative care in hospitals, where policies require the use of heroic measures to prolong life and the transfer of dying patients to intensive care units. This may change, as the Health Care Financing Administration explores ways to reimburse hospitals for palliative care. Also, some nursing homes are now affiliating with hospices in order to offer palliative care, rather than transferring any dying resident to an acute care facility. Palliative care is not the prevailing modality for care of dying patients; it is currently a medical issue, a personal and family issue, and a patients' rights issue.

## MEDICAL ISSUES RELATED TO CARE OF THE DYING

Diagnosis and prescription of therapy are responsibilities of the physician. When the diagnosis of a fatal disease is confirmed, the physician faces several difficult questions:

- Does an adult patient have a right to know the diagnosis?
- Does an adult patient have a right to decide who should be given information about his or her condition?
- Does a physician have a duty to inform a patient that he or she is dying?
- How much information should the patient be given?
- How and when should the patient be told that he or she is dying?

Past medical practice has been to tell the family that the patient is dying, but "protect" the patient by telling as little as possible. This is a departure from ethical practices related to confidentiality. Does a dying patient have less of a right to confidentiality than one who is not dying? Several studies have revealed that (1) most physicians do not make a practice of telling patients that they are dying, and (2) most people believe they would want to be informed.

John Hinton suggests that *how* the information is given is important. It is possible to convey in a tactful and caring manner that the illness will be fatal. People listen selectively, so patients are likely to deal consciously only with as much of the message as they are able to handle at that moment. Hinton offers several reasons why patients should be informed:

- A patient who is not told that she is dying is deprived of opportunities to talk about the illness and dying. This "conspiracy of silence" results in the patient feeling isolated.
- A dying patient needs to get her affairs in order. This pertains to everyone, not just the wage earner or a businessperson. Getting one's affairs in order includes personal as well as business and financial decisions.
- Many dying patients want to deal with spiritual matters in preparation for dying.
- Lack of correct information may lead the patient to seek help from one practitioner after another, until financial resources have been exhausted. A second opinion often is desirable, but a fruitless search for a nonexistent cure may be avoided by honest communication.

**FIGURE 23-5** A warm, supportive relationship is important to a dying patient. *Delmar/Cengage Learning*

Some patients want to have full information about their disorder, the treatment options available, and the probable course of the illness. In general, defense mechanisms provide some protection against being overwhelmed. The patient focuses on some aspects of the illness and ignores others, according to her capacity for coping. Other patients do not want to be told and are willing to delegate control and all treatment decisions to the physician. It would be destructive to try to force such a patient to "face the truth." On the other hand, such patients are likely to ask questions that indicate a need for reassurance. These patients usually suspect the truth, and their questions indicate a need to talk. Active listening may reveal underlying fears and anxieties for which the patient needs reassurance that she will be cared for and that pain will be alleviated.

Many physicians provide information to their patients gradually and try to balance bad news with something positive. Later, they give additional information according to the patient's readiness. How much to tell the dying patient must be decided by each physician, based in part on each patient's situation and emotional stability.

Health care providers involved in care of a dying patient should know what the physician has told the patient so they can respond appropriately to questions from the patient and family. Many patients find comfort in talking about their illness and dying with a sensitive caregiver (Figure 23-5). Frequent contact with caring people who *listen* results in the patient coming to terms with the illness. When there is good communication with family members, relationships improve. Good communication with health care personnel increases the patient's trust.

## ISSUES RELATED TO RIGHTS OF THE DYING PERSON

Some issues discussed in Units 20 and 21 pertain to rights of patients. Rights issues are also concerned with truth, informed consent, control, choices, and protection of personal dignity. The issue of truth has already been discussed as a medical question; but truth is also related to informed consent. A patient who signs an agreement to undergo surgery or certain other treatments should do so only after being given full information:

- What is the probability that the surgery or treatment will help?
- What are the possible side effects?
- Will irreversible body changes result?
- Are alternative treatments available?
- What is the cost of the recommended treatment?

Some patients prefer to delegate decisions to others; that choice should be respected. Many patients wish to retain some degree of control and to participate in decisions; this, too, should be respected. Choices regarding life-maintenance procedures and advance medical directives have already been discussed. Some other choices of patients, especially during the final days, include:

- Solitude versus being surrounded by significant others
- Remaining at home versus being in the hospital
- Remaining alert versus being sedated

Choices made by the patient or family members may conflict with what a health care provider considers to be "best" for the patient. This is a conflict of values. If the patient and family have arrived at acceptance of impending death, and if they are concerned about death with dignity, health care providers may feel frustrated that various available procedures are not being used to prolong life (or prolong the dying process, depending upon one's view). It may help the health care provider to keep in mind that the Patient Self-Determination Act, advance medical directive legislation, and informed consent statutes all resulted from practices that forced unwanted procedures on dying patients.

## ROLES OF HEALTH CARE PROVIDERS

Terminal illness by definition results in death. The goals of care for terminally ill patients, therefore, are different from the goals for patients who have the potential to regain physical well-being. It is difficult for many health care providers to accept any goal other than "getting better." Working with dying patients requires that a health care provider be able to *substitute palliative goals for* **curative** *goals*. Palliative goals include keeping the patient comfortable, being available to listen, providing comforting touch as appropriate, accepting the patient's choices, and respecting the patient as a human being, even if comatose and nonresponsive.

The stages of dying proposed by Dr. Kübler-Ross can help health care providers to understand and accept some of the behaviors manifested by a dying person. For example, anger directed at a caregiver is more easily accepted if it is viewed as one manifestation of a specific stage of the dying process. But attempting to "place" a patient in one stage or another does not serve the patient's needs. Rather, effective care demands the utmost in caring, always keeping in mind that this patient's emotional needs are paramount. Lindemann noted, ". . . one can be surprised at how little actual time expenditure is needed to say the right word at the right time, and not too much. . . ." (Figure 23-6). The "right word" is any word or

**FIGURE 23-6** When diagnosis of a fatal illness has been confirmed, the physician must decide how and when, as well as how much, to tell the patient. *Delmar/Cengage Learning*

phrase that conveys acceptance—of the patient as a human being and of the patient's way of coping with the approaching end of life—a difficult psychological task. Perhaps the patient who is perceived by the staff as "difficult" is a patient who needs help in accomplishing this task.

The health care provider can become the patient's ally in dealing with the process of dying, or the health care provider can ignore the basic humanity of a dying person and become totally preoccupied with the technology used to maintain physical functions.

## GUIDELINES FOR CARE OF A DYING PERSON

These guidelines can be useful as you strive to provide **humane** care consistent with the choices and needs of a dying patient:

- Reassure the patient as needed that you will be there and that you will do all possible to provide comfort. Then keep your word.
- Be aware of the patient's emotional state. Respect the patient's unique way of reacting to the illness and dying.

- Allow the patient to talk about dying; do not deny the fact that the patient is dying with statements such as "Oh, you have lots of time left."
- Allow the patient to express feelings. Anger, crying, remorse, and similar feelings help the patient to deal with the impending loss of life.
- Do not make promises that you cannot keep. Such expressions may make you feel better, but deny the reality of the patient's dying process.
- Let the patient know that you care. Use touch as appropriate and be with the patient as much as your other duties permit.
- Listen—a patient provides clues to her specific needs.
- Do not force your feelings or your beliefs on the patient.
- Whenever appropriate, allow the patient to express a preference about her care.
- Respond to a patient's request for prayer, a religious reading, ritual, or service. Call the hospital chaplain or the patient's spiritual advisor as appropriate.

## REFERENCES AND SUGGESTED READINGS

*Indicates a classic reference that introduced new ideas.

Colby, Bill. (2006). *Unplugged: Reclaiming our right to die in America.* New York: AMACOM. (The author is the lawyer who represented the family of Nancy Cruzan.)

*Duda, Deborah. (1984). *Coming home: A guide to home care for the terminally ill.* Santa Fe, NM: John Muir.

Gruman, Jesse. (2009). *Aftershock: What to do when the doctor gives you—or someone you love—a devastating diagnosis.* New York: Walker.

Hegner, Barbara R., et al. (2008). Death and dying. In *Nursing assistant: A nursing process approach* (10th ed., pp. 540–553). Clifton Park, NY: Delmar, Cengage Learning.

Kiernan, Stephen P. (2006). *Last rights: Rescuing the end of life from the medical system.* New York: St. Martin's Press.

Munoz, Carol, & Luckmann, Joan. (2005). Using transcultural communication to assist people responding to pain, grief, dying, and death. In *Transcultural communication in nursing* (2nd ed.) (pp. 277–295). Clifton Park, NY: Delmar, Cengage Learning.

Tamparo, Carol D., & Lindh, Wilburta Q. (2008). *Therapeutic communications for health* (3rd ed.). Clifton Park, NY: Delmar, Cengage Learning.

Wanzer, Sidney H. (2009). *To die well: Your right to comfort, calm, and choice in the last days of life.* Cambridge, MA: DeCapo.

## SOURCES OF ADDITIONAL INFORMATION

**AARP,** http://www.aarp.org/caregiving

**Contact HospiceNet,** http://www.hospicenet.com

**Family Caregiver Alliance,** http://www.caregiver.org (1-800-445-8106)

**Hospice Foundation of America,** *http://www.hospicefoundation.org (1-800-854-3402)*

## REVIEW AND SELF-CHECK

1. List five fears that a dying person may have.

   fear of the unknown ; fear of being burden to others
   " " " being forgotten ; fear of losing one's mind, fear of
   " " " that loved ones will not be care for  losing control, fear of being
   " " " one's life work will be forgotten  abandoned
   " " about one's possessions, fear of becoming dependent

2. List the five stages of dying, as proposed by Dr. Kübler-Ross, and explain the patient's feelings at each stage.

   denial
   anger - "why me? I don't deserve this"
   bargaining - "if I get well, I will go to church"
   depression -
   acceptance

3. Describe a "healthy" approach to dying.

   Dr. Ross becoming aware of one's identity, communicating one's experience to others, accepting one's life has purpose

4. List seven conditions that contribute to a patient's adjustment to dying.

   Concern to relatives & clergy
   Warm, supportive relationship w/ at least 1 person ; Honesty of from physician
   Relatively good adjustment ; Control of pain
   Strong religious beliefs
   Beliefs that one's life has meaning
   Willingness to talk about approaching death
   Previous contact w/ dying person

5. Name three personal and family issues related to the care of a dying person.

   What, how much, when & how to tell the patient,
   What to tell the family.

6. Name three medical issues related to the care of a dying person.

   Some medical treatment to be used, seek another opinion

7. List five issues related to the rights of a dying patient.

   truth,

   informed consent

   control

   choices

   protection of personal dignity

8. List five guidelines that you could follow to meet the needs of a dying patient.

   to keep the patient comfortable, listen, touch as appropriate, accept patient's choices, respect patient

9. List five advantages of dying at home.

   Assure patient you will be there          Don't force your belief on patient
   You will provide comfort                  Respond to patient's spiritual beliefs
   Be aware of patient's feeling
   Respect patient's way of reacting to illness
   Listen

10. Explain the primary focus of palliative care.

    Keep the patient comfortable w/ pain management

## ASSIGNMENTS

1. Think about your first experience with death. How old were you? Was the deceased an important person to you? If you were a child, what were you told about death? Did you participate in or witness any part of the dying process? Were you involved in any rituals related to the death? Were you encouraged to grieve? Did those closest to the deceased display their grief to you? How was their grief manifested? Did this experience contribute to your fear of death? If it were possible to change that experience, what would you change so that the experience would help you (1) accept the reality of death as a part of life and (2) face your own mortality (that is, your own inevitable death) without fear?

2. Participate in a class discussion to identify various ways health care providers could meet the following needs of a dying person:

    a. Relative freedom from pain and discomfort.

    b. Maintenance of independence, insofar as possible.

    c. Satisfaction of any remaining wishes ("things I wish I had done").

    d. Maintenance of self-esteem when it becomes necessary to yield control to others.

    e. Achievement of emotional adjustment, acceptance of impending death, and a state of inner peace.

3. In a class discussion, consider the following questions:

    a. How can the rights of a comatose patient be protected?

    b. What are the rights of a dying patient whose organs could be used as transplants for patients in the same hospital?

4. List things you have been wanting to do "some day." If you learned today that you have a terminal illness, which of these would you try to do before you die? Set a date and plan to do one of the things on your list.

5. List three people who are very close (either relatives or friends). Beside each name, write out two or more statements that you would want to make if that person were dying. When did you last tell each of these people how important he or she is to you? Plan what you will say to each of these people the next time you are together.

6. Write out a set of guidelines for your next of kin describing the care you wish to receive if you are terminally ill.

Section

# Trends in Health Care

Health care in the United States is in a state of rapid change. As a health care provider, you should be informed about current trends and issues, especially those that affect roles and relationships of health care personnel.

Large segments of the public are now well-informed about health matters; with increasing knowledge, many people want to participate in health care decisions. Lifestyle and stress management are widely recognized as major factors in both treatment and prevention of illness. And more people are using alternative (nonmedical) approaches to health care.

Some patients enter the health care system with a passive attitude: "I'm sick. Fix me. Make me well." These patients are not likely to refuse treatments or seek alternative therapies. But there is a new breed of patient who asks questions and expects answers, may refuse an invasive procedure or specific treatment, and may even question whether or not orthodox medicine can help with his or her health problem. Inadequate answers or a judgmental attitude on the part of a health care provider interferes with establishing rapport or, worse, may alienate the patient. It is essential, then, that health care providers understand and accept those patients who wish to assume more responsibility and actively participate in decisions about their health care.

Section VII is designed to help you learn about selected trends in health care as a basis for working with this "new breed of patient" and for expanding your understanding of holistic health, healing, and the role of stress management in health maintenance. With a broader view of therapeutic alternatives, both medical and nonmedical, you will be better prepared to function in the health care system of the future.

# UNIT 24

# Health Care through the Ages

## OBJECTIVES

Upon completion of this unit, you should be able to:

- State two reasons that some innovations in science and medicine are initially rejected or labeled as quackery.
- Name two beliefs about sickness (or a sick person) that were common in early cultures and are still prevalent today.
- Name five significant scientific or medical advances during the past 400 years that provided the foundation for current health care practices.
- List five differences between holistic and orthodox health care.
- Name three physicians whose innovations contributed to the development of holistic medicine.
- Name a physician who demonstrated that the scientific method can be applied to the study of nonmedical therapeutic interventions.

## KEY TERMS

Allopathic
Alternative therapy
Complementary therapy
Dolorology
Empirical
Herbalism
Holistic health care
Neurotransmitters
Psychoanalysis
Psychopharmaceuticals
Psychophysiological
Psychosomatic
Synergism
Variables

## DEFINITIONS

Before beginning the historical overview that is the subject of this unit, you need to understand certain terms used throughout this section. The literal meaning of **allopathic** is "utilizing drugs." Orthodox medical practice in the United States relies primarily on drug therapy and surgery. *Allopathic medicine* is used in current literature on health care to refer to orthodox medicine as practiced in this country. In this textbook, the terms *conventional* and *orthodox* are used interchangeably, with *allopathic* used to refer to the existing system of medical practice in the United States. *Medical* refers to practices of a licensed medical doctor (M.D.) or osteopath (D.O.); it does not include professional practitioners such as psychologists or chiropractors. The terms **alternative therapy** and **complementary therapy** refer to a wide variety of nonmedical therapies, many of them based on a holistic concept of health and health care. Because "alternative therapy" implies *instead of* medical care, the more inclusive term *complementary therapy* is preferred by many practitioners, most of whom have clients who are also receiving some type of allopathic care. Throughout Section VII "complementary" will be used to describe a nonmedical therapy, and "alternative" will be used to designate a nonmedical practitioner.

A complementary therapy may be provided by someone with a professional level of educational preparation (college degree plus professional training), someone with formal educational training leading to a certificate and/or licensure, or someone who has been trained in a specific therapeutic technique. **Holistic health care** takes into consideration the patient's total being (physical, mental, emotional, spiritual, life context, nutrition, lifestyle) and uses a variety of therapeutic techniques, according to the specific needs of each patient.

## INNOVATIONS IN SCIENCE AND HEALTH CARE

The history of science and health care includes numerous examples of innovative ideas that were rejected initially by those in power at the time. Many of these innovative approaches had merit and were eventually accepted by orthodox medicine. Some innovations were premature—they required changes the culture was not yet ready to accept. Innovations—new ideas—may conflict with existing beliefs and may be perceived as a threat by current practitioners. Many scientists who proposed a new idea or a new method have been subjected to criticism, ridiculed, or even persecuted. Yet some of those innovators who suffered persecution are now recognized as heroes of medicine or a particular field of science.

### The Scientific Model

Today, the scientific model is considered by the medical community to be *the method* for proving the effectiveness of a specific technique, drug, or procedure. Complementary procedures are criticized by members of the medical community because they have not been "proven effective" by the scientific method. Yet many current medical practices have never been subjected to rigorous scientific research. At present a double standard exists, in which complementary practices are rejected or viewed with suspicion by members of the scientific community because of a lack of rigorous research, but certain long-standing medical practices that have never been subjected to such research are accepted without question.

The scientific model requires an approach in which the experimental treatment is administered to certain subjects (the experimental group), whereas an ineffective treatment is administered to other subjects (the control group); sometimes, there is a third group that receives no treatment. The experiment is called a "double-blind study" if neither patients nor caregivers know which subjects are in the experimental group and which are in the control group. A blind study prevents patients' and caregivers' expectations from influencing the outcomes of an experiment.

Studies on the effects of drug therapy have shown that the expectations of those conducting an experiment influence the results. For example, the health care provider who knows that a patient is being given the experimental drug expects it to help the patient. This expectation can affect the patient's response to the drug. Factors that influence the outcome of an experiment are known as **variables.**

The scientific model requires that only one or two variables be manipulated, while all other influences are carefully controlled. After treatment, the experimental subjects (those receiving a specific treatment) are compared with subjects in the control group (who did not receive the treatment). A treatment is considered effective only if there are significant differences between the treatment group and the control group. Research findings are considered valid (proven correct) only if other researchers can repeat the experiment and get the same results.

It is relatively easy to measure and record the effects of a precise amount of a drug on blood pressure. It is more difficult to measure an emotion such as fear and prove that minimizing a preoperative patient's anxiety results in faster postoperative recovery. It is impossible to see or measure a patient's "will to live." Yet emotions, belief systems, and factors such as intention (to get well or to escape one's present life situation by dying) are known to be powerful influences on the course of illness. Health care providers often see two patients who have the same diagnosis and are receiving the same treatment. One recovers, but the other declines and dies. The big question: What made a difference in the outcome of these two patients? The "difficult to measure" variables are ignored by researchers who are committed to the scientific model—that is, precise measurement (quantitative data) of the effects of the specific variable being studied. Some members of the scientific/medical/healing community who are open to alternative approaches are now designing studies that adapt the scientific method to the study of intuitive diagnosis and influences on healing, such as prayer and Healing Touch. No one, however, has devised a method for measuring such powerful factors as the will to live, expectation, or intention.

## Empirical Evidence

**Empirical** refers to experience and observation; *empirical data* are observations collected without the rigorous design of the scientific method. Many alternative therapies involve counseling, meditation, full body massage (also known as "body work"), and other procedures that affect the emotional state, tension level, and perhaps even the beliefs of the patient. Practitioners who use various nonmedical therapies have accumulated a large body of empirical data, but their methods are criticized by members of the scientific community who demand numerical data obtained through research procedures that fit the scientific model. In spite of the difficulties, researchers are now making progress in designing such experiments.

Meanwhile, more and more physicians, seeking better results for their patients, are sufficiently impressed by the empirical data to include certain nonmedical techniques in their practice. Yet most physicians continue to practice allopathic medicine without an awareness of or interest in the potential value of complementary therapies. Some physicians view any therapists other than medical doctors as quacks. Thus, allopathic medicine and holistic medicine represent *two very different belief systems* that have a profound effect on each practitioner's approach to patient care.

## Dilemma of the Health Care Provider

A health care delivery system in the process of significant change presents something of a dilemma for members of the health care team. What is the appropriate response for you, a health care provider, to a patient who is using a complementary therapy in addition to medical treatment? Should you warn the patient about quackery? Should you tell the physician that the patient is not complying with the medical regimen prescribed? Does compliance mean that the patient must follow the medical protocol and forgo any other type of therapy? These questions are less relevant to the average hospitalized patient than to a patient with a chronic health problem, long-term illness, or life-threatening disease. The probability of your caring for such a patient depends on your role, the particular health care setting in which you perform your role, and the extent to which you interact with each patient.

The remainder of Unit 24 describes the historical roots of some current practices. This historical overview also reveals that a holistic approach to health care is not really new, and some therapies considered to be alternative in the United States have been a part of medical practice in other countries for many years.

## HEALING IN EARLY CIVILIZATIONS

Over thousands of years the healing practices of each culture were handed down from one generation to the next. The role of healer was highly respected; possession of the secrets of healing conveyed power second only to the power of the ruler. In ancient civilizations, healers were primarily women and religions centered around worship of the goddess. Large temples erected to various goddesses served as centers of healing, as well as centers of worship. The priestesses performed religious services and were also guardians of healing secrets.

During the second millennium before the birth of Christ, the great goddess, whose power was believed to be derived from Earth, was replaced by a male deity, the god who reigned from above. Thereafter, the goddess religions were condemned as pagan; they either disappeared or went underground to continue their practices in secret. This shift in beliefs about the nature of god was accompanied by a shift in beliefs about healing and healers. The role of *healer* was a *power role*. With the growth of patriarchal religions, power shifted to the father/male figure, and the right to heal was claimed by males.

### Greece and Rome

Although early Greek mythology attributed illness to supernatural causes, it was the Greeks who eventually separated healing from religion and the role of physician from that of priest. Hippocrates, a Greek physician who lived during the period 460–377 B.C., is known as "the father of modern medicine." Hippocrates insisted upon careful observation and the collection of factual information, thereby establishing a systematic approach to diagnosis of illness. His treatments included diet, fresh air and sunshine, and healthful personal habits and living conditions—what we today refer to as "a healthful lifestyle." Hippocrates demonstrated that illness results from natural causes, rather than evil spirits or the anger of the gods. This established medicine as the healing profession. Thereafter religion was the domain of priests, and care of the sick was the domain of physicians. Hippocrates also emphasized a code of behavior for physicians—the beginnings of medical ethics. The Hippocratic oath is still used by many medical schools as part of the graduation exercise for medical students.

### Early Judeo-Christian Period

Jews and early Christians believed in a divine cause for illness and divine intervention as the basis for healing. The Greeks and Romans, with their many gods, could attribute illness to the wrath of one god and healing to the kindness of another god. Jews and Christians, however, believed in one God. This raised an important question: How could the same being who causes illness also heal the sick? This dilemma was resolved by associating illness with sin. If a person became sick, then certainly that person had sinned and was being punished. These beliefs are reflected in some religions today. A current example is the view of some people that acquired immune deficiency syndrome (AIDS) is divine punishment for homosexuality, sexual promiscuity, or drug abuse.

## Biblical References to Healing

Although the Bible does not describe a specific system of health care, there are many references to healing. The healing might be a ritual to cleanse the person of sin, or it might involve touch—the "laying on of hands." Were these biblical healings due to faith? purification? or divine intervention? Did the healers of biblical times utilize energy to bring about instantaneous healing?

Today, a number of healing techniques are based on influencing the flow of energy through the body. There are healers whose ability to heal, either by touch ("laying on of hands") or by "sending energy," has been thoroughly documented. A scientific organization, the International Society for the Study of Subtle Energies and Energy Medicine (ISSSEEM), was established to set up research projects and seek scientific explanations. It is intriguing that early civilizations may have used energy transfer for healing, and that we are now trying to relearn (or to prove by means of the scientific method) what healers of biblical times and earlier civilizations knew and accepted as natural.

## EVOLUTION OF MODERN HEALTH CARE

The Middle Ages, also known as the Dark Ages, lasted over a thousand years, from the fall of the Roman Empire to the Renaissance. Throughout this period, epidemics and plagues recurred, especially in crowded cities. But there was no organized health care system as we know it. Many monasteries had gardens in which various therapeutic herbs were cultivated; the monks performed simple healing procedures. In communities far from a monastery, an older man (the village "wise man") or woman (the village "crone" or "wise woman") served as healer for the community. Perhaps these healers possessed natural healing abilities. It is likely that they possessed secrets of healing that had been passed down from one generation to the next. Eventually, the influence of the wise man or the crone was perceived as a threat to the power of the local priest. A healer who was especially successful might be condemned as a heretic or witch. Many were tortured, then hanged or burned at the stake. Persecution of healers who were neither priest nor physician continued up to the 1800s. Once a system of medicine had become established, natural healers were condemned as quacks.

The Renaissance (a French term meaning "rebirth") followed the Dark Ages and lasted about 400 years. There was renewed interest in science, art, music, and literature and less emphasis on religion. This was a period of discoveries, of new insights and theories, many of which provided the foundation for the scientific methods that are an integral part of modern medical research.

## Developments in Science

During the 1500s, Vesalius studied the human body and made accurate anatomical drawings. Existing beliefs about human anatomy were based on dissection of animals, because it was illegal to dissect a human body. In order to obtain cadavers for his anatomical studies, Vesalius removed bodies from the gallows at night. As a result of these secret studies of human anatomy, Vesalius corrected many misconceptions about the structure of the human body. Vesalius was ridiculed by his colleagues for proposing that their beliefs about human anatomy were erroneous, but today he is credited with establishing anatomy as a science. His book of anatomical drawings is a classic and reprints are available even today.

Just as dissection of human bodies was necessary to identify internal structures, the development of the microscope was a necessary prelude to the discovery of bacteria, the study of cell and tissue structure, and the identification of chromosomes and genes—the basis for modern genetic research. Zacharias Janssen is thought to have invented the compound microscope around 1590. But it would be over 200 years before refinements in lens-making made it possible to magnify objects without distortion. Meanwhile, Anton Van Leeuwenhoek (1632–1723) used a simple microscope to study a wide variety of subjects, including various body fluids. As an amateur scientist, Leeuwenhoek systematically recorded his observations and made detailed drawings. His work provided the foundation for the science of microbiology, even though he was widely criticized when he first published his observations.

## The Germ Theory and Antisepsis

It was not until the nineteenth century, less than 200 years ago, that handwashing was proposed as a means of preventing infections. A Hungarian physician, Ignaz Philipp Semmelweiss (1818–1865), noticed that women who were assisted in childbirth by doctors who had just come from the autopsy room invariably developed "childbed fever." He proposed that doctors should wash their hands after completing an autopsy, to protect their patients. For making this suggestion, Semmelweis was persecuted by his colleagues to the point that he eventually had a nervous breakdown.

Ironically, in the year of Semmelweis's death, Joseph Lister introduced antisepsis to the practice of surgery. The beginning of surgical asepsis was a major event in the history of medicine. Dr. Lister was such a renowned surgeon that his innovation was accepted, and he did not experience rejection and persecution by unconverted colleagues. Lister's use of antisepsis introduced control of infection as an integral part of medical practice. It is noteworthy that Lister's introduction of antisepsis preceded any proof of the existence of microorganisms. Two other scientists, working separately, were to provide proof that microorganisms are present on hands and all objects, thus providing the scientific basis for both handwashing and medical asepsis.

Robert Koch (1843–1910), a German scientist, was responsible for a scientific breakthrough that we now know as the *germ theory*. Through his study of microorganisms, Koch determined the specific cause of several infectious diseases, including tuberculosis. He also established the rules for proving that a specific organism was the cause of a particular infection; this provided the foundation for the field we know today as bacteriology. Development of the germ theory was a major event that established the scientific basis for asepsis, immunization, and modern sanitation.

Many scientists had observed microorganisms under a microscope, but it was Louis Pasteur who established that those tiny objects were living things that reproduced themselves. He demonstrated that wine could be preserved by destroying the microorganisms present. The process he used is known as "pasteurization" and is still used today to ensure that milk and various other foods are safe.

Later, Pasteur developed a vaccine to prevent rabies in people who had been bitten by a rabid animal, thus sparing them a horrible death. Pasteur's contributions are numerous, yet he, too, was subjected to ridicule by his colleagues, even though he was a highly respected scientist. His contributions were recognized prior to his death, however. The Pasteur Institute, founded in 1888 in his honor by the French government, continues to conduct research on the causes, treatment, and prevention of disease.

## Control of Infectious Diseases

The work of Koch and Pasteur led to the development of vaccines to protect people against certain diseases, especially the group of infections known as "childhood diseases." But three of the most devastating diseases are caused by viruses, rather than bacteria: smallpox, poliomyelitis, and, currently, AIDS.

In 1796, an English physician by the name of Edward Jenner developed a method of protecting people from smallpox, a serious disease with a high mortality rate. Smallpox victims were seriously ill for two to three weeks. Those who survived had numerous small scars, known as pockmarks. Widespread use of the smallpox vaccine eliminated the disease in Europe and North America by 1950, but epidemics killed thousands of victims in other parts of the world. Between 1950 and 1970, intensive worldwide efforts to vaccinate the total population of any country where smallpox occurred resulted in eradication of this disease. Because the disease was considered to have been eradicated, vaccinations were discontinued except for persons traveling to remote areas where exposure was a possibility. Meanwhile, the smallpox virus was kept alive in various laboratories, presumably for the purposes of scientific research. Unfortunately, terrorists now threaten to use these stores of smallpox virus as a weapon of mass destruction. With two generations of unvaccinated populations in Europe and the Americas, the potential for a worldwide epidemic now exists.

Up until the outbreak of AIDS, the viral scourge of the twentieth century was poliomyelitis, also called "infantile paralysis" because children were very susceptible and many were left with permanent paralysis. During the 1940s and 1950s, polio epidemics occurred with increasing frequency, especially during the spring and summer months. The mortality rate was high; many survivors were handicapped by paralysis. In 1953 Dr. Jonas Salk's vaccine became available. The Salk vaccine was widely administered and is now required in some states for admission to the public schools. Polio has not been completely eradicated, but cases are now relatively rare. Jenner and Salk made it possible to protect entire populations against two serious viral infections.

Another modern-day threat is the influenza virus. Each year a different strain of the flu emerges, with epidemics occurring in certain regions, especially Asia. During 2008–2009 the emerging flu virus was identified as H1N1, the strain that caused the deadly 1918–1919 flu pandemic that claimed the lives of millions of victims. Once the H1N1 virus was identified, public health officials became concerned about the possibility of another flu pandemic. The public was urged to practice good health habits, especially handwashing, covering the nose and mouth when sneezing or coughing, and wearing a face mask when in areas where flu cases are numerous.

## The Discovery of Radiation

Two physicists in France, Pierre and Marie Curie, laid the foundation for radiation therapies. Together they studied radioactive substances and identified two previously unknown elements: radium and polonium. After her husband's death, Marie Curie discovered that radium had created an image of a nearby key on a piece of film. This discovery revealed what is now basic knowledge—namely, that radioactive materials give off invisible rays that affect nearby substances.

Marie Curie and her daughter, Irene, then only 17 years old, took a portable X-ray machine to the front lines during World War I to make X rays available to doctors treating wounded soldiers. After the war, Irene did research on radioactive substances with her husband and her mother for many years. The dangers of radioactivity were not recognized at that time; both Marie Curie and Irene died of leukemia. The contributions of the Curies are basic to various diagnostic and therapeutic procedures in current medical use.

Concurrently with the work of the Curies in France, a German physicist by the name of Wilhelm Konrad Roentgen accidentally discovered X rays. After conducting some experiments that involved passing an electric current through a special type of glass tubing, Roentgen noticed that some nearby photographic plates had become fogged. His investigation of the cause led to further experiments that resulted in the identification of invisible rays that could pass through soft tissues, but not through bone or metal. This discovery revolutionized diagnostic practices in medicine. Again, the dangers of radiation and X rays were not known in the beginning. Many radiologists died of leukemia before it was recognized that health care providers must have adequate protection when they are working around any type of radiation.

## The Beginnings of Psychiatry and Psychosomatic Medicine

The pioneers just discussed all contributed to medicine as it pertains to physical health. Psychiatry, the medical specialty concerned with mental illness, began with the work of Sigmund Freud, an Austrian physician who first recognized the power of subconscious memories to affect health. Freud developed **psychoanalysis,** a technique for helping patients explore the unconscious part of the mind. Although many of Freud's theories are not accepted by modern practitioners, his writings and those of his students provided the foundation for psychotherapy. He was truly a pioneer, daring to explore territory that had never before been explored by physicians. Freud made the mind and emotions a concern of medicine, which had previously limited its focus to the physical body.

Currently there is a merging of physical medicine and psychiatry, as the powerful influence of mind and emotions on the physical body is acknowledged. **Psychosomatic** medicine is a medical specialty concerned with physical disorders that have a mental or emotional component. Although the term *psychosomatic* (psycho—mind; soma—body) is still in common use, it is slowly being replaced by the term **psychophysiological** (psycho—mind; physiology—body functions).

**Brain Chemistry** The division between physical illness and mental illness has been clouded further by the discovery of a biochemical factor in several "mental" illnesses, especially unipolar disorder, bipolar disorder, and schizophrenia. Several chemicals, known as **neurotransmitters,** are produced by certain cells within the brain. These chemicals affect mental alertness, memory, ability to concentrate, thought processes, judgment, mood, sleep patterns, sexual behavior, irritability, energy, and other factors that influence the ability to perform one's daily activities. An increase or decrease in certain neurotransmitters may have a profound effect on behavior. The discovery of differences in certain neurotransmitter levels of psychiatric patients versus "normal" individuals has led to the development of a new class of drugs. These **psychopharmaceuticals** influence either the production of a specific neurotransmitter or its transmission from one cell to another. The availability of psychopharmaceutical drugs has had a radical effect on the psychiatric field. Many psychiatrists have abandoned "talk therapy" and now limit their practice to diagnostic evaluations and prescription of one or more psychopharmaceutical drugs to manage a patient's symptoms.

Psychologists, clinical social workers, and counselors now provide most of the psychotherapy, often in conjunction with a psychiatrist who prescribes psychopharmaceutical drugs. Individual therapy is often combined with group therapy sessions, which seem to be especially beneficial for those patients who need the interaction and support that group sessions can provide.

**The Genetic Factor** The line between "physical" and "mental" illness has also been clouded by sociological studies and gene research that demonstrate a genetic tendency toward certain mental illnesses. These findings give weight to the hereditary aspect. At the individual level, biorhythms, exposure to light, sleep patterns, REM (rapid eye movement) sleep, and dreams have been found to differ from "normal" in psychiatric patients. One relatively common problem, seasonal affective disorder (SAD), occurs during the winter months, when daylight hours are decreased and cloudy days occur frequently. This disorder is a depressive state precipitated by the seasonal decrease in light. Victims of SAD tend to become depressed in the late fall, then improve as winter draws to an end and spring approaches. These individual patterns and environmental factors further cloud the question of what is a physical illness and what is a mental illness.

**Multiple Causation** The previous discussion indicates the fallacy of the "mental illness stigma," still pervasive in American society. That bias is no more justified than a bias against diabetes, a disorder involving faulty sugar metabolism. But diabetes, hypertension, autoimmune disorders, and many other physical illnesses are now considered to have an emotional and/or stress-related component. Even the infectious diseases, once blamed on the causative bacteria or virus, are now viewed in terms of numerous factors that impact an individual's immune system.

## BEGINNINGS OF HOLISTIC MEDICINE

With increasing evidence of multiple causation of disease, the allopathic approach to treatment of symptoms is being replaced by emphasis on removal or treatment of causes. The search for causes leads naturally to a holistic approach to the care of each patient as an individual with a particular lifestyle, stressors related to occupation and family dynamics, and behavior patterns developed over a lifetime. Any of these could be contributing to the current health problem.

A new breed of physician-pioneer is emerging, calling for treatment of *causes* of illness, rather than management of symptoms. These practitioners focus on the total patient. They insist that treatment must include the mental, emotional, and spiritual aspects of the person, as well as the physical aspects—a *holistic* approach to health care. This approach presents a special challenge. Holistic medicine requires taking time to identify and deal with causes, rather than treating symptoms only. A holistic approach requires taking a detailed history—both family and individual—and conducting a lifestyle inventory.

Genetic clues to the patient's illness may be found in the family history. Individual clues may be found in the individual's own history, such as abuse or neglect on the part of the primary caregiver, or the existence during childhood of attention deficit hyperactive disorder. A description of the patient's home life and work situation may yield clues about whether or not stress is a contributing factor. The lifestyle inventory may reveal additional symptoms, such as sleep disturbances, and may also provide clues to the causation puzzle. Such a detailed study of the patient's individual situation is time consuming. Obviously, a complete study would also include the technological approaches used in allopathic medicine to establish a clinical diagnosis.

Holistic treatment of the patient can begin even before a final diagnosis has been established. If stress is obviously a causative factor, the patient can be taught stress management techniques. If emotional factors are revealed, appropriate therapy for constructive expression of emotions can be planned. Assertiveness training can be recommended to help a patient learn to cope with life problems effectively. If faulty dietary habits are revealed, instruction in healthful eating may be given. Thus, each possible causative factor is dealt with in order to *heal the total patient*. Holistic health care utilizes the skills of many different therapists; it includes the techniques of allopathic medicine as appropriate, but extends the role of the physician into areas beyond orthodox medical practice.

## INNOVATORS AND MODERN MEDICINE

Increasingly, the powerful influence of emotions and stress on health is being recognized. The onset of diseases such as cancer is most likely to occur when the immune system is depressed. It is well known that disorders such as ulcers and high blood pressure have an emotional component, but the emotional component may be the result of long-term stress. Several physicians who acknowledged the roles of stress and emotional factors in the onset and course of illness provided the early foundation for holistic medical practice. They believed that strategies for managing stress and resolving emotional factors must be incorporated into the therapeutic protocol. Their contributions led to changes in cancer therapy, pain control, management of hypertension, and the use of medical intuitives in diagnosis.

### Cancer Therapy

Dr. O. Carl Simonton is an oncologist who noted that the cancer patients who met with him regularly for group counseling seemed to "hold their own" better than cancer patients who did not participate in the group sessions. Some members of the group actually improved. In 1976 the Institute of Noetic Sciences sponsored a project in which Dr. Simonton and his wife, Stephanie (a counselor), provided psychological counseling to cancer patients who had been labeled "terminal" by their own physicians. Only patients who had received orthodox medical therapies for their cancer were accepted into the project. In addition to participating in counseling sessions, each patient was encouraged to write three sets of objectives, one set for three months in the future, one set for six months, and one set for twelve months. Each set of objectives had three components:

1. Meditate for 20 minutes at least twice a day
2. Exercise for 20 minutes five days each week
3. Have one hour of play per day, seven days per week

Play time could not be accumulated; if a patient played two hours on Saturday, there still must be an hour of play on Sunday. Time spent watching television could not be counted as play time. Patients had to specify their play activities in writing. In regard to exercise, the patient would choose something he or she was capable of doing safely. One patient might be able to walk a mile. Another, confined to bed, might be limited to flexing and extending the fingers and arms periodically. Obviously, Dr. Simonton helped his patients *program themselves for living*, as opposed to programming themselves (or allowing others to program them) for dying.

Long-term follow-up of these patients indicated that about one-third lived longer than expected, some experienced complete recovery, and those who did not survive experienced a higher quality of life up until the time of death. "Higher quality" means less pain, increased activity, slower decline, and increased participation in family and community life, as opposed to lying in bed helpless and in pain for weeks prior to dying. According to Dr. Simonton, the patients who improved the most were those who were willing to get in touch with any negative aspects of their lives during the counseling sessions.

Publication of the results of this therapeutic approach met with skepticism and criticism from the medical community. Does this rejection of an innovative treatment sound familiar? Some of the historical figures discussed earlier did not live to see their innovations accepted into common practice. The Simontons are more fortunate. Their approach emphasizing psychological factors was premature. Medicine was not yet ready to give up the notion that cancer is a *physical* disease or to accept the powerful influence of mind and emotions on physiological processes. But within 10 years numerous physicians had accepted the Simontons' approach and were incorporating purposeful, regular counseling into the treatment protocol for cancer patients.

## Pain Management

Dr. C. Norman Shealy is a neurosurgeon who practiced the conventional methods of his specialty until he became aware that many of his patients gained only temporary relief of symptoms, even from extensive surgical procedures that were supposed to correct the problem. Dissatisfied with these results, and especially concerned about the number of neurosurgical and orthopedic patients with chronic pain, Dr. Shealy searched for more effective methods. Collaborating with a young electrical engineer, he spent two years designing a low-voltage electrical unit that could short-circuit pain by preventing the pain sensation from traveling up the spinal cord to the brain. This research led to a device now known as the transcutaneous electrical nerve stimulator (TENS unit; Figure 24-1). It is widely used for control of acute temporary pain and also for long-term, chronic pain. When this technique was first developed, it was an example of "alternative medicine." Because Dr. Shealy was able to demonstrate the effectiveness of TENS to the satisfaction of other neurosurgeons, this example of "alternative medicine" quickly assumed a place within conventional medical practice. Dr. Shealy, the first

FIGURE 24-1 A TENS unit is used to relieve pain. *Delmar/Cengage Learning*

physician to specialize in management of pain, coined the term **dolorology** for this new medical specialty. (*Dolor* is the Latin word for "pain.")

Later, Dr. Shealy introduced the use of microsurgery for intracranial surgical procedures, thus eliminating the need to remove part of the patient's skull to access the brain. He trained many other surgeons in the use of this technique, thereby making another important contribution to conventional medicine. But his search for better results—control of pain, correction of causes, improvement in a patient's well-being—led him to explore other alternatives to conventional medicine. He now advises patients with chronic pain to meditate. Through meditation and identification of unresolved emotions, many of his pain patients gain control over their pain. Some are able to discontinue their long-term use of pain medication.

### Intuitive Diagnosis

Dr. Shealy's search for answers led him to study psychic healers such as Olga Worrall, whose healing ministry in Baltimore resulted in hundreds of documented cures, and Henry Rucker of the Psychic Research Foundation in Chicago. Dr. Shealy's research skills enabled him to design scientifically sound projects to study the performance of these psychics. These studies of healers led him to conclude that there is some type of energy transfer from healer to healee. The patient's body then utilizes that energy for healing. Dr. Shealy's research with the

Rev. Henry Rucker and seven of his associates, none of whom had medical training, showed a high level of accuracy in making an "intuitive diagnosis." These eight psychics were allowed to see, but not speak to, 17 patients for whom a medical diagnosis had already been established. The psychics each wrote their impressions on separate sheets of paper and gave them to Dr. Shealy. All eight gave a correct diagnosis on 11 patients; at least two presented a correct diagnosis on each of the other six patients. As a result of this high level of accuracy, Dr. Shealy continued to explore the potential of gifted "intuitives" to assist in diagnosis. (Note: Dr. Shealy selected the psychics to participate in this experiment according to strict criteria. He now uses the term *intuitive* rather than *psychic*. Because psychic phenomena have recently caught the public interest and become something of a fad, many people claim to have psychic powers for the purpose of making money. Genuine psychics consider their special abilities to be a gift and use this gift selectively to help others.)

Dr. Shealy, pictured in Figure 24-2, believes that physicians who are especially successful in diagnosis are, either consciously or unconsciously, using intuition in addition to their clinical skills.

## Management of Hypertension

Dr. Herbert Benson, a professor at the Harvard Medical School, became concerned about increasing evidence that heart attacks, strokes, and hypertension are occurring in men approximately 13 years earlier than in their fathers. Believing the stress of modern life to exact a high price, both psychologically and physiologically, he studied approaches to stress management outside conventional medicine's use of tranquilizers and/or sedatives. Drugs can control some symptoms related to stress, but do not eliminate *sources* of stress, reverse the physiological effects of prolonged stress, or correct an underlying psychological problem.

**FIGURE 24-2** Dr. C. Norman Shealy is a neurosurgeon and founder of the American Holistic Medical Association. He has developed several innovative approaches to pain management.
*Source: Photo courtesy of Dr. Shealy, Shealy Institute for Comprehensive Health Care, Springfield, MO*

Harvard research studies have shown that control of involuntary body processes, such as blood pressure, heart rate, and flow of blood to a specific part of the body, may be learned through the use of biofeedback. After reviewing research related to conscious control of body functions, Dr. Benson raised the question, "Can we influence our own physiological reaction to stress through individually controlled mental practices?"

Dr. Benson began his search for a practical, *easily learned* means of physiological control. He found that people who used Transcendental Meditation experienced certain body changes within a few minutes after achieving the meditative state. These changes were different from the physiological changes that occur during sleep and hypnosis. Eventually, Dr. Benson and his research team demonstrated that hypertensive patients could lower their blood pressure by using a simple meditative technique twice a day. Many patients were able to discontinue their blood pressure medication and maintain a normal blood pressure simply by incorporating meditation into their daily routines. The choice for hypertensive patients became, "Meditation or medication?"

Three modern medical pioneers—all seeking more effective therapy for their patients—concluded that meditation, practiced at least twice a day for 20 minutes, has therapeutic effects. Dr. Simonton found that this simple practice benefitted cancer patients, even those considered to be terminal by their own physicians. Dr. Shealy found that meditation could be used to manage pain, especially chronic, long-term pain. And Dr. Benson demonstrated that meditation enabled many hypertensive patients to control their blood pressure. Each of these physicians used an alternative practice to enhance the therapeutic benefits of conventional medicine for his patients. Their findings are widely accepted now; in fact, many health care agencies now offer wellness programs that include meditation instruction.

These innovators influenced the practices of some physicians and the breadth of services offered within some health care agencies. The effect on the roles of various health care providers remains to be seen, however. Ultimately, each health care provider's open-mindedness will determine whether or not he can adapt successfully to the role changes required by a holistic approach to health care. Many of these new ideas, some of which are explored in greater detail in the following units, have the potential to enhance each health care provider's performance in patient care; enrich personal and family life; and improve mental, physical, emotional, and spiritual health.

## THE HEALTH CARE SYSTEM—TODAY AND TOMORROW

You are preparing to assume an important role in today's health care system. But that system couldn't exist were it not for the many significant contributions of scientists, physicians, and others throughout history. Some of those contributions were initially rejected and their proponents ridiculed. Today, health care innovations and new theories, or new viewpoints regarding accepted theories, are appearing frequently. Some are rejected by orthodox medicine as quackery or, at best, "not scientifically proven." Some are tried by the more open-minded members of the orthodox medical establishment and, upon proving to be clinically effective, are incorporated into an established medical practice.

Physicians tend to be judge and jury regarding innovations and trends in health care. But what is the appropriate attitude toward such innovations for you in your role as a health care provider? What is an appropriate attitude toward an innovative therapy that is provided by someone whose practice is not under the immediate direction of a medical doctor? Eventually you will need to deal with these questions and decide what will be your attitude toward innovative therapies.

## Technological Advances

Today's health care system is a dynamic (i.e., ever-changing) system. Many current innovations are technological—new, sophisticated equipment for laboratory tests, new techniques for identifying and mapping physical changes in the patient's body, modifications in therapeutic devices, complex machines for maintaining vital functions. These technological innovations tend to be readily accepted into the existing system, though the high cost of some equipment may limit its use to large facilities. Some technological innovations require additional training for health care providers. The expanded role or time-saving feature of some innovations results in ready acceptance. This is especially true of equipment and techniques that contribute to diagnosis.

## Emerging Therapies and Roles

Other innovations—primarily therapeutic approaches—are less readily accepted. Rejection by medical personnel often is based on the fact that a particular technique is performed by someone who is not under the direction of a physician "carrying out doctor's orders." Techniques such as acupressure, Shiatsu, Structural Integration, therapeutic massage, and craniosacral therapy require highly specialized training. Others, such as acupuncture and chiropractic techniques, require completion of a lengthy formal educational program. In addition, professional counselors such as psychologists, social workers, guidance counselors, and pastoral counselors are assuming a greater role in patient care. Many of these have completed a doctoral program (i.e., Ph.D., Ed.D., D.C.) as lengthy as medical education. Some of these nonmedical practitioners are required to be licensed by the state. But education or training, certification, or licensure do not guarantee acceptance by all allopathic physicians.

In fact, some techniques and some therapists may be perceived as a threat to existing roles within the health care system. The usual reaction is to label such practices as quackery, thereby implying that the practitioner is a fraud and the technique worthless. Many patients would testify otherwise, however, having obtained benefits from a complementary therapy that they did not get from orthodox medical treatment. Because public acceptance of these complementary therapies is increasing, you are encouraged to keep an open mind, listen to patients, and withhold judgment until you have enough information to make a rational evaluation.

Actually, many of today's roles within the health care system did not exist 10 or 20 years ago. For the most part, these new roles emerged as a result of fragmenting existing roles, specializing in a specific technique or group of techniques, or specializing in a specific type of patient. In the orthodox system of health care, all of these roles are performed under the direction of a physician. Many of the alternative therapies are performed by practitioners who are not working under the direction of a physician. Yet some of these practitioners are licensed by the state; their practice, therefore, is completely legal. This makes it all the more important that health care providers be informed and are able to evaluate a given therapy without arbitrarily labeling any unfamiliar therapy as "quackery."

Also, keep in mind that some of these complementary therapies are "innovative" only from the perspective of health care in the United States. The Chinese have been using acupuncture for at least 5,000 years. Homeopathic medicine has been practiced throughout Europe for 200 years. Chiropractic techniques were developed in the early 1900s. Being over 90 years old, chiropractic no longer qualifies as "innovative." It is a form of therapy now widely accepted by the American public, though not by many allopathic physicians, especially orthopedic surgeons.

## SCIENTIFIC STUDY OF COMPLEMENTARY THERAPIES

Another physician who has applied the scientific method to the study of "difficult to measure" variables is Dr. Larry Dossey. Many people believe that the power of prayer has a direct effect upon healing, and some can offer anecdotal evidence as "proof." The scientific community, however, does not accept anecdotal evidence. Dr. Dossey's interest in identifying various influences on the course of an illness has led him to explore alternative healing. Influenced by his scientific training, he used research methodology to study the effectiveness of prayer under a variety of conditions. His conclusions: prayer can and does have a measurable effect, regardless of whether or not a patient knows that prayers are being offered on his behalf. Thus, Dr. Dossey successfully demonstrated that the scientific method can be adapted to the study of some nonmedical healing variables.

## ISSUES IN HEALTH CARE

The conflict between orthodox medical practice and complementary therapies is especially evident in several areas: pharmaceuticals versus natural remedies, herbal remedies, nutrition, and nutritional supplements. A full discussion of each of these topics is beyond the scope of this book, so the following paragraphs are intended only to introduce each topic as an area of concern for health care providers. Many books and journals are available to those who want to become informed about any of these topics. Because of the wealth of information now being published, ongoing study will be necessary to keep up with new developments.

### Pharmaceutical Drugs

Pharmaceutical companies constitute a multibillion-dollar industry. The industry justifies the high prices of drugs in the United States on the basis of costs involved in research and obtaining approval from the Food and Drug Administration (FDA). Yet those same drugs sell for much lower prices in other countries. Some cost factors that pharmaceutical companies do not reveal to the public include incentive programs (all-expenses-paid trips, hospitality rooms at professional meetings) to influence doctors' prescription choices, financial support to researchers in university settings, payments to public figures (models, actors, a former vice president of the United States) to promote a particular drug, and the costs of advertising in the mass media. Company representatives visit doctors' offices regularly with gifts for doctors and the office staff, as well as literature and free drug samples.

Not satisfied with the results of these expensive public relations efforts directed to the medical profession, drug companies now promote specific drugs to the public, with the FDA's approval. Television commercials and full-page advertisements with beautiful, smiling people tout the benefits of specific drugs for common ailments, such as arthritis and osteoporosis. The risk of side effects is presented with rapid-fire dialogue on television or in the fine print of an advertisement. The purpose of mass advertising is to sell drugs—by priming patients to pressure their doctors for a specific drug prescription. Although the marketing tactics of drug companies are a major factor in the escalating costs of health care, a more serious concern is risk—the dangerous side effects of many drugs that have been marketed aggressively.

Many drugs available today save lives, control symptoms, and prolong life. But the long-term effects of many new drugs are unknown; most drugs receive FDA approval on the basis of short-term research. Adverse reactions to prescription drugs are among the 10 most frequent causes of hospital admissions. More than 100,000 deaths per year are due to prescription drugs: unexpected side effects, incorrect dosage, drug interactions, allergic reactions, or damage to vital organs, especially the heart, liver, or kidneys. For example, the diabetes drug Rezulin was approved by the FDA in 1997; it was withdrawn from the market in 2000 after being linked to numerous fatalities due to liver damage. With increasing public awareness of these problems, many people are using herbs, natural remedies, homeopathic remedies, nutritional healing, and other alternatives to pharmaceutical drugs.

## Herbalism

**Herbalism,** the medicinal use of plants, is perhaps the oldest form of healing. Healers throughout the ages have used the roots, stems, leaves, flowers, nuts, and fruits of plants to treat illnesses and injuries. This knowledge was passed down from generation to generation by word of mouth, although certain ancient cultures recorded their healing practices on papyrus or clay tablets. Following development of the printing press, Culpeper published the *London Dispensary* in 1653 and, later, his *Complete Herbal*, a book that is still available today. In regard to these early records of herbalism, Dr. Norman Shealy states, "Globally, herbal lore is a treasure chest beyond price" (Shealy, 2006, p. 104). He considers herbalism to be a holistic system that has a completely different philosophy than that of orthodox medicine, as reflected in the following basic tenets:

> *The whole plant is better than an isolated extract.*
>
> *Treat the whole person, not just the symptoms.*
>
> *Practice minimum effective treatment and minimum intervention.*
>
> *Strengthen the body and encourage it to heal itself (Shealy, 2006, p. 104).*

In Germany, herbal remedies are available only by prescription from a medical doctor or professional herbalist. In the United States, herbalism is practiced both as a profession and as a self-help and home remedy system. A professional herbalist must have extensive training that may include several years' study in Europe, India, or the Orient. Only a professional herbalist should diagnose and prescribe an herbal prescription for a patient. But for a self-help program, preparations from professional herbal pharmacies are available through mail order and in health food stores, holistic pharmacies, wellness centers, and holistic medical offices. Herbal remedies are available in various forms: as a tincture, essential oil, ointment, cream, tablet, capsule, powder, or tea. Essential oils are concentrated and must be diluted in a carrier oil (almond, sesame, light olive) before being applied directly to the skin.

Anyone who wishes to include herbalism in a personal self-care or family care program should acquire basic information about herbs and various types of preparations, learn the therapeutic actions of various forms of the most useful plants, and then use herbal remedies appropriately. The fact that plants are natural does not mean that they are harmless. Plant materials can have powerful effects, and some plants are poisonous. *One should use an herbal remedy only with knowledge and understanding of its therapeutic effects and appropriate use.*

Herbal preparations can be applied externally to the affected area by soaking, rinsing, rubbing, or applying a compress or poultice; they may be taken internally in the form of a tea, powder, or liquid; some part of the plant may be added to boiling water to produce healing vapors that the patient inhales.

Correctly used, an herbal remedy can affect the cause of illness, rather than merely suppress symptoms. Herbal treatment requires more time than most drugs. For example, St. John's wort, currently popular as a natural treatment for depression, may require up to three months for the full benefit to become apparent. An antidepressant drug may become effective within a month, but antidepressant drugs can have serious side effects. St. John's wort has few, if any, unpleasant side effects. The active ingredient in St. John's wort is hypericin, but other ingredients in the plant also contribute to its mood-altering effects. Hypericin alone is not as effective.

Plants contain many different components that work together. Even when the active ingredient has been identified, it is probable that other components of the plant support and facilitate the effects of the primary active ingredient. The enhancement of an effect by a combination of ingredients is known as **synergism,** which is considered by herbalists to be a major advantage of herbs over prescription drugs.

## Nutrition and Health

Traditionally, nutrition education has focused on the components of a balanced diet—proteins, fats, and carbohydrates—and the major food groups from which they are derived. As the health movement developed over recent decades, with its emphasis on exercise and healthful eating, greater attention has been directed to other components of the diet: vitamins, minerals, trace minerals, amino acids, and fiber. Vitamins are organic nutrients that serve numerous functions in the body; a severe deficiency results in a medically recognized condition, such as scurvy or rickets, but symptoms of a mild or moderate deficiency may not be recognized and correctly diagnosed. Minerals are inorganic substances that the body needs in relatively large amounts (e.g., calcium); trace minerals are those the body needs in tiny amounts (e.g., copper). Amino acids are the building blocks of the body; there are 20 amino acids, of which 8 are essential and 12 are nonessential. An essential amino acid must be obtained from foods, whereas a nonessential amino acid is one the body can synthesize from other nutrients. The body must have an adequate supply of these various components in order to build and repair tissues—an ongoing process throughout life—and to carry out various body processes.

Nutrition has recently become a national concern. Obesity and diabetes are epidemic, indicating that large numbers of people do not eat healthful meals. Instead of a home-cooked dinner, prepared from homegrown vegetables, many people eat at fast-food restaurants or serve a dinner of convenience foods. Corporate farming provides stores with fruits and vegetables of questionable nutritive value and, possibly, contamination with chemical herbicides and pesticides. The food industry is using chemical additives whose effects on health are unknown. Many meats contain antibiotics and hormones. These and numerous other factors contribute to growing concern about practices within the food industry that alter or modify a food from its natural state.

Anyone who wishes to have a healthful diet must find a source of organically grown foods or grow their own. Range chickens and eggs and organic meats are available, although more expensive. The grocery shopper must read labels to avoid foods that contain chemical additives, usually as preservatives, artificial ingredients, unhealthful forms of fat, or dyes. These choices are not possible for everyone. Nor are most people concerned enough to focus on healthful eating. So the adverse effects of unhealthful eating have significance for health care providers. Holistic practitioners consider diet to be an important factor in health, and possibly a contributing cause of any chronic illness. But healthful eating may require more than wholesome food.

A mild or moderate deficiency of a vitamin or mineral can result in symptoms that are not recognized by allopathic medicine. The holistic practitioner, however, obtains a dietary history from new patients and is alert for indications of any nutritional deficiency. Sometimes a patient's therapy is directed primarily to ensuring that the diet contains the needed amount of each nutrient. Some medical doctors are now addressing nutritional concerns with their patients. A leader in nutritional medicine is Jonathan Wright, M.D., who has had a nutritional medical practice for about 30 years. Dr. Wright also publishes a newsletter to educate the public about nutrition and has formulated a variety of nutritional supplements for therapeutic use and health maintenance. For example, a supplement offered by Dr. Wright's clinic facilitates blood sugar metabolism, thereby enabling some diabetics to manage their condition nutritionally, without pharmaceutical drugs.

Healthful eating is a primary requirement for maintaining health and for treating illness, but diet alone may not be enough to protect one's health against stress and the many pollutants to which we are all exposed. Full protection and a therapeutic plan for healing requires supplementation.

## Nutritional Supplements

Although obstetricians and pediatricians have recommended vitamins to their patients for many years, most allopathic practitioners do not. Medical schools that offer a short course in nutrition usually make it an elective rather than a required course. There are indications of change, however, as professional conferences focus on nutrition, many jointly offered by a center for mind-body medicine, a major university, and a medical school.

Naturopathic schools and chiropractic schools emphasize nutrition in accordance with their holistic philosophy. Nutritionists who are associated with holistic health centers are more likely to counsel patients about all aspects of nutrition, including the use of supplements, than dietitians in an allopathic agency. Herbalists also are knowledgeable about nutrition; many substances prescribed by herbalists are found in the kitchen, some on the spice rack! Anyone seeking guidance about nutrition should find a qualified counselor and/or embark on a self-education program. If *nutrition therapy* is needed, then professional consultation is essential.

Vitamin, mineral, and amino acid supplements are all available as tablets, capsules, and powders. Natural products sold in health food stores and holistic centers are preferable to the synthetic products marketed through chain stores. For example, vitamin C made from rose hips is preferable to ascorbic acid (the chemical name for vitamin C), for the same reason that herbal products differ from pharmaceutical drugs—the whole is better than a single primary ingredient. A multivitamin is preferable to taking several vitamins separately, which can lead to an imbalance. The B vitamins should be taken in the form of B complex, again because the ratio of the different vitamins should be balanced. Selection of a brand is important; analytical studies of some brands have shown that their labels are misleading.

As a health care provider, you will find it beneficial to become knowledgeable about nutrition, healthful eating habits, and supplements. This will help you maintain a high level of wellness and enable you to protect yourself against health risks to which you may be exposed in your work. It will not be within your role to prescribe, but it will be appropriate to suggest sources of information if a patient asks you about nutrition or supplements. You may occasionally have an opportunity to suggest a change in eating habits that could enhance a patient's nutritional status. Your best approach to becoming informed about nutrition is to read a journal related to holistic healing regularly and subscribe to a nutrition newsletter written by a medical doctor or a naturopath.

## STAYING INFORMED

Many issues now confront society and the health care system: abortion, AIDS, organ transplants, prolonged use of life-support systems, patients' rights (including the right to refuse treatment), a patient's right to die, advance medical directives, and malpractice litigation. Some of these are moral and ethical issues; some have direct implications for certain roles, and therefore are of special concern to health care providers. Many of these issues are highly emotional; the proponents of one side or the other may base their arguments on catch phrases that arouse strong emotional reactions in the listener.

A full discussion of these issues is beyond the scope of this book; they are mentioned here because every health care provider should be informed about them. Being informed makes it possible to avoid emotionalism and examine an issue thoughtfully. Read, attend meetings, consider various viewpoints, and use every opportunity to become informed; then decide what *you* believe instead of blindly adopting the opinion of someone else. Strive to keep an open mind, combined with a healthy dose of skepticism.

For a large segment of the population, the major issues in health care are *accessibility* and *cost*. For providers of health services, the major issue relates to the patient-physician relationship and *who should make decisions about health care options*. For third-party payers (insurance companies), the major issue is maintaining greater income (through insurance premiums) than is paid out for health care services—*making a profit*. There is currently no national health care policy that adequately resolves the many issues related to costs. Any national health care policy must resolve such questions as:

- Who is entitled to health care?
- What is *essential* health care and what is *nonessential*?
- Who should decide whether a specific service for a specific patient is essential or nonessential?
- What is a reasonable cost for each type of service?
- What is a reasonable income for each health care provider?
- Who will pay for essential services?
- Who will pay for services that are deemed nonessential, but are desired (or demanded) by a patient?

You may be wondering why you should be concerned about accessibility and costs. These two issues are of personal concern to you and your family, even though you, as a health care provider, will probably have ready access to health care. These issues are of great concern to many of your patients, however. As you interact with a patient who is dissatisfied with his health care plan, you may be the object of that patient's displaced anger. Do not take it personally. Be a good listener, and be aware that the complaints you are hearing may be all too true. Meanwhile, we can all hope that eventually everyone will have access to affordable health care.

# REFERENCES AND SUGGESTED READINGS

> **Note:** In the following list, * indicates a "classic" reference, meaning that the author introduced one or more concepts related to holistic health care; ** following an entry indicates a comprehensive reference illustrated with color drawings and photographs.

Balch, James E., & Stengler, Mark. (2004). *Prescription for natural cures.* Hoboken, NJ: John Wiley.

*Balch, Phyllis A. (2002). *Prescription for herbal healing.* New York: Penguin Putnam. **

*Balch, Phyllis A. (2002). *Prescription for nutritional healing: The A-to-Z guide to supplements* (2nd ed.). New York: Avery.

*Benson, Herbert. (2000). *The relaxation response.* New York: Morrow/Avon.

*Dossey, Larry. (1999). *Prayer is good medicine.* New York: HarperCollins.

*Dossey, Larry. (1999). *Reinventing medicine: Beyond mind-body to a new era of healing.* New York: HarperCollins.

Kasper, S., et al. (2006, September). Superior efficacy of St. John's wort extract WS(R) 5570 compared to placebo in patients with major depression. *Alternative Medicine Review, 11*(3), 247–248.

Khalsa, Dharma Singh. (2003). *Food as medicine: How to use diet, vitamins, juices, and herbs for a healthier, happier, and longer life.* New York: Atria Books.

Lininger, Schuyler (Ed.), et al. (2002). *The natural pharmacy.* Rosedale, CA: Prima. **

MacPherson, Hugh, et al. (2009, October 3). Closing the evidence gap in integrative medicine. *British Medical Journal, 339*(7724), 763–764.

Shealy, C. Norman. (2006). *Life beyond 100: Secrets of the fountain of youth.* New York: Penguin.

*Shealy, C. Norman, & Myss, Caroline M. (1993). *The creation of health: The emotional, psychological, and spiritual responses that promote health and healing.* Walpole, NH: Stillpoint.

Simontacchi, Carol. (2007). *The crazy makers: How the food industry is destroying our brains and harming our children.* New York: Jeremy P. Tarcher.

*Simonton, O. Carl, Matthews-Simonton, Stephanie, & Creighton, James. (1992). *Getting well again.* New York: Bantam Books.

# REVIEW AND SELF-CHECK

1. State two reasons that innovations in science and medicine are often rejected or labeled as quackery.

   a. Conflict w/ existing beliefs - Perceived as threat to current practitioners

   b. Empirical - based on experience & observation  Scientific - clinical trials

2. Name two beliefs about sickness, or a person who is sick, that were common in early cultures and are still prevalent today.

   Illness

3. Name five significant scientific or medical advances during the past 400 years that established the foundation for today's health care practices.

4. List five major differences between holistic health care and orthodox medical care.

   Hollistic
   All disease is psychosomatic
   multiple causation
   Healing - psychosomatic

5. Name three physicians who introduced ideas and practices that are basic to holistic health care.

6. Name a physician who demonstrated that the scientific model can be used to study some complementary therapies.

7. Place the letter of each discovery listed below beside the appropriate name in the column on the right.

   a. The germ theory              _e_ von Leeuwenhoek
   b. Handwashing                  _b_ Semmelweis
   c. Use of antiseptics           _a_ Koch
   d. Rabies vaccine               _h_ Roentgen
   e. Microscope                   _g_ Salk
   f. Smallpox vaccination         _i_ Curie
   g. Polio vaccine                _c_ Lister
   h. X rays                       _j_ Freud
   i. Radium                       _a_ Pasteur
   j. Role of the unconscious mind _k_ Vesalius
   k. Accurate human anatomy       _f_ Jenner

## ASSIGNMENTS

1. Select a topic from this chapter and prepare an oral report to present in class, as scheduled by the instructor.

2. Participate in a discussion of one of the following topics:

    a. Beliefs about the causes of illness and recovery.

    b. Innovations that have been introduced into your local health care system within the past five years.

    c. A complementary therapy that you have heard someone label as "quackery."

    d. A complementary therapy that someone you know is using.

3. Participate in a role-play where you are a health care provider; your patient has just told you that she is enrolled in a class to learn how to meditate.

# UNIT 25

# What Is Healing? Who Is the Healer?

## OBJECTIVES

Upon completion of this unit, you should be able to:

- Explain *placebo* as used in orthodox health care systems and in a holistic health care system.
- Describe the relationship of emotional states to the immune system.
- Compare *curing* and *healing*.
- List six factors that influence healing (holistic view).
- Explain the importance of love to the healing process.
- Explain *intention* as a factor in healing.
- Name five characteristics of patients who survive despite diagnosis of a life-threatening condition.
- List five differences between the holistic approach to health care and the orthodox approach.
- Explain the importance of stress management to health.
- State two challenges for health care providers who wish to contribute to a patient's healing process.

## KEY TERMS

| External locus of control | Internal locus of control | Placebo effect |
| Intention | Placebo | |

Every health care provider has wondered at times why one patient recovers from a serious illness, while another patient with the same disease and therapy slowly declines and eventually dies. What triggers the healing process in some patients, even when the prognosis is grim? Is there some subtle, unseen influence that makes a difference in the course of illness?

## PLACEBO EFFECT

Another puzzle is **placebo effect**—improvement or recovery when the "drug" administered to a patient is actually a **placebo,** an inert substance such as a sugar pill. Why does the patient improve, even though the "treatment" administered is not medically acknowledged as having therapeutic value? Studies of placebo effect have led to recognition that "expectation" or "being special" (i.e., being part of a research project) may influence the outcome of treatment. Expectation applies to both patients and health care providers; if either or both believe that a treatment or drug is going to cure the patient's illness, improvement is more likely to occur. Placebo effect is a problem for researchers who are trying to test the effectiveness of a new treatment, because it is difficult to control. This is why double-blind studies are used to test the effectiveness of a new drug. Placebo effect is used by some people as a defense against accepting an innovative therapy. Anyone who does not want to give serious consideration to a new therapy may simply dismiss any positive results of the innovation as "just placebo effect."

## THE IMMUNE SYSTEM—PROTECTOR AND DEFENDER OF THE BODY

Despite years of discussion, there is no satisfactory explanation for *why* placebo effect occurs. Also puzzling is the fact that in an epidemic, some people get sick and others, even members of a victim's family, do not contract the infection. This raises questions about the immune system. Why does it protect sometimes, but not always?

It is now known that all of us have cancer cells in our bodies, but certain components of the immune system destroy those abnormal cells with great efficiency until . . . what? Why does the immune system stop destroying those abnormal cells? What change permits those cancer cells to reproduce and form a tumor?

These questions have led to a number of discoveries about what affects the immune system. Physicians in ancient cultures observed that a grieving person was likely to develop cancer within a year or two following a significant loss. But at that time, the existence of the immune system was completely unknown. Modern clinicians and researchers have established the validity of that ancient observation. Certain emotional states, especially grief, depress the immune system and render it less capable of destroying abnormal cells present in the body. The result is a favorable climate for the growth of cancer cells.

This particular body/mind/emotions relationship is now widely accepted. Yet much research on cancer still involves searching for an external intervention. This type of thinking denies the powerful mind/body relationship, clinging instead to the "old" way of attributing both the cause and the cure of disease to external influences. Much of our knowledge of the immune system has been gained during the past 40 years. Even though today's research techniques enable scientists to study the immune system more effectively, there are still many unanswered questions.

## THE MIND/BODY HEALING SYSTEM

Dr. Andrew Weil has spent many years studying people who experienced healing despite pessimistic medical predictions. The medical profession labels these incidents as "spontaneous remission" and makes no effort to determine the factors that keep such patients from succumbing to their illnesses according to medical expectations. Dr. Weil believes there should be more research to identify the factors that enable some people to reverse the course of an "irreversible" disease.

In *Spontaneous Healing*, Dr. Weil describes the human body's innate potential for maintaining health and overcoming illness. Chapter 5 of his book contains a description of the body's system for healing at various levels: the most basic healing is at the DNA level (the molecule that carries the genetic blueprint on chromosomes and genes), with other healing processes occurring at cellular membranes, tissues, and organs. Dr. Weil's detailed explanation of this multilevel process provides a basis for understanding the complexity of the body's system for repairing damaged cells and tissues. Emphasizing that the healing process is an innate function, Dr. Weil explains:

- The body has within its DNA all of the information needed to repair itself.
- The healing system can recognize damage.
- Healing processes operate continuously.
- The body's healing mechanism can replace damaged cells with healthy cells to maintain normal structure and function.

Dr. Weil believes that this healing process is the body's spontaneous response to cellular injury. The challenge for medical researchers is to identify the switches that turn on the body's healing mechanism, so that therapy can be directed to stimulating the healing response if it does not occur spontaneously. Dr. Weil also suggests the mind as one source of triggers that activate the body's healing system. The prevailing view of disease as an enemy leads naturally to thinking of treatments as "weapons" and hoping for new ways to "fight" a disease. His work with patients has convinced him that "fighting this thing" is less effective than *acceptance of the illness*. Once a patient accepts the illness and *improves his or her lifestyle*, possibly to enjoy "what time I have left," energy may increase and symptoms may diminish. Dr. Weil believes that such improvement indicates the body's innate healing response has been triggered, rather than that the disease has gone into spontaneous remission.

Dr. Weil takes a detailed social history from each new patient to identify eating habits, sleep patterns, exercise, family relationships, sexuality, hobbies, relaxation activities, and spiritual beliefs and practices. With this overview of the patient's lifestyle, he is better prepared to identify roots of the patient's problem and potential solutions. Often the most significant clue within the social history is evidence of major stressors. With certain life changes that enable the patient to decrease and/or manage stress, health improves. A patient's healing depends on the body's healing response to a specific illness or injury. In the case of illness, Dr. Weil emphasizes promotion of healing by addressing *causes*—the reasons some people get sick and others, exposed to the same circumstances, do not. His approach is compatible with the concept of *multiple causation* of disease.

## WHO GETS SICK? WHO GETS WELL?

Some clinical practitioners and researchers are proposing new ways of looking at the causes of disease. One theory is that there are *several* contributing causes in any illness, rather than a single cause. Some of the causative factors lie *within* the individual:

- Immune system function (specifically resistance and susceptibility)
- Emotional states, which we now know to have powerful effects on the immune system
- Physiological changes due to chronic stress
- Subtle factors—beliefs, attitudes, will to live, and, possibly, an unconscious desire to escape one's life situation

In *The Creation of Health*, Dr. Shealy lists six major causes of illness and death:

- Smoking
- Consumption of alcohol
- Obesity
- Consumption of excessive fat, salt, and sugar
- Lack of exercise
- Failure to wear a seat belt and speeding

All of the above contributors to illness or injury involve *choices*, and the choice each individual makes is based on a combination of beliefs, values, and attitudes that influence behavior. From a holistic perspective, persons who choose unhealthful practices are also choosing to be sick or injured at some time in the future.

The concept of multiple causation leads naturally to the view that *healing* requires thinking of the patient as an entity (a whole being) within the context of family life, occupational setting, community, and culture—the holistic approach. In order for healing to occur, one must modify beliefs and attitudes and make healthful life choices.

As a health care provider, you need to provide a therapeutic environment that will facilitate the healing process. You have already learned that a therapeutic climate includes physical comfort and correct technique in performing procedures. But is something else required for a truly therapeutic climate?

Perhaps you have noticed that the patients of some physicians and some therapists seem to recover more readily than the patients of other physicians and therapists. Perhaps the same surgery was performed, the same drugs prescribed, the same therapeutic techniques used. What makes the difference in results? Does the difference lie within the patient, or can it be attributed to some characteristics of the health care providers?

Dr. Shealy believes that some physicians are "natural healers." In addition to their medical skills, they unconsciously convey healing energy to their patients. Perhaps this "energy" is a natural love for humanity, especially for those who are suffering. Dr. Shealy's emphasis on the healing power of love is now reflected in numerous books by other physicians who have found that loving, caring relationships, especially in group therapy settings, have a positive effect on their patients. It is possible that many health care providers, not only physicians, are "natural healers."

## THE POWER OF LOVE

Love is essential to healing. *Love for self* influences the patient's body response to illness; a *loving attitude on the part of health care providers* establishes a healing climate. And *loving relationships* provide the emotional support that facilitates healing. Dr. Bernie Siegel gained much public attention following the publication of his book *Love, Medicine and Miracles: Lessons Learned about Self-Healing from a Surgeon's Experience with Exceptional Patients*. Numerous other publications emphasize the importance of love—self-love as well as love from others—to health and well-being.

## HEALING VERSUS CURING

There is a clear distinction between healing and curing. *Healing* refers to what patients (or their bodies) do for themselves to improve their condition. *Curing* refers to treatment provided to the patient by physicians or therapists.

Many healing systems and techniques facilitate the patient's self-discovery, which promotes self-healing. Effective techniques include meditation, nutritional therapy, herbal therapy, homeopathy, acupuncture, Rolfing, chiropractic techniques, Alexander-Feldenkrais technique, rebirthing, counseling, and biofeedback. If you are like most health care providers, many of these terms are totally new to you. It is not necessary to know about them all, but you need to know that these methods, among others, are found effective by a large segment of the public. When you encounter a patient who has used or is using one of these methods, view it as your opportunity to learn about the technique from your patient.

## INTENTION

Current thinking, then, emphasizes both the role of the patient and the role of loving, supportive relationships in determining the outcome of illness. This presents a *new dimension* to the role of health care provider. Patient care that consists of carrying out the physician's orders or performing assigned procedures is a limited role. The challenge to health care providers is to perform patient care with the *conscious* **intention** of helping the patient to heal. This does not require additional time or effort. It does require concentration—*giving full attention to the patient* and *focusing on loving, positive thoughts throughout a procedure* for the purpose of providing a healing climate.

Would this make a difference? A wealth of literature provides extensive evidence that *intention does make a difference*. Each health care provider must make a personal decision about whether or not to strive for creating a truly healing climate in each contact with a patient. Be aware also that healing occurs only if the patient has the *intention* to get well. Intention, in turn, is affected by such factors as belief systems, faith, and will to live. A newly recognized challenge for health care providers is acceptance—*nonjudgmental acceptance*—of a patient who does not intend to get well.

## WHO SURVIVES?

"When you are hit by adversity or have your life disrupted, how do you respond? Some people feel victimized. . . . Some shut down. They feel helpless and overwhelmed. . . . A few, however, reach within themselves and find ways to cope with the adversity." With these words, Dr. Al Siebert, a psychologist, introduces his book *The Survivor Personality*. Dr. Siebert believes that survivors differ from other people only in their ability to "*reach within* themselves and *find ways to cope.*" For many years, he has studied people who survived various types of life crises, including the diagnosis of an incurable disease. In the chapter entitled "Self-Managed Healing," Dr. Siebert discusses the reluctance of the medical profession to acknowledge that some patients survive despite medical predictions of imminent death. As noted earlier, when such patients improve and no longer exhibit symptoms of their "fatal" illness, most doctors label the improvement as "spontaneous remission" and make no effort to determine the factors that may have contributed to the patient's improvement.

Dr. Siebert's research led to the identification of several common factors in the stories of people who survived medical diagnosis of a terminal illness; such patients:

- Develop their own strategy for survival after finding that they cannot get guidelines for survival from their physicians.
- Recognize that they must search and experiment to find the survival strategy that is unique to their own situation.

**FIGURE 25-1** Patients who are characterized by an external locus of control may see help from outside sources as their only hope, whereas patients characterized by an internal locus of control may become actively involved in making lifestyle changes and developing their own potential for healing. *Delmar/Cengage Learning*

- Perceive their health crisis as a wake-up call—something in their lifestyle is contributing to the illness, and survival requires change.
- Accept that survival may require modifying one's belief system.
- Decide to make changes in ways of living, relationships, thought patterns, beliefs, and/or expression of feelings in order to improve the quality of life.

A factor that Dr. Siebert believes differentiates survivors is a psychological concept known as locus of control (Figure 25-1). People with an **external locus of control** believe that their lives are controlled by factors external to themselves: illness is caused by some outside force (germs, an accident, punishment for one's sins), and any cure will also be an external force (e.g., the physician, a drug, a special treatment). This type of person looks to the doctor to make her well or, if that is not possible, to manage her illness. She does not want advice about what she can do for herself.

People with an **internal locus of control** feel responsible for what happens to them; consequently, they are likely to seek ways of dealing with any adversity, including a serious illness. This type of person seeks information and wants to know what worked for others. People characterized by a strong internal locus of control want to participate in treatment decisions and may seek complementary types of therapies, learn to meditate, and make extensive changes in lifestyle. Also, they are likely to view the adverse situation as a learning experience or "wake-up call." Some survivors refer to a past adversity as "the best thing that ever happened to me," meaning that the experience led them to examine their life situation and make significant changes in their lives.

## THE HOLISTIC APPROACH TO HEALTH CARE

You have learned about many of the factors that influence a person's health, including individual choices. The belief that illness is the result of outside influences (e.g., germs, accidents that "just happen") affects the choices people make. Thinking, "Other people get sick or have accidents, but I don't," may result in carelessness. How people feel about themselves influences their choices and self-care. Behaviors that indicate lack of self-care and unhealthy choices include:

- Being a workaholic
- Not allowing oneself time to play (not using leisure time for re-creating oneself)
- Eating "on the run" or eating mostly convenience meals
- Ignoring bodily sensations that may be early warning signs of illness
- Ignoring the effects of stress on the body, mind, and emotions
- Ignoring safety precautions in the workplace
- Driving fast or recklessly
- Not wearing a seat belt

Life choices are increasingly recognized as contributing causes of illness or accident. Modern living exposes us to many stressors not known by earlier societies. Each day we encounter air pollution, food additives, building materials and home furnishings that give off toxic fumes—the list is almost endless. But the greatest stressors for many people are time pressures and interpersonal relationships.

Job responsibilities plus home responsibilities plus commuting time plus errand-running leave little leisure time for many people. Time pressures interfere with the development of satisfying and mutually supportive relationships, even within a family setting. Relationship problems may continue for years because "there just isn't time to work on it." People are risking their health when they fail to make time to cope with stress and improve relationships. As a counselor stated after talking with a highly stressed client, "The people who need meditation the most are the ones who say they don't have time. Yet taking 20 minutes a day to meditate could make a world of difference in how their day goes."

## The Mind/Body Connection

Dr. Kenneth Pelletier works with chronically ill patients in a hospital-based clinic. In addition to clinical expertise developed through the years, Dr. Pelletier has extensive knowledge of stress and psychosomatic disorders, based on a comprehensive review of the literature and research reports. He summarizes this voluminous body of literature in *Mind as Healer, Mind as Slayer*. According to Dr. Pelletier, illness is the result of "a complex interaction of social factors, physical and psychological stress, . . . personality . . ., and the inability of the person to adapt adequately to pressures." With this broad view of causation, he then presents evidence for classifying most of today's major health problems as psychosomatic and/or stress-related disorders.

In orthodox medicine, an illness is generally labeled psychosomatic when no organic pathology has been found. In holistic medicine, according to Dr. Pelletier, *psychosomatic* is defined as *a fundamental interaction between mind and body that is involved in all diseases and health maintenance.* Such a definition mandates that diagnosis and treatment of illness take into consideration the mind/body relationship.

Another term that has different meanings under these two systems of health care is *placebo*. In orthodox medicine, *placebo* refers to a treatment or procedure that has no therapeutic value. In the holistic view, placebo effect includes factors that do affect the healing process:

1. The patient's belief system
2. The patient's will to live
3. Patient/health care provider relationships
4. Family relationships
5. Changes in lifestyle
6. Ability (or willingness) to make changes in order to reduce and manage stress

Dr. Pelletier cites several conditions under which stress (the general adaptation response or the fight-or-flight reaction) becomes chronic, rather than serving as an alarm response that is dissipated once the emergency has passed:

1. The source of stress is ambiguous, meaning that the individual is not really clear about what stressors exist in his or her life situation.
2. The stress continues over a prolonged period of time.
3. There are several sources of stress in the individual's life situation.

The prolonged semi-alert physical state that results from this combination of circumstances eventually produces physical and/or physiological changes—a disease or, in the holistic view, a psychosomatic disorder.

Our modern lifestyle includes a wide variety of stressors, many of which we cannot escape. Dr. Pelletier maintains, therefore, that *every individual must develop a regular pattern of stress-reducing activities as a means of health protection.* The alternative is psychosomatic illness or dependence on a crutch such as alcohol or tranquilizers. In his practice, Dr. Pelletier uses biofeedback to help patients learn to control certain body processes and minimize or reverse the effects of stress. The clinic also emphasizes the use of meditation as a stress-reducing activity.

Patients must learn to differentiate between a healthful level of stress and a pathogenic level that can lead to disease. Because some stressors cannot be eliminated, the only healthful choice is to learn how to minimize the effects of those particular stressors. Dr. Pelletier believes the health care system must focus on teaching people to identify stressors, make lifestyle changes to eliminate as many stressors as possible, develop body awareness, and learn effective stress management techniques *before* the onset of symptoms.

## Characteristics of Holistic Health Care

It is generally acknowledged, even within orthodox medicine, that approximately 85% of the patients seen in a physician's office have a psychosomatic disorder. Yet orthodox medicine continues to rely heavily on drugs and surgery as the primary treatments. Table 25-1 contrasts philosophical differences between orthodox medicine and holistic medicine.

The holistic philosophy recognizes that each individual is unique. Health, sickness, and healing are related to a balance or imbalance among body, mind, emotions, and spirit. The holistic philosophy also emphasizes that disease is the result of multiple factors, not just one. When a patient's treatment is based on a single cause and other contributing factors are

### TABLE 25-1

**Basic Philosophical Assumptions**

| HOLISTIC MEDICINE | ORTHODOX MEDICINE |
|---|---|
| All disease is psychosomatic in origin. | Disease is generally caused by external factors, such as pollution or germs. |
| Disease has multiple causation; each person has a "weak point" (i.e., respiratory system, heart, lower back); when that person is subjected to stress over a long period of time, disease or disability is most likely to appear at the weak point. | Most diseases have a specific cause. Infections are caused by microorganisms; there are no other causative factors. |
| The healing process is psychosomatic; a person's will is a primary factor in getting sick or getting well. | Good medical care produces better health. |
| A single-factor approach to health (to healing, to prevention of illness) is too narrow. | A specific therapeutic agent can cure most diseases. |
| Patients have some responsibility for the course of an illness. | Healing is the responsibility of health care providers. |
| All states of health (including sickness) are psychosomatic. | If you are not sick, then you are well. |

Excerpted from Kenneth Pelletier, 1987, *Mind as Healer, Mind as Slayer,* New York: Dell Publishing.

ignored, the patient is likely to experience a sequence of illnesses. The ultimate example is the patient who has undergone one surgical procedure after another, until no more internal organs can be spared. Then the patient develops a systemic disorder, such as diabetes, arthritis, hypertension, or systemic lupus erythematosis. In such a case, symptoms were treated but the underlying causes of illness were ignored. A *partial cure* was effected with each surgery, but the patient was not *healed*.

## Diagnosis and Therapy from a Holistic Perspective

Preventive medicine recognizes *unmanaged stress as a major contributor to illness*. It also recognizes that *healing* in modern society requires the learning of stress management techniques. In Unit 24, you learned that Dr. Simonton, Dr. Shealy, and Dr. Benson have all recognized the importance of stress management. The Simontons' research with cancer patients revealed *a distinctive personality profile that includes habitual repression of anger*. For that reason, each patient's therapy also includes counseling, to assist the patient in dealing with suppressed anger and other negative emotions. Patients are taught to meditate and incorporate at least two, but preferably three, meditations into their daily routines.

At his pain rehabilitation center, Dr. Shealy teaches patients to meditate and take responsibility for their health. A high percentage of his chronic-pain patients, most of whom have been on pain medication for many years, eventually are able to manage their pain through meditation and other self-regulatory techniques. Dr. Shealy also emphasizes good nutrition and an exercise program appropriate for each patient.

Dr. Benson teaches hypertensive patients to meditate as an integral component of their treatment. Because meditation requires considerable self-discipline, a certain percentage of patients will become "dropouts"—they do not make meditation a part of their daily routine. Of those who do practice meditation regularly, many are able to reduce their dosage of antihypertensive drugs, and some are able to discontinue it completely. The potential of meditation to lower blood pressure is so powerful that Dr. Benson emphatically warns new meditators to let their physicians know that they have started meditating. The blood pressure should be monitored, so that the antihypertensive drug can be reduced as blood pressure approaches normal levels, usually within a period of two to six months.

From these few examples, several approaches emerge as essential to healing:

1. Concern for the patient's total being: emotional, mental, and spiritual, as well as physical aspects
2. Having the patient participate in a planned program of health care, including lifestyle changes
3. Teaching the patient stress management techniques
4. Helping the patient face and resolve emotional issues
5. Helping the patient assume responsibility for his or her illness, health, and well-being

It may take weeks or months to make all the changes needed, to deal with emotional issues that may underlie the illness, or to experience the full benefits of therapy. Many patients are not willing to take responsibility for their own health. And therein lies the problem. Even those who are willing to take some responsibility may find it hard to change their lifestyle, deal with painful issues, or even to persist in a long-term plan until the benefits become apparent.

There is also a problem from the standpoint of health care delivery. The holistic approach is time consuming. It requires going beyond the physical examination and related diagnostic studies to study the "whole patient" and the life context within which that patient lives and works. It involves *teaching people*, rather than providing a quick cure. It requires patience and persistence to help people identify underlying causes of illness and make significant lifestyle changes. It also requires that health care providers maintain a loving, caring attitude toward their patients.

## FUTURE HEALTH CARE SYSTEMS

It is possible that we will someday have two health care systems:

1. The existing system for two types of patient:
    a. Those whose illness requires orthodox medical care
    b. Those who are not willing to take responsibility for their own health
2. An alternative, holistic system for people who want to participate in their care, are willing to make lifestyle changes, and are willing to practice health maintenance techniques

Regardless of the delivery system, it is desirable that health care encompass the holistic concepts that (1) each patient is an individual who lives and works within specific settings that impact that person's health, and (2) therapy must address all dimensions of that individual's being: emotional, mental, and spiritual as well as physical. In addition, the information provided in this unit makes it apparent that stress management must become an integral part of health care for prevention and health maintenance, as therapy for chronic conditions, and as a significant part of the treatment protocol for persons recovering from serious illness or injuries. Because of growing recognition of the importance of stress management within the medical community, Unit 27 is designed to help you, as a future health care provider, learn several techniques for managing stress. *Only as a practitioner of stress management will you be prepared to help others learn about the importance of managing their own stress.*

But there will always be patients who prefer orthodox medical care to holistic care, and there will be health care providers who find greater job satisfaction in one system than in the other. As a health care provider, you may eventually have the opportunity to pursue your career in either type of health care setting. Your own beliefs about health and healing should be considered when you are faced with such a choice.

## REFERENCES AND SUGGESTED READINGS

> **Note:** In the following list, * indicates a "classic" reference, meaning that the author introduced one or more concepts related to holistic health care in the listed book or its earlier edition.

*Benson, Herbert. (1999). *Timeless healing*. New York: Simon & Schuster.

*Borysenko, Joan. (2007). *Minding the body, mending the mind*. New York: DaCapo.

*Carlson, Richard, & Shield, Benjamin (Eds.). (1990). *Healers on healing*. Los Angeles, CA: Jeremy P. Tarcher.

Hegner, Barbara R., et al. (2008). Caring for the emotionally stressed patient. In *Nursing assistant: A nursing process approach* (10th ed.). Clifton Park, NY: Delmar, Cengage Learning.

*Keegan, Lynn. (2000). *The nurse as healer*. Clifton Park, NY: Delmar, Cengage Learning.

*Locke, Steven, & Colligan, Douglas. (1986). *The healer within: The new medicine of mind and body*. New York: Dutton.

*Pelletier, Kenneth R. (1992). *Mind as healer, mind as slayer: A holistic approach to preventing stress disorders*. New York: Delta/Seymour Lawrence.

*Siebert, Al. (1996). *The survivor personality*. New York: Berkley Publishing Group.

*Siegel, Bernie S. (1986). *Love, medicine, & miracles*. New York: Harper & Row.

Tamparo, Carol D., & Lindh, Wilburta. (2008). The therapeutic response to stressed and anxious clients. In *Therapeutic communication for health care* (3rd ed., pp. 102–123). Clifton Park, NY: Delmar, Cengage Learning.

Weil, Andrew. (2006). *8 weeks to optimum health: A proven program for taking full advantage of your body's natural healing power*. New York: Knopf.

Weil, Andrew. (2008). *Spontaneous healing*. London: Sphere.

> **Note:** Appendix C lists resources and organizations related to holistic health care and specific disorders.

## REVIEW AND SELF-CHECK

1. Compare the meanings of *placebo* and *placebo effect* as used in orthodox health care and as used in holistic health care.

2. What is the effect of extreme emotional states on the immune system?

3. Name one or more differences between *curing* and *healing*.

4. List six factors that influence healing, according to a holistic view of health care.

5. Explain the importance of love to the healing process.

6. Explain the importance of intention (a) of the patient and (b) of the health care provider.

7. List five differences between orthodox and holistic health care.

8. Explain why stress management is important to health.

9. Name two ways a health care provider can contribute to a patient's healing process.

## ASSIGNMENTS

1. Participate in a class discussion of one or more of the following statements:
   - Love, including self-love, is essential to health and well-being.
   - Harmony among body, mind, emotions, and spirit is essential to health and well-being.
   - Life choices can increase the probability of illness.
   - Life choices can increase the probability of an accident.
   - Life choices can promote health and well-being.

2. List stressors in your life situation (include your various roles as student, health care provider, family member).

3. Beside each stressor listed in Assignment 2, indicate with a checkmark those stressors that could be eliminated by a relatively minor life change. (Example: getting up 15 minutes earlier in order to prepare for the day in a leisurely manner.)

4. Review the list and checkmarks, then select one stressor to eliminate; state a specific life change you will make, beginning not later than tomorrow.

5. The next time you encounter a difficult situation involving a patient (or co-worker, teacher, friend, family member), consciously project positive feelings for that person. Continue to think and feel positively as you deal with the situation. Afterward, when you are no longer in that person's presence, consider the following questions:
   a. What was the effect on you of your positive thinking? Were you calmer, less angry than you might have been? What was your physical condition—relaxed or uptight?
   b. What was the effect on the other person? Was there an improvement in attitude or behavior as you projected positive feelings?

6. Your classmate comments, "That love stuff is stupid. It's all I can do to complete my assignment. I don't have time to go around feeling love for my patients." How would you respond?

7. Drawing on your personal experience (relatives, friends, acquaintances) and your clinical experience, list examples of people who:

   a. Recovered from a life-threatening illness, contrary to the expectation of their physicians.

   b. Recovered from a serious illness through medical intervention, such as surgery, only to develop symptoms of another serious illness within a year.

8. Refer to one example in Assignment 7a and consider: What factors may have contributed to recovery? What traits characterize that person?

9. Refer to one example in Assignment 7b and consider: What traits characterize that individual?

# UNIT 26

# Broadening Your View of Health Care

## OBJECTIVES

Upon completion of this unit, you should be able to:

- Compare the behavior of a legitimate health care provider and one whose practice and/or qualifications are questionable.
- List two steps for evaluating a health care provider.
- Explain the primary characteristic of a holistic approach to health care.
- State the focus of psychoneuroimmunology and energy medicine.
- State one characteristic of osteopathy, chiropractic therapy, psychotherapy, homeopathy, traditional Chinese medicine, and Ayurvedic medicine.
- Name a complementary therapy that influences energy flow through the body.
- Name three therapies that use specific points to stimulate energy flow and relieve energy blockage.
- Name five effects of therapeutic massage.
- State two responsibilities of a health care provider to someone who asks advice about a complementary therapy.

## KEY TERMS

| | | |
|---|---|---|
| Dosha | Pitta | Vata |
| Holism | Potentiation | Yang |
| Invasive | Prana | Yin |
| Kapha | Subluxation | |

As pointed out in previous units, numerous changes are occurring in medical practice and the delivery of health care. Some of these changes affect the roles and responsibilities of health care providers. Many people are using complementary therapies to assist in stress reduction or to alleviate a specific health problem. Unit 26 is designed to help you learn about legitimate complementary therapies, identify some of the changes occurring within orthodox medicine, and know the characteristic features of selected complementary therapies.

## WHAT IS LEGITIMATE THERAPY?

A legitimate health care provider does not make false promises (Figure 26-1). A legitimate health care provider employs appropriate therapies and encourages each patient, even in the presence of serious illness, to maintain hope and a positive attitude. On the other hand, one should be suspicious if practitioners:

1. *Promise* a "cure."
2. Claim to have a *secret method* not available to other practitioners.
3. Demand a large payment "up front."
4. Become defensive or evasive about their qualifications.

Recognizing unrealistic claims of curative power is the first line of defense in protecting oneself from a fake healer. The second line of defense is determining the qualifications of the practitioner.

### Education and Credentials

Many roles in health care services require formal education. Qualified *professional* practitioners display in their offices at least two college or university degrees and a license from the state or a certificate from a recognized professional organization. Qualified practitioners of a complementary therapy also have documentation. Educational programs that prepare a specific type of practitioner issue a certificate or diploma to those who successfully complete the program of study. In some states, certain complementary practitioners must be licensed by the state.

**FIGURE 26-1** The patent medicine salesmen of the past were salesmen—not healers. *Delmar/Cengage Learning*

If such documentation is not displayed, ask to see written evidence of a practitioner's qualifications. A potential client has the right to know the qualifications of a practitioner, especially when a fee is involved. If questions regarding licensure, certification, or educational preparation make the practitioner defensive, evasive, or even uncomfortable, seek help elsewhere.

**Psychic and Energy Healing**

A field that does not require educational preparation and licensure is psychic healing. Dr. Shealy and Dr. Elmer Green at the Menninger Institute have studied psychic healers, such as Olga Worrall. They were able to demonstrate in a scientifically controlled experiment that Mrs. Worrall could affect another person by what she called "sending energy." Actual changes in body structure or function resulting from "energy transfer" from one person to another have now been demonstrated, but the *how* and *why* are not fully understood. The Reverend Rosalyn Bruyere is an intuitive healer who has been the subject of research studies at the University of California, Los Angeles (UCLA). Her ability to facilitate healing has earned her an international reputation. Rev. Bruyere helps other healers extend their skills through personal instruction and workshops. Gifted healers are relatively rare, and most are quite spiritual. Believing that their power to influence healing is a divine gift, they use that gift with humility, love, and compassion to benefit others. Some healers do not charge a fee, but accept contributions to a church or charitable organization that sponsors their work.

**Implications for Health Care Providers**

As a health care provider, you may be asked for a recommendation or opinion about an alternative therapy or a particular practitioner. Exercise caution in responding to such a request. Your best and safest approach is to help that person obtain the information needed for (1) evaluating the proposed therapy or practitioner, and then (2) making his or her own decision. Do not make such a decision for someone else. Instead, point out the educational, licensure, or certification requirements for the therapy being considered. You should also know what constitutes a legitimate title. Anyone may call themselves "counselor," "therapist," or "healer." But the terms *licensed* and *certified* can be used legally only if the practitioner has been granted that title by the state, an educational program, or a professional association.

Each person who considers the services of a nonmedical therapist has a responsibility to evaluate the qualifications of the practitioner, then make a *conscious decision* based on information about that specific therapy and that particular practitioner. After a reasonable trial period, another *conscious decision*—to continue or not continue—should be based on whether or not the therapy is beneficial. The need for careful evaluation of a therapy and provider is less critical if the therapy is offered through a holistic health center headed by a physician or other health-related *professional* practitioner. The employing agency has a responsibility to check credentials and determine if the practitioner is competent.

## HOLISTIC MEDICINE

Changes in health care during the past two or three decades include changes in medical practice and roles. Health care was once the sole domain of the medical doctor and the dentist, but numerous other professional practitioners now provide health care. The growth in holistic medicine has contributed to greater involvement of nonphysicians (psychologists, counselors, nutritionists, and various other practitioners) in health care, with increasing emphasis on responsibility of the patient to participate in decisions regarding his or her health care program.

A holistic approach to healing requires that the patient's mental, emotional, and spiritual aspects be considered, in addition to the physical functions that are the focus of orthodox medical practice. Further, the patient's total life situation is considered, with special attention to stress factors and to any dysfunctional (not functioning effectively) attitudes and beliefs. Treatment includes whatever orthodox medical interventions are indicated, plus measures to decrease the effects of stress and to correct any dysfunctional attributes that have been identified. The total treatment plan may include one or more complementary therapies provided by nonmedical practitioners.

Box 26-1 lists some characteristics that may be considered a theoretical foundation for holistic health care. Note that the patient's willingness to assume responsibility for his or her health is viewed as essential to healing. This *involvement of the patient in decision making* is difficult for many allopathic physicians, who are accustomed to a *dominant* role in the doctor/patient relationship. The holistic physician, however, is comfortable in a *cooperative* doctor/patient relationship.

---

### BOX 26-1

### Theoretical Basis for Holistic Health Care

- Every illness or physical malfunction is complex and has multiple causation.
- Illness is the result of mental, emotional, physical, attitudinal, and spiritual stress, in addition to environmental, chemical, electrical, and cosmic forces.
- Spiritual stress arises from fear, anger, guilt, frustration, anxiety, and depression.
- A healthy attitude and healthful habits are essential to a healthy body.
- Unhealthy habits represent a deficiency in love, wisdom, reason, and will.
- Resistance to disease is the result of heredity, maternal habits and nutrition, and lifetime exposure to various environmental influences.
- Treatment must be directed toward healing emotions and spirit, in addition to treatment of physical symptoms.
- Thoughts, feelings, and beliefs of the patient are tools that can rebuild the body.
- The patient is actively involved in decisions: treatment, changes in lifestyle, changes in beliefs and attitudes.
- The patient is responsible for the healing process.
- Denial blocks the healing process.
- The therapist's task is to facilitate the healing process.

*Source:* Based on C. Norman Shealy & Carolyn M. Myss, 1993, The Creation of Health: The Emotional, Psychological, and Spiritual Responses That Promote Health and Healing *(Chapters 1 and 2), Walpole, NH: Stillpoint.*

In emphasizing the spiritual aspects of illness and health, Dr. Shealy is not speaking of religion, but rather of the subtle aspects of *being human,* such as feelings, beliefs, will, intuition, compassion and tolerance for other beings, and beliefs regarding the cosmos and/or the divine. Dr. Shealy believes that science and technology, which currently characterize the health care system, must begin to encompass spirit in order to humanize the practice of medicine. When the delivery of health care services does embrace these holistic concepts, the roles of all health care providers are affected. There is greater emphasis on *therapeutic interaction* as patient care procedures are performed. Box 26-2 lists some characteristics of the future health care system, as perceived by Dr. Shealy.

The belief that patients must assume greater responsibility for their health is reflected in the current activities of former U.S. Surgeon General Everett Koop. As Surgeon General, Dr. Koop represented allopathic medicine. During 1996, he began a project to develop a medical video series for the public. Explaining the need for this series, Dr. Koop stated that the best way for a patient to face a medical condition is to *take responsibility and become knowledgeable.* Only two or three decades ago doctors considered information about diseases to be their exclusive domain! This example of greater openness of allopathic medicine to patient involvement is encouraging to proponents of the holistic approach.

A startling wake-up call to orthodox medicine was delivered when a special article of *The New England Journal of Medicine* was printed in the January 1993 issue. A group of health professionals associated with several medical schools and major hospitals conducted a survey during 1990 to determine the extent to which the American public was using unconventional therapies. The findings clearly indicated that the American public was seeking and using numerous unconventional therapies, either in conjunction with medical care or as an alternative. Some of the major findings of this study include:

- *One in three* U.S. adults used an unconventional therapy in 1990.
- Visits to providers of unconventional therapies *exceeded* the number of visits to primary-care medical doctors nationally.
- Out-of-pocket expenditures for unconventional therapies were comparable to out-of-pocket expenditures for all hospitalizations.
- About one out of every four Americans under the care of a medical doctor for a *serious health problem* also used an unconventional therapy.
- Of unconventional therapy encounters, 7 out of 10 *occurred without the knowledge of the medical doctor.*

This article in a prestigious medical journal received much attention in the medical community and was brought to the attention of the public by articles in the mass media. Subsequently, a number of significant changes began to occur. Some medical practices and health care agencies broadened their scope to include one or more complementary therapies as an option for patients. The U.S. Congress directed the National Institutes of Health to establish an Office of Alternative Medicine. Two journals of alternative medicine were established. Numerous books by physicians and other professionals with a holistic perspective have been published. Newsletters that emphasize the holistic approach and/or the use of natural remedies are now available.

The remainder of this unit is devoted to preparing you to understand and accept some of these changes: several emerging areas in medicine, some nonmedical systems of therapy, and

> **BOX 26-2**
>
> **Characteristics of a Holistic Health Care System**
>
> - Patient care is provided by a team.
> - The *minimum* team consists of a physician (M.D. or D.O.), nurse, physical therapist, psychotherapist, and the *patient*.
> - Team members consciously develop their intuitive skills as an aid to identify each patient's needs.
> - Spinal manipulation and massage may be an integral part of the treatment plan.
> - Acupuncture and electromagnetic forms of therapy may be used, in association with music and sound, to balance the patient's energy system.
> - The patient is taught the elements of a healthy lifestyle, including principles of good nutrition.
> - The use of relaxation techniques is considered an essential part of a healthful lifestyle.
> - An exercise program is an essential part of the patient's healthy lifestyle.
> - Naturopathic concepts and homeopathic remedies are incorporated into medical practice.
> - Spiritual healing is encouraged to provide the framework for physical, chemical, emotional, and behavior therapies.
> - Various forms of energy therapy are accepted.
> - Holistic health education is part of the school curriculum, beginning in kindergarten.
> - Parents attend classes to improve parenting skills and learn to incorporate holistic health practices into family living.
> - Patients are expected to confront their negative beliefs and attitudes and change unhealthy habits.
>
> Source: Based on C. Norman Shealy & Carolyn M. Myss, 1993, The Creation of Health: The Emotional, Psychological, and Spiritual Responses That Promote Health and Healing *(Chapter 2)*, Walpole, NH: Stillpoint.

specific therapeutic techniques. Some were among the "unconventional therapies" included in the 1990 survey; all would be included, or at least accepted as having potential value, in a holistic health care system today.

## PSYCHONEUROIMMUNOLOGY

It has long been accepted in conventional medicine that emotional factors may affect various body functions, even to the point of changing body structure, as in an ulcer. There is now compelling evidence that mental/emotional states affect the immune system. The "mind/body connection" is being studied extensively by researchers such as Dr. Pelletier, Dr. Joan Borysenko, and her husband, Dr. Myrin Borysenko, an immunologist. This area of research is called psychoneuroimmunology (PNI), an interdisciplinary field involving such disciplines as psychology, biophysics, biophysiology, and medicine. Dr. Shealy considers PNI to be "one of the most exciting and innovative fields today." PNI includes the study of mental factors (i.e., attitudes, thoughts, beliefs) and stress on the immune system. PNI research is also identifying neurochemicals that are released in association with anger, hostility, guilt, and other negative emotional states.

Dr. Elliott Dacher believes that PNI research is demonstrating the capacity of individuals for self-healing. Attaining competence in self-healing requires learning and using several techniques for regulating and directing one's life. Two essential components of self-healing are mindfulness and self-regulation. Mindfulness, achieved through meditative practices, may lead to insight and creativity, which in turn may lead to self-regulation and healing. Dr. Dacher has incorporated training in these powerful techniques in his medical practice; as a result, his patients learn how to participate in their own healing. Dr. Dacher also conducts workshops to teach these techniques to groups, especially health care providers, and has published a text/workbook for helping people learn mindfulness and self-regulation through independent study and practice.

## ENERGY MEDICINE

Dr. Elmer Green, the first president of the International Society for the Study of Subtle Energies and Energy Medicine (ISSSEEM), says that in 1964 he discussed with a prominent psychiatrist the kind of scientific program presented 27 years later at ISSSEEM's 1991 conference. The psychiatrist, a leading researcher in psychiatry and mental health, believed that the scientific world would not be ready to accept the mind/body relationship before the year 2000.

The pioneers of holistic healing, many of whom are quoted in this book, have been far more influential than that psychiatrist expected. Research related to energy medicine is providing a new and different knowledge base for study of the body and for developing energy-based therapies. The development of techniques and instruments sensitive enough to measure the body's "subtle energies" has stimulated interest among many researchers. The energy pathways, or meridians, of the body have been mapped, thereby scientifically validating their existence. The electromagnetic fields of the body are being studied. Knowledge that is just beginning to accumulate may well be the basis for new therapies involving body energies. Energy medicine is a new frontier in medicine; the discoveries that emerge will very likely have a profound effect on health care and therapeutic procedures.

## OSTEOPATHY

The first school of osteopathic medicine was established in Missouri in 1892. Originally, osteopathy was fiercely opposed by the medical establishment but was widely accepted by the public. The basic theoretical foundation for osteopathic practice is that musculoskeletal disorders, especially any changes in the vertebral column, interfere with circulation of blood, flow of body energies, and other functions essential to good health. Osteopathic technique originally consisted of manipulations to relieve tension around the spinal column. The educational preparation of osteopaths was gradually extended until it became as lengthy as medical education, the primary difference being instruction in manipulation of the spine as a therapeutic tool. Eventually, osteopaths were accepted by teaching hospitals for specialization in such areas as surgery and obstetrics. Most general hospitals now grant staff privileges to osteopaths. In addition, there are 180 osteopathic hospitals in the United States; some general hospitals have an osteopathic wing. There are now 15 colleges of osteopathic medicine. All states and Canada have licensure requirements for osteopaths. The osteopathic physician uses the legal title "D.O." (doctor of osteopathy) instead of "M.D." (doctor of medicine).

## CHIROPRACTIC

The basic theory underlying the practice of chiropractic is that any **subluxation** of a vertebra creates pressure on one or more nerves where they emerge from the spine. A subluxation may involve rotation of a vertebra to the right or left or dislocation of the vertebra in a posterior or anterior direction. This pressure interferes with proper function of the nerve, which then affects the functioning of the body part served by that nerve. The purpose of a chiropractic treatment, then, is to remove pressure from the nerve by restoring each vertebra to its proper alignment. A chiropractor uses X-ray films, various tests of body movement and muscle strength, measurements (e.g., length of the legs, level of the hips, level of the shoulders), and palpation to locate problem areas.

A subluxation may result from normal daily activities. Sitting for long periods of time, poor posture, and poor body mechanics when bending or lifting have an adverse effect on spinal alignment. Any fall, a car accident, even a sudden stop, can result in a subluxation or damage to the soft tissues surrounding the spine. The most frequent symptoms are low back pain, headache, pain in the temporomandibular joint (TMJ), and pain that radiates down a leg or down one arm. The injury known as whiplash involves the muscles of the neck and shoulders; once the swelling and pain of whiplash have subsided, subluxation of one or more cervical vertebrae may be found.

The underlying philosophy of chiropractic is that correction of any problem that interferes with nervous system functioning enables the body to heal itself. Chiropractic treatment consists of adjustments at specific points to correct subluxations and relieve nerve pressure, plus a number of other techniques as needed by the individual patient: traction, cold, heat, massage, acupressure, ultrasound, or electromagnetic stimulation. As muscle spasm diminishes and spinal alignment improves, the chiropractor may recommend exercises to strengthen the affected area or to improve posture. Many chiropractors do a nutritional analysis and recommend dietary changes. Chiropractors do not recommend either prescription or over-the-counter (OTC) drugs because of the risk of side effects. Many chiropractors do recommend herbal or homeopathic remedies, especially for management of pain during the acute phase.

Chiropractic education is a four-year postbaccalaureate program, so it is equal in length of time to medical and osteopathic education. Licensure, required in every state, is based on a National Board Examination. Some states permit chiropractors to use acupuncture; other states limit acupuncture to medical practitioners. The legal title for a chiropractor is D.C. (doctor of chiropractic).

## NATUROPATHY

Naturopathy is a healing system that evolved from the popular spas of Germany and Austria, which used water, fresh air, sunshine, and exercise to promote health and healing. Naturopathy was introduced into the United States around 1890 and was widely practiced until the 1930s, with emphasis on nutrition added to the other natural approaches to therapy. At that time, new drugs and advances in surgical techniques overshadowed naturopathy and became the predominant forms of health care for several decades. In the 1960s there was a resurgence of interest in naturopathy, and it is now widely practiced.

The leading schools of naturopathy in the United States are Bastyr College, located in Seattle, Washington, and National College of Naturopathic Medicine, in Portland, Oregon.

The doctorate of naturopathic medicine is a four-year graduate program. Bastyr College also offers a master of science degree in nutrition and acupuncture, a bachelor of science degree in natural health sciences, and certificates in traditional Chinese herbal medicine and midwifery. Graduates of a naturopathic school use the title doctor of naturopathy (N.D.).

The basic belief of naturopathy is that the body has "vital force," the power to heal itself. The naturopathic physician searches for causes of a client's health problem and develops a plan for stimulating the body's own vital force and restoring a state of homeostasis, or balance. Diagnosis includes assessment of the client's physical condition, emotional status, and lifestyle. The vital force can be weakened by unhealthful diet, lack of exercise, inadequate rest and sleep, stress, emotional issues, negative attitudes, and exposure to pollutants. When the vital force has been weakened, the individual is susceptible to infectious agents and allergens. Symptoms such as fever are indications that the body is attempting to heal itself; therefore, symptoms should not be suppressed. Instead, the body should be supported in its self-healing effort.

Naturopathy uses two different approaches. Cleansing the body of toxic buildup may require a period of fasting, a juice fast, detox teas or foods, and perhaps a special procedure, such as a liver flush. Following the cleansing procedures, the focus is on strengthening the vital force with a nutritional diet, supplements as indicated, plus healing practices such as breathing exercises, relaxation techniques, and physical exercise (Figures 26-2 and 26-3). The naturopathic physician performs therapeutic interventions such as acupressure and is qualified to prescribe both herbal and homeopathic remedies. In some states, naturopathic physicians may qualify to perform acupuncture. Naturopathic physicians often refer clients for massage therapy, reflexology, chiropractic adjustments, or to a class for learning yoga, meditation, or movement therapy. If the patient's condition indicates a need for a pharmaceutical drug or surgery, the naturopathic physician would refer the patient to an allopathic physician.

## PSYCHOTHERAPY/COUNSELING

The area of practice known as psychotherapy originated with the work of Freud, beginning around 1880. Freud's concern with the mind—a radical new approach in medicine—eventually resulted in a new medical specialty, psychiatry. Initially, the specific concern of psychiatry was mental illness. But during the last 40 years the *human potential movement* emerged. People became aware that developing their full potential was hindered by such problems as poor adjustment, lack of assertiveness, inability to cope with life problems, poor interpersonal skills, and addiction. The demand for services to help people deal more effectively with their life situations led to rapid growth of the mental health field.

As a result of this expansion, mental health ceased to be the domain of the psychiatrist. Professional counseling emerged as a field of practice, related to but different from psychiatric practice. Most psychotherapists work with clients who are not mentally ill, but need help in learning to cope with some type of life problem: to release suppressed emotions, correct faulty thought patterns, improve interpersonal skills, or modify the dynamics within a family or work setting.

Mental health is now an interdisciplinary field involving psychologists, social workers, counselors, ministers, recreation therapists, occupational therapists, music therapists, and art therapists. The educational preparation varies from about six years (for a master's degree) to eight or more years (for a doctorate) in such fields as psychology, social work, pastoral counseling, family therapy, and counseling. Titles of professional workers in the field include licensed clinical psychologist, licensed clinical social worker (LCSW), licensed marriage and

**FIGURE 26-2** Herbs are potent natural substances with medicinal properties. *Delmar/Cengage Learning*

family therapist (LMFT), certified rehabilitation counselor (CRC), and certified addiction counselor (CAC). If a practitioner uses a term such as "licensed counselor" or "certified counselor" rather than one of the above legal titles, it would be wise to ask: (1) Licensed (or certified) by whom? and (2) What is the special area of licensure (or certification)? Unless a license was issued by the state or a certificate was issued by an educational program or professional association, the term *counselor* is meaningless.

**FIGURE 26-3** Many people use natural substances and practices as an alternative to traditional health care. *Delmar/Cengage Learning*

## HOMEOPATHY

Homeopathy was developed as a therapeutic system by Samuel Hahnemann, a German physician who had become dissatisfied with medical practices of the early 1800s. The basic principle of homeopathy is that "like cures like." For example, the tears and runny nose of a new cold are like the tears and runny nose produced by close contact with raw onions. Therefore, allium (Latin for "onion") in *very small* doses could be used to treat a cold. Over a period of many years, Dr. Hahnemann used volunteers to determine the effects of a large amount of many substances—plant, mineral, and animal. He then matched these effects to the symptoms of various disorders and experimented to find the dilution (i.e., the minimal amount) of that substance that would control those specific symptoms. Determining the effects of a specific substance is known as a "proving." After many years of research and clinical trials, Dr. Hahnemann's use of homeopathic remedies was so effective that he developed a large following of patients and physicians throughout Europe.

Homeopathy has been practiced in Europe and India for over 200 years. In England, there are two levels of homeopathic medical practice. At one level, the homeopathic physician has been trained in diagnosis and treatment according to the methods of Dr. Hahnemann and his followers. Another level of homeopathic physician has completed orthodox medical training, then specialized in homeopathy. Homeopathic hospitals were included in the British National Health Service when it was established in 1947. The royal family of Great Britain has used homeopathic physicians for several generations.

Homeopathic remedies are prepared according to very precise measurements and procedures. The original solution, usually an alcoholic extract, is diluted repeatedly to produce the dilution used as a remedy. *The more dilute a remedy is, the more powerful its effects.* This is known as **potentiation.** The extreme dilution of homeopathics is the basis for rejection of homeopathy by many allopathic physicians. Extreme dilutions are the basis for desensitization procedures used by allopathic physicians to treat allergies! The manufacture of homeopathics is regulated by the Food and Drug Administration. The *Homeopathic Pharmacopoeia of the United States* is the official source of detailed information about every homeopathic medication. Homeopathics are available without a prescription. Consultation with a homeopathic physician is the preferred approach to using homeopathics but is difficult to obtain in many communities.

Homeopathy was popular in the United States during the 1800s. In 1900, there were 22 homeopathic colleges and 56 homeopathic hospitals. There were also homeopathic sanitariums, mental asylums, and children's hospitals. Increasing opposition from conventional medicine during the early 1900s led to the decline of homeopathy; the last homeopathic college closed in 1930 (Campbell, 1996). Currently, there is renewed interest in homeopathy in the United States. The National Center for Homeopathy teaches postgraduate courses for physicians, so acceptance and use of homeopathy is slowly spreading throughout the medical community. The National Center for Homeopathy also offers workshops for anyone interested in learning about homeopathy, either for personal and family use or as the introductory phase of a career path. Numerous advanced workshops are required to obtain credentials as a homeopathic practitioner. Graduate-level workshops are offered for health professionals who wish to include homeopathy in their health care practices.

Homeopathy has already gained a large following among those who wish to take responsibility for their own health. Many people prefer homeopathy because they have found it effective and because of its safety, a notable contrast to the risk of side effects from many pharmaceuticals. Most health food stores carry a variety of homeopathics, and some pharmacies now have a homeopathic section.

Homeopathy differs from conventional medicine in many respects. In homeopathic medicine, the totality of symptoms is considered before selecting an appropriate medicine. The individuality of the patient is important, and the individual characteristics of each illness are considered in detail. No one symptom determines the treatment; rather, the complex of symptoms presented indicates which homeopathic remedy to pursue. Table 26-1 shows how each aspect of a headache indicates one or more homeopathic remedies, but the total picture presented by the patient's symptoms would determine the specific remedy of choice. Usually, a remedy is used every three to four hours, but only as long as symptoms are present. Sometimes, one or two doses clear up all symptoms. If the patient has not recovered after two days, symptoms are reviewed and another remedy is started, based on the total picture at that time. Table 26-1 illustrates an important point: not all headaches (or sore throats, coughs, or colds) are the same; each illness is considered in regard to many specific factors before selecting a homeopathic remedy.

Administration of a homeopathic remedy is different from that of pharmaceuticals. A homeopathic remedy should be taken at least 20 minutes before eating or 30 minutes after eating or drinking. Homeopathics come in the form of small globules, tablets, and liquids. The *globules or tablets must not be touched; the desired number should be poured into the lid or dispenser top of the vial, then dropped under the tongue.* They are very soluble, so absorption usually requires a minute or less. Liquids are dispensed in a dropper bottle; the drops should be placed on the tongue and left there until absorbed.

The practice of homeopathic medicine is regulated by the states. Most states allow the use of homeopathy by licensed health care professionals: medical doctors (M.D.), osteopaths (D.O.), naturopaths (N.D.), dentists (D.D.M. and D.D.S.), chiropractors (D.C.), and veterinarians (D.V.M.). Interestingly, because homeopathic remedies are inexpensive, safe, and easy to use,

## TABLE 26-1

### Matching Symptoms to Homeopathic Remedies: Headache

| | SYMPTOMS | PREFERRED HOMEOPATHIC REMEDY* |
|---|---|---|
| PAIN: | Intense, throbbing | Belladonna, Sanguinaria |
| | Sharp, knifelike | Sanguinaria |
| | Stinging, burning | Spigelia |
| | Band around the head | Gelsemium |
| | Steady ache | Bryonia |
| ONSET: | Sudden | Belladonna |
| | In morning | Bryonia, Nux vomica |
| | In back of head | Gelsemium, Sanguinaria |
| END: | Sudden | Belladonna |
| FOCUS: | Forehead | *Belladonna,* Bryonia, Pulsatilla |
| | Right eye | Sanguinaria |
| | Right side of head | Belladonna, Gelsemium, *Sanguinaria* |
| | Left eye | *Bryonia* |
| | Left side of head | Belladonna, Spigelia |
| | Changes frequently | Belladonna, Pulsatilla, Sanguinaria |
| OTHER: | Hands and feet cold | Belladonna |
| | Face flushed, hot | Belladonna |
| | Recurrent pattern | Sanguinaria |
| | Visual disturbances | Gelsemium |
| | Fatigue, looks tired | Gelsemium |
| | Nausea | Nux vomica |
| | Sensitive to light | Belladonna |
| | Sensitive to noise | Belladonna, Spigelia |
| | Sensitive to movement | Belladonna, *Bryonia,* Nux vomica, Sanguinaria, Spigelia |
| | Sensitive to touch | Belladonna |
| | Sensitive to strong smells | Belladonna |
| | Irritable | Bryonia, Nux vomica |
| | Wants to be left alone | Bryonia, Gelsemium |
| | Wants to be comforted | Pulsatilla |
| MADE WORSE BY: | Warmth or cold | Spigelia |
| | Motion | Belladonna, *Bryonia,* Nux vomica, Gelsemium, Sanguinaria, Spigelia |
| | Going down steps | *Belladonna* |
| | Walking briskly | Pulsatilla |
| | Blowing nose | Pulsatilla |
| MADE BETTER BY: | Firm pressure | Belladonna, Bryonia, Pulsatilla, Sanguinaria |
| | Sitting | *Belladonna* |
| | Being up and about | Nux vomica |
| | Gentle motion | Pulsatilla |
| | Walking slowly in open air | Pulsatilla |

*Italics indicate preferred remedy for that symptom.
*Source:* Adapted from Cummings, Stephen & Ullman, Dana. (2004) *Everybody's Guide to Homeopathic Medicines.* New York: Penguin.

a layperson can learn to select appropriate medications for many common illnesses. Several hours of study and one or more good references can be used to cope with numerous health problems. The ideal, for anyone who wishes to use homeopathy personally or within the family, is to attend a workshop. Homeopathy is an inexpensive therapy, but its effectiveness depends upon *selection of the best remedy* for a specific health problem and *correct use* of homeopathic substances. Obviously, any acute illness or an illness that does not respond to home treatment should be evaluated by a licensed health practitioner.

## TRADITIONAL CHINESE MEDICINE

Traditional Chinese medicine (TCM), which is becoming popular in the United States, differs from Western medicine in many ways. The licensure designation for the U.S. practitioner is doctor of oriental medicine (O.M.D.). Many practitioners are trained in both oriental medicine and Western medicine and integrate these two systems into their practice. TCM, the prevalent form of medicine throughout Asia, uses a wide range of remedies, with herbalism being the predominant therapy. The earliest written records of the medicinal uses of herbs are from China and date from the second century; the first encyclopedia of herbal remedies is also Chinese, dating from the sixteenth century (Woodham & Black, 1997). In China, the larger hospitals have two sections, one for TCM and the other for Western medicine; patients choose the type of care they wish to receive. TCM is based on the concepts of **holism** (i.e., wholeness) and balance of **yin** and **yang** (Figure 26-4). The basis of yin/yang theory is that everything is either yin or yang and is balanced by its polar opposite. Yin embodies feminine characteristics: the moon, night, passivity, coldness, blood, and body fluids. Yang is masculine: the sun, day, activity, heat, energy, growth, and metabolism. Both yin and yang embody some degree of the other; the ideal is perfect balance, but the relationship is flexible. Perfect balance leads to health, wholeness, and harmony.

A problem in one part of the body affects the whole, so treatment must restore the body to a state of wholeness. The perfect balance of yin and yang is disturbed when either yin or yang becomes excessive; each organ is either yin or yang. Excessive yang is indicated by acute pain, spasms, and headaches; excessive yin is indicated by coolness, dull aches and pains, and fatigue. Illness is viewed as evidence that a state of imbalance exists, so treatment is aimed at restoring balance.

The TCM practitioner looks for a pattern of symptoms, rather than for the symptoms of a specific diagnosis. Eight patterns of disharmony provide the framework for classifying symptoms and identifying the therapy needed to restore balance and wholeness. Diagnosis and treatment are based on characteristics of the five elements: wood, fire, earth, metal, and

**FIGURE 26-4** Chinese medicine and philosophy emphasize unity and harmony among parts of the whole. *Delmar/Cengage Learning*

water. Each element has specific yin and yang organs, one of the seasons, specific tastes, and emotional states. All of the characteristics of a specific element support each other, so disease of a specific organ is treated in accordance with that organ's classification: either yin or yang and a specific element. It is apparent from this brief description that diagnosis and treatment in TCM differ greatly from those in Western medicine. For the U.S. public, the best-known aspect of Chinese medicine is acupuncture, a technique that is at least 5,000 years old.

Acupuncture is based on the theory that life energy, known as Ch'i, flows through channels located throughout the body. Twelve major channels, known as meridians, are associated with specific internal organs. There are numerous branches and connections, so that the cells in every portion of the body receive this flow of energy. Any blockage in the flow of energy results in disease until such blockage is removed or clears up spontaneously. Each meridian has its own pulse, which is different from the arterial pulses of the circulatory system. The acupuncturist uses these 12 pulses to locate any blockage in energy flow. The location of the blockage determines what organ or body part is affected.

Modern researchers are now using sensitive electronic equipment to trace these energy pathways and locate the points of energy concentration, thus using scientific methodology to validate the underlying theory of acupuncture. Such research is a major focus of "energy medicine," an emerging specialty in medicine. The energy pathways and significant points located throughout the body provide the basis for a number of complementary therapies, such as Shiatsu, kinesiology, acupressure, trigger point therapy, and reflexology, some of which are discussed in this unit.

Acupuncture was relatively unknown in the United States until 1971, when an American surgeon reported to the American Medical Association his observations of acupuncture in China. At about the same time, an American journalist who was traveling in China developed appendicitis. His postoperative pain was controlled by acupuncture, rather than by drugs. His report of this experience, published in the *New York Times*, brought acupuncture to the attention of the American public. Although acupuncture had been an established medical specialty in France for about 25 years, the initial reaction of the medical community in the United States was unfavorable. In spite of that initial rejection of acupuncture, there is growing acceptance by the general public and by some members of the medical community.

## AYURVEDIC MEDICINE

Ayurveda has been practiced in India for several thousand years. *Ayurveda* is a Sanskrit word that means "science of life," and the focus of this approach to health care is on various factors that affect one's life: diet, **prana** (the breath), exercise, spiritual practices, and one's relationship to nature based on body type (**dosha**).

Doshas are three types of vital energy that exist throughout nature: **vata, pitta,** and **kapha.** Each dosha is a combination of two of the five elements: ether, air, fire, water, and earth. Each human body is primarily one type of dosha, but may also exhibit some characteristics of one or both of the other two doshas. In the human body, doshas are affected by foods, the time of day, seasons, emotional states at any given time, stress, and the elements of that specific dosha. *Prana* refers to life energy that is taken into the body through breathing and food.

Imbalance in the dosha or any blocks to the flow of prana result in a toxic condition and illness. Ayurvedic healing emphasizes detoxification of the body. A cleansing routine is followed by specific therapeutic modalities: strict dietary regimen that includes a prescribed eating schedule appropriate to the patient's dosha, herbs, and various approaches to improving the flow of prana, such as massage, yoga, meditation, and specific exercises. Therapy is designed to restore balance to the dosha and improve the flow of prana.

Ayurveda was introduced to the United States in 1984 by Dr. Deepak Chopra, who was born in New Delhi, India, but received his medical education in the United States. While practicing medicine as an endocrinologist in the Boston area, Dr. Chopra studied Transcendental Meditation under an Indian Yogi and became interested in Ayurvedic medicine. He went back to India to study health care practices there. Upon returning to the United States, he incorporated Ayurvedic principles into his medical practice. His first book, *Quantum Healing: Exploring the Frontiers of Mind/Body Medicine* (1989) proposed an integrated system of health care and quickly became a best seller. The principles of Ayurvedic medicine and health guidelines for vata, pitta, and kapha body types appealed to many people who were seeking a systematic approach to taking more responsibility for their own health and well-being. In *Quantum Healing*, Dr. Chopra also explained the health implications of quantum physics research: that *everything is energy vibrating at a specific frequency*. Those findings were compatible with the basic principles of Ayurvedic medicine and also provided the scientific basis for studying the role of energy in health and healing.

Needless to say, scientists and representatives of orthodox medicine were quick to challenge these new ideas, issuing warnings and derogatory critiques. But Dr. Chopra's popularity with the public steadily increased as he conducted workshops and seminars all over the United States. He has written numerous books, produced videotapes, and conducted seminars and workshops to teach about holistic healing. He established the Chopra Center for Well-Being in La Jolla, California, where he offers educational programs, and health care is available through the Ayurvedic clinic.

## COMPLEMENTARY THERAPIES

Many complementary therapies involve a hands-on technique (as in massage), the application of pressure at specific points (as in acupressure and reflexology), or influencing the flow of body energies (as in Healing Touch). Other therapeutic approaches in common usage include hypnotherapy; biofeedback; polarity therapy; movement therapies; and the use of color, light, and aromas for specific therapeutic benefits. Further information on these therapies is available in the references listed at the end of the unit. Some alternative practitioners use a variety of techniques, according to a patient's specific problem. Others specialize in one particular technique and use it exclusively. Some complementary therapies can be learned readily by a health care provider and used to enhance basic patient care. Some are useful to enhance a practitioner's own health and well-being. Some offer a career path, which would require training and certification in preparation for establishing a private practice as an alternative practitioner. A full explanation of all complementary therapies is beyond the scope of this textbook, but sources of information on education, licensure, and certification may be found in several references listed under "References and Suggested Readings." The remainder of this unit describes six popular therapies that are accepted by increasing numbers of physicians.

## HEALING TOUCH

Healing Touch is an energy-based system of therapy developed by Janet Mentgen, RN, who began practicing in 1980. The goal of Healing Touch is to facilitate self-healing by restoring harmony and balance in the body's energy system, as pictured in Figure 26-5. A clear energy

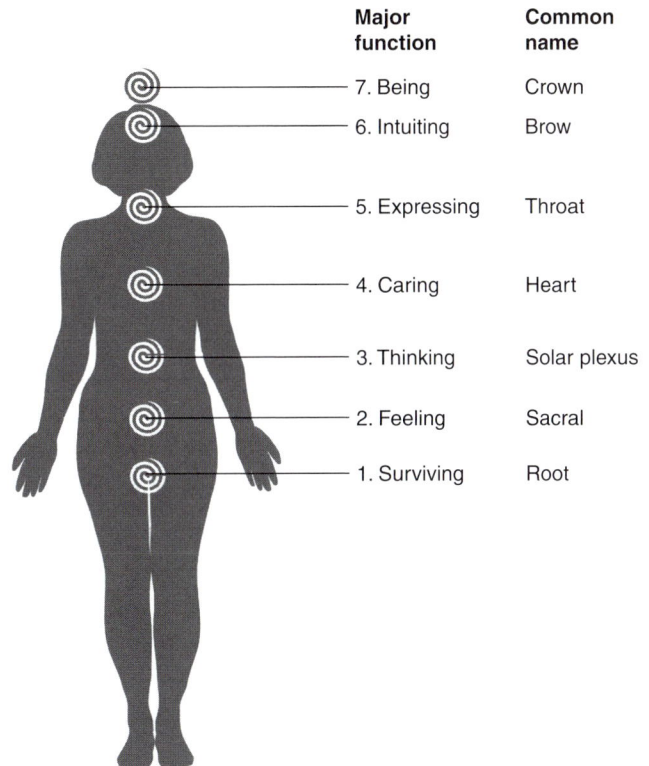

**FIGURE 26-5** Location of the seven major energy centers. *Source:* From Dorothea Hover-Cramer, 2002, *Healing Touch: A guidebook for practitioners* [2nd ed.], Clifton Park, NY: Delmar, Cengage Learning.

field and balanced flow of energy through the body have both relaxing and energizing effects. Healing Touch is effective in treatment of chronic illness, acute illness, and injury, often as an adjunct to allopathic medical care. Surgery patients benefit from receiving energy work either preoperatively or postoperatively; the ideal is to have energy work before surgery and as soon as possible after surgery. Healing Touch is now used extensively in all clinical areas of nursing and can be incorporated into the practice of health care providers who are in direct contact with patients. The procedures can also be learned by persons without a medical background who wish to develop their healing abilities.

Healing Touch is taught through five levels of weekend workshops. In Healing Touch Level 1, workshop participants learn the theoretical basis of energy healing, use the hands to assess a person's energy field, then practice and experience 10 to 12 different healing interventions with a partner. This workshop is a revelation for first-time participants. *Experiencing the power of energy work tends to convert even the most skeptical participant into a believer!*

Interventions learned in Healing Touch Level 1 are easily incorporated into patient care in hospitals and nursing homes; some can be used in a clinic, office, or home setting. All of the interventions can be learned by lay healers, and all can be used with friends and family members. Participants are encouraged to use one or more procedures daily for balancing and maintaining their own energy, either to maintain health and vitality or to facilitate healing.

In Healing Touch Level 2, students learn how to perform a full Healing Touch session: interviewing the client, assessing the client's energy field (Figure 26-6), and selecting one or more appropriate interventions to remove energy blocks and balance the flow of energy. Several interventions specific to the back are practiced and experienced. How to conclude

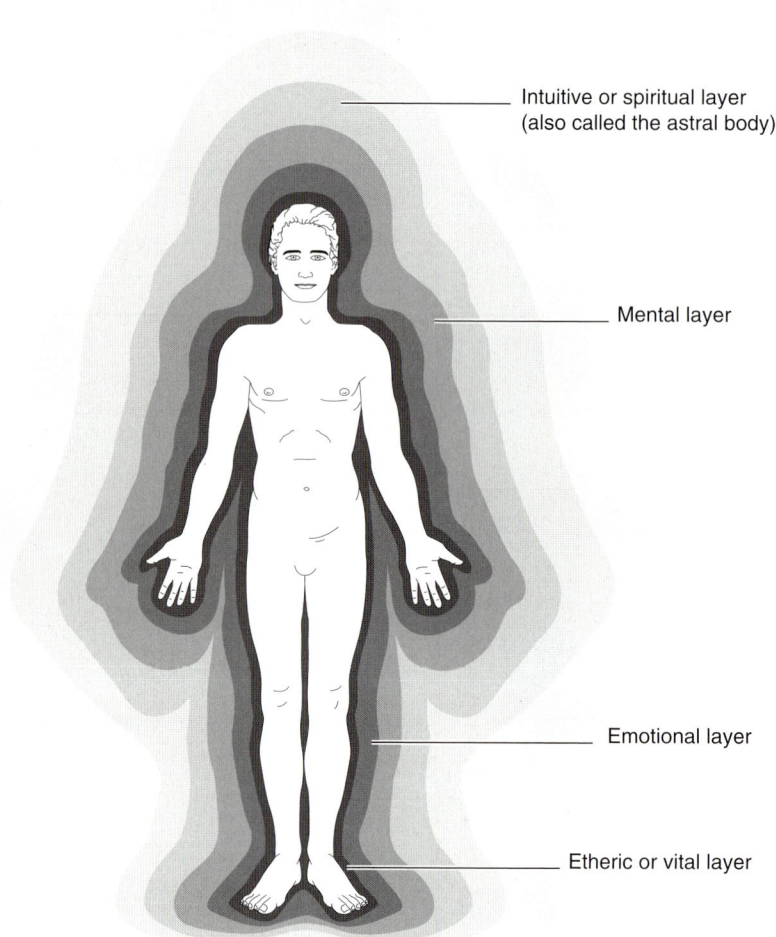

**FIGURE 26-6** Four major layers of the human energy field extending beyond the physical body. *Source:* From Dorothea Hover-Cramer, 2002, *Healing Touch: A guidebook for practitioners* [2nd ed.], Clifton Park, NY: Delmar, Cengage Learning.

a session includes: teaching the client a self-help technique, recommending a healthful lifestyle change, or referring the client to another health care provider for a specific type of problem. Healing Touch Level 3 involves advanced procedures related to the client's entire energy field, which extends out about 18 inches from the body. Serious students of Healing Touch repeat each of these workshops, learning more from each repetition. Serving as a workshop assistant after completing Level 3 also is a valuable learning experience.

Healing Touch Levels 4 and 5 are for students who wish to qualify for certification as a Healing Touch practitioner (CHTP). Healing Touch can be learned by attending weekend workshops. Many nurses find that Level 1 interventions provide them with additional tools for effective patient care. For lay healers, Healing Touch provides structure, specific techniques, and a systematic process for healing sessions.

## ACUPUNCTURE

A number of complementary therapies utilize specific points for stimulating energy flow or releasing a blockage. Acupuncture is an **invasive** procedure, in that the skin is penetrated, as shown in Figure 26-7; the theory is discussed in the section on traditional Chinese medicine.

**FIGURE 26-7** Acupuncture is used to treat many different conditions by correcting energy imbalances. The needles are left in place from 5 to 20 minutes. *Delmar/Cengage Learning*

Acupressure, Shiatsu, and reflexology utilize many of the same points as acupuncture, with the advantage of being noninvasive.

Acupuncture is a good example of new knowledge (new at least to U.S. physicians until the early 1970s) that was rejected because it conflicted with existing beliefs of the medical community. But acupuncture is widely practiced in other countries and is gaining acceptance in the United States. Dr. Shealy believes that acupuncture has great potential for relief of chronic pain. Others see it as a desirable alternative to the numerous risks of general anesthesia.

Many acupuncture practitioners in the United States went to Asia or England for training. Some medical centers in the United States now offer training in acupuncture for medical personnel. The Traditional Acupuncture Institute in Columbia, Maryland, offers a three-year course leading to the master of acupuncture degree. Many of the students and some faculty members are nurses.

Some states limit the practice of acupuncture to medical doctors; others license trained acupuncturists with or without a medical degree. Anyone considering acupuncture treatments should determine the qualifications of the practitioner—educational preparation *and* licensure.

## ACUPRESSURE AND SHIATSU

Acupressure is widely practiced throughout China and is now gaining followers in this country. Acupressure is a noninvasive alternative to acupuncture for relief of pain or muscle tension and for boosting one's energy level. When acupressure successfully stimulates the flow of energy (i.e., relieves a blockage), it stimulates self-healing by the body. Acupressure may be learned and used by anyone, may be self-administered, and is safe. The technique involves using the fingers, knuckles, or even an elbow to apply pressure at specific locations. Points that are relevant to the problem are tender. After locating a tender point, the acupressurist applies pressure for several seconds, then releases. The pressure-release sequence is repeated for several minutes until tenderness at that point disappears.

There are numerous books from which one may learn acupressure. There are also several centers where health practitioners may learn advanced techniques. The practice is not regulated, meaning that a practitioner does not have to be licensed. Those who complete a course or workshop are awarded a certificate from the school or center that offers such training. Word-of-mouth recommendations and personal experience are about the only means of determining the effectiveness of the procedure or a particular practitioner.

Shiatsu is the Japanese adaptation of acupressure. In Japanese, the word *shiatsu* means "finger pressure." Shiatsu consists of a rhythmic application of pressure at specific points, using the thumbs, fingers, or palms. Detailed charts show the points at which pressure should be applied for a specific purpose. For areas above the neck, pressure is applied for no more than three seconds. In other areas, pressure is applied for seven seconds. If a particular point is painful, pressure should be light; every few minutes, pressure can again be applied to the painful spot. The point becomes less painful with each application of pressure until, eventually, deep pressure can be applied. Shiatsu can even be self-administered to relieve a headache, toothache, or other pain in a specific area. Performed by a therapist, Shiatsu is a form of whole-body therapy. Many massage therapists use selected Shiatsu points to enhance the effectiveness of a therapeutic massage.

Some schools of massage therapy include Shiatsu in the curriculum. New York State requires completion of a course in Shiatsu to qualify for the massage therapy licensure examination. Although Shiatsu is complex and best learned through formal training, the basic technique may be learned from a well-written textbook. Any therapist who wishes to use the technique on clients should participate in a workshop, enroll in a Shiatsu course, or obtain one-on-one instruction from a qualified Shiatsu practitioner. States do not regulate the practice of Shiatsu.

## REFLEXOLOGY

It has been suggested that the footwashing mentioned in the New Testament was actually foot reflexology—a ritual in which a host or hostess made a newly arrived guest comfortable by washing and massaging the feet. Reflexology uses specific pressure points on the hands and feet that correspond to specific organs or body areas, as shown in Figure 26-8. For example, a line along the arch of the foot corresponds to the spine. A person with neck pain has tender points toward the front of the arch; one with low back pain, toward the heel end of the arch. The reflexology points have been mapped; charts show the points on the feet and hands that correspond to specific body areas. Reflexology may be used therapeutically, but it is especially effective if used once a week as a preventive measure. At the end of a reflexology session,

FIGURE 26-8 Foot reflexology chart. *Source:* From Dwight C. Byers, 2001, *Better Health with Foot Reflexology: The Original Ingham Method.* St. Petersburg, FL: Ingham. Used by permission of Dwight C. Byers.

the client is usually completely relaxed. One reflexologist says her clients always leave with "happy feet."

Massage schools include reflexology in their curriculum. The International Institute of Reflexology in St. Petersburg, Florida, offers a two-week course and certifies graduates as "reflexologists." Faculty from the institute offer workshops throughout the world, including numerous sites within the United States. Although learning the basics of reflexology from a good textbook may be adequate for self-use or for working on friends and family, anyone who claims the title "reflexologist" should be certified by an educational program. The states do not regulate the practice of reflexology. The illustration on this page shows reflex points on the feet from the therapist's view (i.e., the left foot is on the right side of the diagram).

## THERAPEUTIC MASSAGE

Massage is an ancient therapeutic technique. Swedish massage, probably the best-known type, consists of several basic techniques and specific procedures for manipulating the soft tissues. Swedish massage was originally developed as a medical treatment, performed only by a masseur (male) or masseuse (female) with extensive training. At one time, massage was the primary technique used by physical therapists; today, however, most physical therapists use a variety of techniques but very little "hands-on" massage.

Most massage therapists use some of the basic techniques encompassed by Swedish massage. Some massage therapists incorporate polarity therapy and pressure point therapy into the massage routine. A neuromuscular massage therapist also uses pressure at certain points to stimulate nerve function, which then improves muscle activity in the area. Certain techniques are especially effective for specific problems, such as sports injuries, tension headaches, whiplash, or muscle spasm. Swedish massage utilizes long strokes, kneading, and friction to relax the superficial layer of muscles and improve circulation. Variations on this basic technique include deep tissue massage to release muscle spasm; neuromuscular massage that uses concentrated finger pressure to break up the pain/spasm cycle; lymphatic massage to increase lymphatic flow and remove toxins; Thai massage to relieve spasms and improve flexibility by gently stretching tight muscles, tendons, and ligaments; and Structural Integration (also known as "Rolfing") to improve posture and balance by stretching muscle fascia, thereby realigning the body so that the ear, shoulder, hip, and ankle form a straight line. A weekly massage is a pleasant way to release tension and an excellent stress management technique (Figure 26-9).

The advantages of massage therapy are numerous, regardless of which particular method is used. Some specific benefits include:

- Improved performance and increased stamina (for athletes)
- Accelerated healing (following muscle or joint injuries)
- Correction of body alignment (especially in conjunction with osteopathic or chiropractic adjustments)
- Improved circulation to the soft tissues
- Improved elimination, as increased flow of blood and lymph through the muscles removes accumulated waste
- Improved balance and coordination as posture, alignment, and muscle function improve
- Decrease in anxiety, as excess lactic acid is removed from muscles and blood
- Release of suppressed emotions that may be the basis of long-term muscle spasm
- Increased energy as muscle tension is released, because tight muscles tend to trap energy
- Relief of pain and/or muscle spasm associated with such conditions as arthritis, chronic neck or back pain, asthma, multiple sclerosis, and other chronic disorders

**FIGURE 26-9** Massage therapy has numerous benefits.
*Photo courtesy of Chicago School of Massage Therapy; Robert K. King, President.*

A certified massage therapist (CMT) has completed a formal course of instruction. Available courses vary in length from about 100 hours to several thousand hours. A legitimate massage therapist is completely professional and respects the modesty of the client at all times. The massage therapist does not diagnose or prescribe, but does need information about any existing health problem and the reason for seeking massage therapy.

Licensure requirements vary from one state to another. In those states that do not require a license, learn the educational qualifications of any practitioner you are considering as a therapist. Qualified massage therapists are willing to discuss their educational preparation. The best recommendation for a massage therapist (or any health care provider) comes from satisfied clients.

## THE SELF-HELP TREND

Public interest in holistic health evolved out of the self-help movement that focused on freeing oneself from psychological and mental blocks. That movement resulted in a flood of "pop psychology" self-help books on such topics as assertiveness, self-esteem, communication, interpersonal relationships, and sexuality. The result was a marked change in attitudes toward responsibility for increasing one's effectiveness in coping with life situations and improving relationships. Various health organizations began to emphasize exercise and a healthful diet, further encouraging individual responsibility for health and well-being.

The current interest in complementary therapies seems to be a natural outgrowth of these earlier movements. Also, more and more people recognize that modern life involves high levels of stress. One can seek escape from stress and life problems through such crutches as tranquilizers or alcohol. Or one can utilize stress reduction techniques and modify lifestyle to eliminate some sources of stress. If a chronic health problem exists for which allopathic medicine offers only symptomatic relief, one can choose that approach or seek an appropriate complementary therapy.

The person who is seeking techniques for self-help probably has already assumed some degree of responsibility for health management. That does not mean that the individual fully understands all that is involved in achieving optimal health. If you have the opportunity to help such a person, encourage the individual to learn about wellness rather than to seek help for a single problem. That means considering lifestyle, stressors in the life situation, stress management techniques, nutrition, exercise, and any mental/emotional factors that may be affecting physical health. By now you surely recognize that this is the holistic approach. High-level wellness (and, in the case of chronic diseases, recovery) cannot be achieved without a holistic approach. Remember the difference between "curing" and "healing"? The goal for every patient should be true healing, so that optimal health, whatever that might be *for that individual,* can be achieved.

Some self-help techniques can be learned from books and articles. Others, such as identifying emotional factors that need to be resolved, may be accomplished more readily with professional help. The person who begins a self-help program alone may experience improvement, then become aware of the need for help. Whatever the approach, most of the following will contribute to improvement in one's overall health:

- Awareness of choices that affect health
- A *conscious* choice to modify lifestyle
- Daily use of a stress management technique

- Self-study, workshops, and/or counseling to release feelings related to old traumas, unmet needs, and/or unresolved conflicts
- One or more techniques for directing the flow of body energies and releasing blockages

## ROLE OF THE HEALTH CARE PROVIDER

Increasingly, medical doctors are open to holistic health care and some complementary therapies. Numerous medical doctors are writing books about their expanded approach to therapy, some providing anecdotal reports of their patients' healing experiences. Some patients are writing about how they took responsibility for their own healing and recovered from a supposedly irreversible disease. The cover of the January 20, 2003, issue of a leading weekly publication stated, "Special issue: How your mind can heal your body." Over half of that issue was devoted to the role of the mind in health and healing (*Time*, 2003). The cover of another leading weekly for that same week proclaims in bold print, "New targeted medicines promise breakthrough cures" (Fischman, 2003, pp. 50–58). This illustrates two opposing views of health care in two major weekly magazines, one reporting on mind/body healing, the other on pharmaceutical drugs as the solution for health problems! Increasing numbers of people are accepting responsibility for their own health, but a large percentage of the population still embraces the notion that there is, or some day will be, a drug for every health problem.

As a health care provider, you have a responsibility to encourage patients to believe in their doctors and in their prescribed therapies. Inevitably, however, you will encounter a patient, relative, or friend who asks your advice about a complementary therapy. It would be appropriate for you to help such a person obtain information, but that person should make the decision to use or not use a specific therapy. Use your best judgment in each situation without exerting influence in either direction. An open mind combined with healthy skepticism is a good combination. Do not deny someone the potential benefit of a complementary therapy simply because you are ignorant about it or because it is not offered in your particular health care agency at this time.

## REFERENCES AND SUGGESTED READINGS

> **Note:** *Indicates a "classic" publication that introduced information and ideas basic to holistic health care.

Balch, Phyllis A. (2008). *Prescription for nutritional healing*. Garden City Park, NY: Avery.
*Byers, Dwight C. (2001). *Better health with foot reflexology*. St. Petersburg, FL: Ingham Publishing.
Castleman, Michael. (2009). *The new healing herbs*. Emmaus, PA: Rodale Press.
*Chopra, Deepak. (1989). *Quantum healing: Exploring the frontiers of mind/body medicine*. New York: Bantam.
Chopra, Deepak. (2009). *Reinventing the body, resurrecting the soul*. New York: Harmony/Crown.
*Dacher, Elliott S. (1996). *Intentional healing: A guide to the mind/body healing system*. New York: Paragon.

Dale, Cyndi. (2009). *The subtle body: An encyclopedia of your energy anatomy.* Boulder, CO: Sounds True.

Feingold, Ellen. (2008). *The complete self-care guide to homeopathy, herbal remedies, and nutritional supplements.* Troy, NY: Whitson.

*Gach, Michael Reed. (1990). *Acupressure's potent points: A guide to self-care for common ailments.* New York: Bantam.

*Gach, Michael Reed, & Henninh, Beth Ann. (2004). *Accupressure for emotional healing.* New York: Bantam.

Graedon, Joe, & Graedon, Teresa. (2006). *Best choices from the people's pharmacy.* New York: New American Library.

Hickey, Steve, & Roberts, Hilary. (2007). *The cancer breakthrough: A nutritional approach for doctors and patients.* Henderson, NV: LivOn Books.

Hoffman, David. (2007). *Herbal prescriptions after 50.* Rochester, VT: Healing Arts Press.

*Hover-Kramer, Dorothea. (2002). *Healing touch, a guidebook for practitioners* (2nd ed.). Clifton Park, NY: Delmar, Cengage Learning.

Hyman, Mark. (2007). *The ultrasimple diet.* New York: Pocket Books.

Hyman, Mark. (2008). *The UltraMind solution: Fix your brain by fixing your body first.* New York: Scribner.

*Lansky, Amy. (2003). *Impossible cure: The promise of homeopathy.* Portola Valley, CA: R.L. Ranch Press. (The author describes curing her child of autism, using homeopathy.)

*Lininger, Schuyler W. (Ed.) (2002). *The natural pharmacy: From the top experts in the field, your essential guide to herbs, vitamins, minerals, and homeopathic remedies.* Rocklin, CA: Prima.

Mars, Brigitte. (2007). *The desktop guide to herbal medicine.* Boulder, CO: Basic Health.

*Murray, Michael, & Pizzorno, Joseph E. (2002). *Encyclopedia of natural medicine.* Collingdale, PA: Diana Publishing. (Contains useful addresses in the appendix.)

Nauman, Eileen. (2004). *Homeopathy for epidemics.* Flagstaff, AZ: Light Technology Publications.

Nestle, Marion. (2006). *What to eat.* New York: North Point Press/Farrar, Strauss, and Giroux.

Neustaedter, Randall. (2005). *Flu: Alternative treatments and prevention.* New York: Random House.

Pelletier, Kenneth R. (2002). *Best alternative medicine.* New York: Fireside.

Perko, Sandra J. (2005). *The homeopathic treatment of influenza: Special bird flu edition.* San Antonio, TX: Benchmark Homeopathic Publications.

Petersen, Melody. (2008). *Our daily meds.* New York: Farrar, Strauss and Giroux.

Roizen, Michael F., & Oz, Mehmet C. (2007). *You: Staying young.* New York: Free Press/Simon & Schuster.

Schmukler, Alan V. (2006). *Homeopathy: An A to Z home handbook.* Woodbury, MN: Llewellyn.

*Shealy, C. Norman. (1998). *The illustrated encyclopedia of natural remedies.* Boston, MA: Element Books. (Useful addresses are given on pp. 486–489.)

*Shealy, C. Norman, & Myss, Carolyn M. (1993). *The creation of health: The emotional, psychological, and spiritual responses that promote health and healing.* Walpole, NH: Stillpoint.

Snyder, Mariah, & Lindquist, Ruth. (Eds.) (2006). *Complementary/alternative therapies in nursing* (5th ed.). New York, NY: Springer Publishing Company.

Somers, Suzanne. (2008). *Breakthrough: Eight steps to wellness.* New York: Crown.

Spreen, Allen, & Euten, Roni. (2009). *Tomorrow's cancer cures today.* Baltimore, MD: Health Sciences Institute.

*Ullman, Dana. (2002). *Essential homeopathy: What it is and what it can do for you.* Novato, CA: New World Library.

Walker, Marsha Jelonek, & Walker, Johnathan D. (2003). *Healing massage: A simple approach.* Clifton Park, NY: Delmar, Cengage Learning.

Weil, Andrew. (2007). *Healthy aging.* New York: Anchor.

## SOURCES OF ADDITIONAL INFORMATION

**Alternative Medicine Foundation,** http://www.amfoundation.org

**American Association of Naturopathic Physicians,** 1-866-538-2267

**Amy Lansky,** http://www.impossiblecure.com

**David G. Williams. (Ed.). Alternatives for the Health Conscious Individual.** Mountain Home Publishing, 2700 Cummings Lane, Kerrville, TX 78028. Monthly newsletter.

**Homeopathic Educational Services,** http://www.homeopathic.com

**Jonathan V. Wright. (Ed.). Nutrition & Healing. Agora Health,** LLC, 819 N. Charles St., Baltimore, MD 21201. Monthly newsletter, http://WrightNewsletter.com

**National Center for Complementary and Alternative Medicine (NCCAM),** http://www.nccam.nih.gov, 1-888-644-6226

**National Center for Homeopathy.** Homeopathy Today. 801 North Fairfax St., Suite 306, Alexandria, VA 22314. e-mail nchinfo@igc.org.

**University of Pittsburg:** Folk Library of Health Sciences, www.pitt.edu/cbw/altm.html

**Weston Price Foundation,** http://www.westonaprice.org/abcsofnutrition

## REVIEW AND SELF-CHECK

1. Compare legitimate health care providers and those of questionable qualifications by listing four possible behaviors of each.

2. Name two steps for evaluating a health services practitioner.

3. What is the primary characteristic of a holistic approach to health care?

4. State the focus of the two following areas of health care:
   a. Psychoneuroimmunology

b. Energy medicine

5. Name two complementary therapies that influence the flow of energy through and around the body.

6. Name three therapies that use specific points to stimulate the flow of body energies.

7. Name five benefits of therapeutic massage.

8. Describe appropriate behavior for you, as a health care provider, when someone asks your advice about using a complementary therapy.

## ASSIGNMENTS

1. Participate in a class discussion about how a health care provider should respond to a request for advice about using a specific complementary therapy for a chronic problem.

2. Participate in a class sharing session. Those who have experienced a complementary therapy may share their experiences. Those who have *observed first-hand* (hearsay is not acceptable) the effects of a complementary therapy on a family member or close friend may share their observations.

3. As a class project, planned with your instructor, find out what complementary therapies are available in your community. Present findings to the class as oral reports or, with the approval of your instructor, invite an alternative therapist to speak to the class and demonstrate one or more therapeutic techniques.

# UNIT 27

# Managing Stress with Relaxation/Meditation

## OBJECTIVES

Upon completion of this unit, you should be able to:

- Define *mind-talk* and *mindfulness*.
- Define *Relaxation* as a process.
- State two reasons a recreational activity is not adequate as a stress management technique.
- Describe the primary physiological change that occurs during Relaxation.
- Name the primary physiological change that occurs during meditation.
- State three psychological changes that may occur as long-term effects of meditation.
- Name two reasons a health care provider should use a stress management technique at least once a day.
- Name the major disadvantage of meditation as a therapeutic tool.
- Use a specific technique for Relaxation.
- List five positive statements that could serve as affirmations.
- Use a specific technique for meditation (optional).

## KEY TERMS

Affirmation
Blood lactate
Visualize

You have now learned that most health care providers acknowledge the role of stress and psychosocial factors in the onset of illness. It is not within the role of nonphysician health care providers to *prescribe* stress management for a patient, because diagnosis and prescription of a therapeutic plan are the domain of medicine. In some circumstances, however, it is appropriate for any health care provider to talk with a patient about the importance of stress management. Your participation in helping a patient learn about stress management is more likely if you are working with a holistically oriented medical practitioner. In the meantime, you, as a health care provider, have a responsibility to yourself and your family to maintain the best possible state of health. That includes learning about stress management and modifying your daily routine to include one or more specific stress management techniques. This unit, then, is for *you*.

## STRESS MANAGEMENT

This unit presents two specific techniques for managing stress: Relaxation and meditation. The word *Relaxation* is capitalized to remind you that we are discussing a *specific process* with *specific effects*. This is quite different from the customary use of the word *relaxation*.

There are many ways of coping with stress. Some people have a daily exercise program that significantly reduces their stress level. Others participate in a sport at least once a week. Sports may or may not reduce stress, depending upon one's level of competitiveness. If winning is important, then losing a game may increase stress, rather than reduce it.

Certain activities that people think of as "relaxing" do *not* have stress management value. For example, watching television, partying, going to the beach, a weekend skiing trip, and other such recreational activities are diversions—escapes from the daily pressures of the job and home responsibilities. Though pleasant and possibly self-renewing, recreational activities do not bring about the physical and psychological changes that are essential to managing stress effectively.

## MIND-TALK AS A SOURCE OF STRESS

Dr. Elliott Dacher describes two basic activities, mind-talk and mindfulness, that cannot occur simultaneously. When one is active, the other is inactive. Mind-talk is active most of the time and involves thoughts, feelings, mental images, and various sensations. It is the ongoing mental chatter that we all experience, especially when engaged in an activity that does not require conscious mental effort. Household tasks, many job tasks, walking, riding an exercycle—these types of activities are accompanied by a stream of mind-talk *unless it is consciously controlled*.

Stored memories provide the content for mind-talk; it may be factual or psychological, useful or destructive. When mind-talk arouses negative feelings associated with a past experience, we relive a bad experience that cannot be changed. Thus, mind-talk may be the source of ongoing stress. Mind-talk can be so engrossing that a person is out of touch with what is happening at the moment. By taking conscious control, however, an individual can learn to avoid stressful feelings associated with past experiences and anxiety related to some anticipated future event.

## MINDFULNESS

In contrast to mind-talk, *mindfulness* must be learned, is self-initiated, and requires conscious effort. Mindfulness has three aspects that occur in sequence: attention, concentration, and meditation. One *consciously chooses* to enter a state of mindfulness, primarily by giving full attention to what is happening at the present moment. Full attention to an ongoing activity quickly becomes concentration. A state of mindfulness may be experienced while reading, enjoying some aspect of nature, being involved in an artistic pursuit, cruising the Internet, or being totally absorbed in relating to another person. By shifting from mind-talk to mindfulness, then, one attends to what is happening at present.

Dr. Kabat-Zinn, director of the stress management clinic at the University of Massachusetts Hospital in Boston, describes mindfulness as a means of fully living in the present, which is all we have. The past cannot be changed; the future is yet to be. So we should make the most of the present, which is best done through mindfulness. Dr. Kabat-Zinn teaches mindfulness and meditation to patients as a means of coping with the stress of their illnesses.

## RELAXATION AND MEDITATION

The physical and psychological effects of Relaxation and meditation have been thoroughly documented by clinical practitioners and researchers. Although the therapeutic value of these two techniques is now widely accepted, the preventive potential has only been explored in limited settings, such as psychosomatic medical practices, psychological services, and corporate health maintenance programs.

### Background

Historically, meditation has its roots in various religions, especially those of the East (i.e., India, China, and Japan). There are numerous references to meditation in the Bible, and many people use a prayerful form of meditation. The monks of various religious traditions use meditation as one means of spiritual development. But meditation is not prayer. In fact, many meditators do not consider their meditations to be a religious activity. Each meditator determines the extent to which his or her meditation has religious significance.

The technique known as Relaxation is a relatively new therapeutic procedure. It seems to have originated around 1929 with Dr. Edmund Jacobson, a Chicago psychiatrist who believed muscle tension and anxiety to be significant factors in the onset of illness. He developed a technique known as *progressive relaxation*.

Concurrently with Jacobson's research on muscle tension, a German psychiatrist, Dr. J. H. Schultz, developed a therapeutic technique for helping patients learn to control certain autonomic functions. This technique is known as *autogenic training*, or AT. The work of these two physicians has led to the development of numerous Relaxation techniques based on either progressive relaxation or AT.

### Physical and Psychological Effects

Relaxation and meditation are two different processes. You can practice a Relaxation technique without meditating. However, meditation brings about physiological changes and, for habitual meditators, has long-term effects that do not occur with Relaxation alone.

Both Relaxation and meditation result in feeling rested; the 20-minute procedure may dissipate fatigue or sleepiness as much as a two-hour nap. Many people not only feel rested, but also experience increased energy at the completion of either procedure.

The primary physiological change that occurs with Relaxation is *release of tension in the skeletal muscles*, accompanied by a *decrease in* **blood lactate**. A high level of blood lactate is associated with anxiety. Relaxation training emphasizes learning to *control* muscle tension. The Jacobson method emphasizes learning to *recognize* the presence of muscle tension, then *consciously let go of the tension*. Most other methods focus on the "letting go" phase, on the assumption that the individual is already able to recognize the presence of muscle tension. Those who have achieved heightened awareness of muscle tension through the Jacobson method believe that learning to recognize the presence of muscle tension, or the onset of muscle tension, is essential to successful use of Relaxation.

Some of the benefits of Relaxation can be experienced within a few practice sessions, but the full benefits are realized after the procedure has been performed at least once a day over a period of several weeks. One who has mastered the technique can recognize muscle tension as it begins (usually around the eyes or in the neck), then can quietly use Relaxation to relieve that tension within a few minutes. Obviously, anyone who works or lives in a stressful situation benefits from using Relaxation intermittently throughout the day, to avoid a buildup of muscle tension.

In contrast to Relaxation, meditation affects various body processes, essentially slowing the pace of bodily activity: respiratory rate and pulse rate decrease, blood pressure lowers, and the metabolic rate, as measured by the body's oxygen consumption, slows. Some therapists believe the meditative period helps the body establish balance and harmony among the various systems, a state that promotes healing and optimal functioning of the immune system.

Meditation is also characterized by a change in brain activity. In 1929, Dr. Hans Berger, a German psychiatrist, published a report in which he described a distinctive pattern of brain waves (9–13 cycles per second) that occurs when a person is in a quiet state, not actively thinking or reacting to various stimuli. Dr. Berger labeled this pattern *alpha rhythms*. Subsequent research confirmed Dr. Berger's findings and identified other brain wave patterns. Beta rhythms (13–18 cycles per second) predominate during the fully conscious state. Theta rhythms (5–8 cycles per second) and delta rhythms (less than 5 cycles per second) occur during sleep.

Sleep researchers have found that brain wave patterns during sleep go through cycles, with the deepest stage of sleep characterized by delta rhythms and the lightest stage of sleep by alpha rhythms. Dreaming occurs during light sleep and is accompanied by rapid eye movements (this stage is often referred to as *REM sleep*). Although alpha rhythms occur during REM sleep and also during meditation, the meditator is awake, conscious of surroundings but not interacting through sensory, mental, or emotional responses. The meditator can return to full beta consciousness at will.

The benefits of continued meditation over a prolonged period are mental, emotional, and spiritual. The latter term is used here not in the religious sense, but to refer to that mysterious aspect of being human that is beyond body and mind and emotions. For many people the spiritual aspect is related to the divine; for others, it is being in touch with the collective unconscious, cosmic forces, or other metaphysical concepts. Whatever one's personal belief regarding the spiritual, it does appear to be an aspect of individuality that must be in harmony with mind and emotions in order for the body to experience optimal well-being. The long-term effects of daily meditation include:

- Changes in perception of self, others, and life events
- Re-evaluation of values and beliefs
- A freeing of emotions, especially suppressed emotions
- Greater compassion
- Increased capacity for self-love and love for others
- Greater readiness to accept love
- Improved ability to cope with life situations
- Increased awareness of "self"

### Advantages and Disadvantages

Relaxation and meditation can be viewed in the light of an investment and its dividends. For an investment of about 20 minutes a day, the potential dividends include prevention of stress-related illness, therapy for an existing illness or injury, and increased energy for daily activities as chronic muscle tension is relieved. The long-term meditator does risk the pain of dealing with suppressed emotions and of changing beliefs, values, and perceptions as a result of meditative insights. But one who completes the process of dealing with such unresolved issues is thereafter free of their restrictive, negative influence.

The disadvantages pertain to the learning process, the length of time required to experience full benefits, and competing demands for one's time. It is not easy for a busy person to incorporate a 20-minute routine into an already full day. But it is very easy to rely on the "I just don't have time" excuse. Dr. Simonton dealt quite effectively with this excuse when he asked a conference group, "What is so important that it cannot wait 20 minutes for you to do your meditation?" Most of us, trying to answer that question honestly, cannot list anything other than a true emergency.

It takes time to learn Relaxation. It takes even more time to learn to meditate. After about two weeks of consistent practice, you begin to experience the benefits. But it takes persistence over a period of months, perhaps even one or two years, to experience the long-term benefits. Many people who learn a meditation technique do not use it consistently or for a long enough period of time to experience the long-term payoff. It is too easy to give in to competing demands on one's time.

The remainder of this unit introduces you to three different Relaxation techniques, then to two types of meditation. Information about each is followed by a step-by-step procedure. You may want to tape-record each procedure; use the tape to learn the steps of one specific procedure until you can practice without the tape. An alternative approach is to read through the instructions several times, then practice the procedure. Afterward, reread the instructions. Thereafter, read the instructions before and after each Relaxation. Soon, you will be able to go through the procedure on your own. *Learn one procedure thoroughly before going on to another.*

## RELAXATION TECHNIQUES

You already know that a skill is developed through practice. *Mastery* of a task or technique is achieved by continuing to practice a skill regularly over a period of months or years. Relaxation is a special type of skill that involves control of muscle tension throughout the body. You can develop skill in controlling muscle tension only by practicing at least once a day for about 20 minutes; skill will be achieved more quickly by practicing twice a day.

One who has *mastered* Relaxation can release tension within a minute or two just by thinking, "Relax." Achieving that level of mastery enables one to manage the stress of modern living.

Some people find that Relaxation alone meets their needs. Others, after experiencing the benefits of Relaxation, develop an interest in learning to meditate. The primary emphasis here is on learning Relaxation, which requires less time than meditation. An introduction to meditation and two examples of a simple meditation follow, for those who wish to go beyond Relaxation.

### Principles

There are many techniques for achieving Relaxation. No one method is right for everybody. Some people find that one method is more comfortable or more effective than others. To find the technique that works best for you, try a specific method once a day for at least two weeks. Then try another method once a day for two weeks (Figure 27-1). After you have tried

**FIGURE 27-1** Some people like to use music during Relaxation and meditation. *Delmar/Cengage Learning*

the three methods described next, select the one with which you are most comfortable and practice it daily for a month. At that point, you should be able to recognize muscle tension as soon as it develops. Then, you can withdraw from a stressful situation and devote two to five minutes to "letting go." You will no longer need a full 20 minutes to reduce muscle tension. This does not mean that you discontinue your daily use of the full 20-minute procedure; the short procedure helps you get through a stressful day with less tension buildup. Continue your daily routine for total Relaxation—a time for re-establishing balance and harmony—and accept it as a healthful part of your daily routine for the remainder of your life.

## Preparation

It is important to make certain preparations before starting a Relaxation procedure.

1. Decide on the time of day and the location for your Relaxation. Then, be consistent so that time and location become associated with Relaxation. The location should be a particular room and chair (or pillow, or area of the floor) that is used only for Relaxation. Select a time when you can be alone for at least 20 minutes, preferably before eating a

meal. Early morning is a good time—it gets your day off to a good start. Late afternoon is also good, to release the day's accumulated tensions before you have dinner.

2. Inform anyone in the area that you are not to be disturbed for the next 30 minutes. (Actually, you will probably use only 15 to 20 minutes.) If you are alone, turn off the phone or let incoming calls go to voice mail.

3. Prepare the environment by closing the door, dimming the lights, and eliminating distractions. Put the dog and cat out.

4. Loosen any tight clothing, such as a belt or necktie; remove your shoes.

5. Assume a comfortable sitting position with the spine straight from head to hips, feet flat on the floor, hands resting on the thighs. If you have back or neck problems you may lie down. But be aware that in the lying position you may fall asleep as you become relaxed. Sleep is not the same as Relaxation! If you do choose to lie down, use the floor (your bed is for sleeping); keep the legs parallel (not crossed at the ankles); keep the arms parallel to the body but not touching it. The tendency to fall asleep passes after you have practiced the procedure several times.

6. Take several deep breaths, allowing the abdomen to expand as you inhale and to contract as you exhale.

7. Feel your body "letting go." Feel your hips and buttocks settling into the chair or floor.

8. Consciously put aside your thoughts and feelings, your worries and concerns of the day, as the final step in preparing for Relaxation.

After about 20 minutes, the body seems to signal that it is ready to resume activity. If you do not trust your ability to recognize this signal, include setting a timer in step 3. Use a timer that sounds only once, rather than repeatedly. Then, if you choose to continue to enjoy Relaxation after the timer sounds, you can do so without having to get up and turn the timer off. With practice these preparation steps become automatic. Now it is time to learn Relaxation.

## Methods

Three different Relaxation procedures are presented next. Each has its particular advantages. With practice, each will result in the release of muscle tension throughout your body.

**Progressive Relaxation** The following steps are based on a method developed by Dr. E. Jacobson, a physiologist and physician. This method is designed to help you become aware of the feeling that accompanies muscle tension, then become aware of how a relaxed muscle feels. Learning to differentiate these sensations—tension versus relaxation—increases body awareness and prepares you to recognize the need for Relaxation during the day. With practice, you will be able to relax almost anywhere (even without sitting or lying down) and get results within a few minutes. As you do the following steps, keep the rest of your body relaxed while you work on a specific body part.

1. Flex the toes of both feet; observe how the toes and feet feel in this tightened state. Now, let go and observe the feeling that accompanies this release.

2. Tighten the legs (calves and thighs) and observe the tension; let go and observe the feeling of relaxation.

3. Tighten the buttocks, hips, and abdominal muscles and observe. Relax these areas and observe.
4. Tighten the muscles of the chest and upper back and observe. Relax these areas and observe.
5. Tighten the hands by making a fist and the arms by flexing at the elbow; observe the tension. Relax the hands and arms and observe.
6. Tighten the shoulders (raise them toward the ears) and observe; let go and observe.
7. Tighten the entire head area—throat and neck, jaw, face, eyes, forehead, scalp—and observe the feeling. Relax and observe the difference as tension flows out of these areas. Let the jaw relax until the lips part slightly.
8. Raise and lower the eyebrows several times. Pull the eyebrows together, as though you are frowning, then release and observe.
9. Tighten the entire body, from toes to scalp. Hold the tightness as long as you can. Let go. Become as limp as a rag doll. Observe.
10. Say to yourself, "I am relaxed. I am relaxed. I am relaxed."
11. Scan your body for any areas of tightness. If you find such an area, mentally "look at" the area and send it an order, "Relax." Repeat for any other areas of tightness.
12. Conclude the procedure by sitting (or lying) quietly for several minutes. Enjoy your state of Relaxation.

As you get up to resume activity, try to maintain the feelings of peace and relaxation. When you do feel a group of muscles beginning to tighten, think "I am relaxed." You may find it more effective to send the order "Relax" to the specific part of the body where you tend to hold tension, such as the jaw or neck muscles. Your goal is to be able to control stress-related muscle tension just by telling yourself, "I am relaxed" several times. But that goal can be achieved only if you have your body practice "letting go" regularly over a period of time.

**Autogenic Training** Autogenic training was developed by a German physician, Dr. J. H. Schultz. It is usually referred to as "AT" or "the Schultz method." With his patients in a state of deep relaxation, Dr. Schultz used positive statements to "program" his patients for healing.

Dr. Schultz emphasized that each step be practiced until the desired effect occurs; then and *only then* should the learner go on to the next step. The procedure includes the repetition of one or more positive statements, such as "I am at peace" or "I am in a state of well-being." A person who has learned to go through all the steps of AT reaches a state of *deep relaxation*. The combination of deep relaxation and **affirmations** (positive statements) is especially beneficial.

The following steps are based on the Schultz method. Initially, you will practice only steps 1 and 2, then terminate the procedure. For that reason, the termination step (step 9) is presented after step 2 as well as following step 8. Regardless of how many steps you perform, *always terminate the session by performing step 9*. Now, after making the usual preparations, do the following steps:

1. Think, "I am relaxed." Repeat several times.
2. Think, "My right arm is heavy." (If you are left-handed, substitute "left" for "right" throughout this step.) Continue to think, "My right arm is heavy" while focusing your attention

on your right arm. When you begin to experience heaviness in the right arm, think, "My right arm is heavy and warm." When you experience both heaviness and warmth in the right arm, think, "My arms are heavy and warm." Focus your attention on both arms. Experience the heaviness and warmth. When both arms are warm and heavy, think, "My arms and legs are heavy and warm." Mentally focus on your arms and legs; consciously experience the heaviness and warmth. Terminate your practice by performing step 9.

3. Bring yourself out of the relaxed state by opening your eyes, yawning, and stretching for about 10 seconds; flex and extend your arms several times.

    Practice steps 1 and 2 for several days. *Do not go to step 3 until you feel heaviness and warmth in both arms and both legs.*

4. Think, "My heartbeat is strong and regular. My heartbeat is strong and regular."

    *Proceed to step 4 only after you have practiced steps 1 through 3 for several days. Remember to terminate the procedure with step 9.*

5. Think, "My breathing is free and easy. My breathing is free and easy." Be aware of your breathing, but do not try to control it. As you become more relaxed, your breathing will be shallow and the rate will slow. Your body is using less oxygen, but you will not experience air hunger.

    Practice steps 1 through 4 for several days before adding step 5. Terminate the procedure with step 9.

6. Think, "My abdomen is warm. My abdomen is warm." Focus your attention on the abdominal area. Be aware of the warmth. You may feel this warmth spreading to the hips and around to the low back.

    Practice steps 1 through 5 for several days, always ending with step 9.

7. Think, "My forehead is cool. My forehead is cool." Envision a cool breeze blowing lightly across your forehead.

    This is a difficult step for many people. It is an important step, however, so *practice steps 1 through 6 for several days until you do experience coolness over the forehead.* End with step 9.

8. Think, "My mind is still and quiet. My mind is still and quiet." Experience a period of mental blankness; if any thoughts pop into your mind, mentally repeat, "My mind is still and quiet."

9. Think one or more positive statements related to peace, serenity, health and well-being, or happiness or joy; if you prefer, use a statement related to your religious beliefs.

10. When you are ready, bring yourself out of the relaxed state by opening your eyes, yawning, and stretching; flex and extend your arms several times. Sit quietly for a few minutes before returning to your day's activities.

Remember, *never terminate autogenic training without performing step 9.* The circulatory system changes during deep relaxation. It is important that you perform step 9 to *restore normal circulation to the muscular system before you become physically active.*

**Self-Directed Relaxation** The most widely used technique for Relaxation is probably some variation on this third method. While learning the procedure, allow at least one full minute for each step; eventually, you will be able to go through steps 1 through 8 in one to three minutes. After making the usual preparations, mentally direct the process as follows:

1. Think, "My toes and feet are warm." Repeat until you experience warmth in the toes and feet.
2. Think, "My legs are warm." Experience the warm sensation creeping up from the toes and feet.
3. Think, "My hands and arms are warm." Repeat until you can feel the warmth in your hands and arms.
4. Think, "A warm feeling is moving up my spine." Experience this sensation.
5. Think, "The warmth is spreading up the back of my neck and into my scalp." Experience the spreading warmth.
6. Think, "My forehead, face, jaws, and throat are getting very warm." Experience and enjoy this warmth.
7. Think, "My chest is warm." Experience the warmth spreading across your chest and around to your upper back.
8. Think, "My abdomen is warm." Experience the warmth spreading over the abdomen and around to the lower back.
9. Think, "My entire body is warm and totally relaxed."
10. At this point, simply enjoy Relaxation for 20–30 minutes. If you wish, use an affirmation to accomplish some positive result, such as healing or good feelings about yourself.

After mastering steps 1 through 9, you will experience deep relaxation for almost the full 20 minutes. Afterward, you will be refreshed and energized as you resume your activities.

## MEDITATION METHODS

Meditation is a process for achieving a state of mental quietude. It is accompanied by brain waves that are significantly slower than in the thinking/sensing state, but not as slow as in sleep. The meditator is alert and aware of the immediate surroundings, but not actively engaged in thinking, planning, analyzing, or other mental activities. Regular meditators find a sense of peace, increased awareness, a greater sense of self, and guidance toward solutions for current problems.

For health care providers, a significant aspect of meditation is its potential as a therapeutic tool. Meditation has a calming effect, which is itself therapeutic. Drs. Shealy, Simonton, Benson, and other clinical practitioners and researchers have found that patients who make meditation a part of their daily routine improve their quality of life. Some of them get well. Many of those who do not become completely free of disease do show marked improvement. Some can be maintained on a lower dosage of medication, whereas others improve enough to discontinue medication. Needless to say, no patient should abandon medical therapy in order to take up meditation. Rather, meditation is best used as an adjunct to other therapies prescribed by the patient's physician.

The therapeutic value of meditation may be enhanced by combining the meditative state with mental imagery (visualization). Cancer patients can be taught to meditate, then mentally visualize the cancer cells being destroyed by the immune system, or visualize a tumor gradually shrinking in size. A patient with an ulcer can visualize the edges of the ulcer healing, gradually decreasing the size of the ulcer until it no longer exists. Some patients learn to control chronic pain through meditation. Meditation and visualization may be learned through reading, recordings, or one-on-one instruction accompanied by daily practice.

## Principles

Because physical tension is a deterrent to achieving the meditative state, the first task of a beginning meditator is to learn Relaxation. Otherwise, a beginning meditator may spend the first 10 to 15 minutes releasing muscle tension, with only a few minutes spent in meditation.

There is no point in doing a meditation only once. Meditation is a *learning process*, one that must be continued for at least several weeks to experience the desired effects. One reason for this lengthy learning period is that meditation requires concentration. The beginning meditator quickly discovers how hard it is to keep attention focused on the meditation itself. After a momentary "good" beginning, various thoughts or feelings surface and suddenly the meditator is thinking, planning, or remembering instead of meditating. These random thoughts and feelings are sometimes referred to as the *inner dialogue* that must be controlled in order to achieve the meditative state. Because complete control comes slowly and *only with practice*, the first challenge is learning to concentrate. This is also one of the early benefits of meditation—increased powers of concentration.

As you begin your first meditation, you will quickly experience this intrusion of thoughts. As soon as you recognize that some thought has captured your attention, gently dismiss it and return to your meditation. Some teachers of meditation suggest ways to avoid the trap of becoming involved with a particular thought. One such technique is considering these thoughts to be leaves floating on the surface of a river or creek. You, sitting on the bank, simply note each passing leaf (thought), but do not become absorbed in observing any one of them.

Do not expect immediate or dramatic results. Meditation is a discipline. Some beneficial effects will be apparent after a month or two of consistent practice. A therapeutic meditation, used faithfully two or more times a day, may begin to have effects after two or three weeks. The full benefits of meditation are experienced by those who make it part of their lifestyle and meditate at least once, but preferably twice, a day over a period of months. An experienced meditator came into the office on a Monday morning and exclaimed, "I have finally found out what meditation can do for you! I had a breakthrough this weekend. I feel good about myself. I see my life and the world differently. Even the sky is bluer and the grass is greener." The keys to success as a meditator seem to be consistency and persistence over the long term.

## Types of Meditation

There are several types of meditation and many meditative techniques. No one technique is suitable for everyone. The best approach for a beginner is to try a simple meditation for at least two months, and then try a different method for two months. After learning several types of meditation and trying various methods, the beginning meditator will find one approach that seems "right."

The test of whether or not a meditation is right for you is how you feel afterward. Following a meditation, sit quietly for several minutes, being aware of how you feel. If you feel better than before the meditation, then that method is right for you. If you feel tired or sense that something is not right, then do not use that particular technique again. Simple meditations seldom have an adverse effect, but be aware of the possibility. Certain advanced meditative techniques are more likely than the simple meditations to prove inappropriate for some people.

Meditation methods can be classified as structured or unstructured. A structured meditation requires the meditator to attend to only one thing at a time: a particular thought, word or phrase, or object. The purpose of this focus is to develop one's powers of concentration. Often, an additional effect is some new perception or new understanding. A structured meditation clearly defines what the meditator is to work on; any mental wandering is corrected and attention is returned to the prescribed task.

An unstructured meditation is one in which the meditator identifies facts pertaining to a chosen subject, then focuses on *feelings* about those facts. This type of meditation primarily affects emotions. It is especially useful in a counseling situation, where the meditator can receive professional guidance in dealing with a troublesome area.

## Procedures

Both of the meditations described next are structured meditations. The first is designed to build the powers of concentration; the second is a guided imagery meditation that should result in a sense of well-being.

*Do not try a meditation until you have learned Relaxation*; otherwise, you will not get the full benefit of the meditation experience. If you begin to slump during the meditation, pull yourself erect. If you have an itch and cannot ignore it, then scratch. It is better to take care of such a distraction than to spend your entire meditation trying to ignore it.

### Breath-Counting Meditation

1. Follow the preparation instructions for Relaxation. Set a timer and place it where you cannot hear the ticking or sit where you can see a clock.

2. Sit in a comfortable position. This may be the cross-legged position of yoga shown in Figure 27-2. Otherwise, sit in a straight-backed chair with both feet flat on the floor. Place your hands on your thighs; palms may be down or up. The spine should be straight from head to low back.

3. Take three or four deep breaths. As you inhale, let your abdomen expand, then let the chest expand. As you start to exhale let the chest contract, then let the abdomen contract. Feel your body beginning to relax.

4. Now, give your full attention to counting. Do not try to regulate your breathing; let your body regulate the depth and rate. Inhale, then as you start to exhale, think "1." As you start the next exhalation, think "2." Continue up to 4, then start over with 1. You may think "and" during each inhalation if that helps to keep your attention on counting. Do not focus on the breathing itself. *Focus on counting, but coordinate the count with exhaling.*

5. Continue breath counting for 5 to 10 minutes the first time, gradually increasing the total time to 20 minutes. As your concentration improves, you will have fewer distracting thoughts and the time will pass more quickly. When you have achieved a high level of

**FIGURE 27-2** One meditation posture.
*Delmar/Cengage Learning*

concentration, you will be surprised when the timer sounds—"I can't believe 20 minutes have passed already!"

6. Sit quietly for a few minutes. As you get up to resume your activities, try to maintain the meditative sense of peace and harmony.

## A Guided Imagery Meditation

The purpose of this meditation is to balance body energies and promote a sense of well-being. Follow the preparation steps for Relaxation to put yourself into a relaxed state, then use the following steps:

1. Imagine that you have a pipeline running from the end of your spine down through the chair, through the floor, and through the ground right to the center of the earth.

2. Now focus your attention on your feet and their contact with the earth. (Actually, they are probably in contact with the floor, but think of this as being in touch with Mother Earth.) **Visualize** energy rising through the pipeline from the earth and passing through your feet and up your legs. Feel this energy passing into your body, up the abdomen and chest, up the face and over the head, then down the spine and into the pipeline. Visualize this flowing energy picking up any aches and pains, any anger or grief, any and all negativity as it flows through you and into the pipeline. (Yes, you are "flushing" the negativity out of your body!) Continue to run earth energy until your body begins to feel lighter; this could take from one to five minutes.

3. Now visualize a brilliant white light coming from above and entering the top of your head. Let this light flow through your torso, down your legs, and into your feet and toes. Let more light flow into your neck and shoulders and down your arms into the hands and

fingers. Feel this light filling your entire body and spreading out from your body about 18 inches, so that you are within a capsule of healing, protective light. Experience the light until you are ready to end your meditation.

4. Open your eyes and sit quietly for several minutes. You should feel refreshed and energized. Try to maintain the meditative sense of peace and harmony as you resume your activities.

## USING POSITIVE AFFIRMATIONS

Tension, stress, anger, anxiety—all of these may be due to negative thoughts and feelings. Self-criticism and the memory of a bad experience, lived over and over in the mind, create and maintain a state of stress. Mindfulness is one approach to controlling negative mind-talk. Another approach is the use of affirmations to enhance the effectiveness of Relaxation and meditation.

An affirmation is a positive thought or statement that provides an alternative to negative self-talk. An affirmation should be short, positive, and related to feelings or beliefs. It should be stated in the present tense: "I am . . ." rather than "I will be . . ." The affirmation can be repeated silently during a Relaxation or in a quiet moment at the beginning or completion of a meditation. The affirmation can also be written on a card that you carry with you, tape to your mirror, or place in any location where you will see it frequently. Repeat your affirmation mentally at intervals throughout the day to maintain a positive state of mind and reinforce the positive feeling or belief.

You have now learned several methods for managing stress. As students in a health care educational program, you experience the stress of assignments and tests. As you carry out clinical assignments, you experience the stress of the health care setting, which may be somewhat overwhelming to you at first. In addition, you experience the stress associated with your other life roles. Recognize that you are subject to many stressors and be good to yourself. Eat right, sleep right, take time to play, and use a stress management technique at least once each and every day!

## REFERENCES AND SUGGESTED READINGS

> **Note:** *Indicates a "classic" reference that introduced new ideas.

Buchanan, Jim. (2007). *Labyrinth for the spirit.* New York: Sterling.
Davis, Martha, et al. (2008). *The relaxation and stress reduction workbook* (6th ed.) Oakland, CA: Harbinger.
Gawain, Shakti. (2002). *Creative visualization: Meditation exercises to enrich your life.* New York: Simon & Schuster.
Hoffman, Elizabeth. (2006). *Staying focused in the age of distraction.* Oakland, CA: New Harbinger.
*Jacobson, E. (1938). *Progressive relaxation.* Chicago, IL: University of Chicago Press.
*Jacobson, E. (1991). *You must relax.* New York: National Foundation for Progressive Relaxation.
Jacobson, James. (2005). *How to meditate with your dog: An introduction to meditation.* Kihei, HI: Maui Media.
Kabat-Zinn, Jon. (2005). *Wherever you go, there you are.* New York: Hyperion.
Novak, Jyotish. (2009). *How to meditate: A step-by-step guide to the art and science.* Nevada City, CA: Crystal Clarity.

## REVIEW AND SELF-CHECK

1. Explain the difference between *mind-talk* and *mindfulness*.

2. Explain the difference between Relaxation, as explained in this unit, and the common meaning of relaxation.

3. State two reasons that recreational activities are not fully adequate for management of stress.

4. Name the primary physiological change that occurs during:
   a. Relaxation
   b. Meditation

5. Name three psychological changes that are experienced by long-term meditators.

6. Name two reasons a health care provider should use one or more stress management techniques daily.

7. Name the major disadvantage of meditation as a therapeutic tool.

8. List five statements related to feelings or beliefs that you could use as positive affirmations.

## ASSIGNMENTS

1. For one week, list the stressors you experience in class, in the clinical area, at home, and in your various relationships.

2. Indicate with an "A" the stressors that arouse anxiety.

3. Use the following two procedures, adapted from exercises in Dr. Dacher's book *Psychoneuroimmunology*. Use a clock or watch, preferably with a second hand, to time certain steps as indicated below.

    a. To become aware of the power of mind-talk to control your mind:

    - Settle into a comfortable position, note the time, close your eyes.
    - For three minutes, be aware of any thoughts that occur to you.
    - Notice how one thought leads to another, in endless procession.
    - Begin to label each thought as it occurs: a memory, expectation about a future event, a judgment about an event or someone, something you like or dislike.
    - Become aware of any feelings that arise as certain thoughts occur: fears, anxieties, anger, guilt, pleasure.
    - For the next two minutes, count the thoughts that occur. Open your eyes and note the position of the second hand and the minute hand. Now, give your full attention to your breathing, excluding all thoughts of any type. As soon as a thought occurs, note the positions of the second hand and minute hand. How long were you able to focus on your breathing without any thought occurring? You probably maintained the focus on your breathing for only a few seconds, certainly for less than a minute. This illustrates the power of mind-talk.

    b. To learn how mindfulness can control mind-talk:

    - Observe your breathing—the movement of air in and out of your nostrils, the movement of the chest wall, or the expansion and contraction of the abdomen during inspiration and expiration.
    - When a thought occurs, be aware that your attention has shifted from focusing on the breath to focusing on mind-talk. Without trying to control it, just quietly observe your mind-talk. *Note that as you observe without getting involved*, your body becomes more relaxed.
    - Gently return to focusing on the breath. Each time a thought occurs, repeat these two steps. The length of time you can maintain your focus on the breath will increase with practice. Now, you should also be more aware of how mind-talk automatically controls your attention, *unless you take conscious control*.

> **Note:** The previous exercise introduces you to the first stage of mindfulness—attention. The next two stages, concentration and meditation, may be achieved as you practice Relaxation and, if you choose to do so, one or more meditation exercises.

4. For the next two weeks, use a Relaxation technique before breakfast or dinner.

5. For the following two weeks, try a different Relaxation technique.

6. After you have completed Assignment 5, try a third method. Then plan a long-range stress management program using the method you prefer.

7. Optional: After you have mastered one or more Relaxation techniques, try a simple meditation once a day for at least one month. If you find meditation beneficial, read about meditation as you continue to practice. You may eventually outgrow simple meditations and want to explore some of the more complex types of meditation. Many of the references listed under References and Suggested Readings in Units 24, 25, and 26 provide guidance and/or meditation procedures.

# Glossary

**abstinence:** voluntary avoidance of a specific substance or behavior.
**abuse:** improper treatment; may be verbal or physical, resulting in injury to the victim; also, may be sexual, involving a child or unwilling adult.
**abuse, drug:** misuse or overuse of a drug, legal or illegal.
**acceptance:** approval or belief in an idea, someone, or something.
**ADD:** acronym for *attention deficit disorder.*
**addiction:** physiological dependence on a substance; cessation results in withdrawal symptoms.
**ADHD:** acronym for *attention deficit hyperactivity disorder.*
**adjustment:** the degree to which one is dealing successfully with life situations.
**adrenalin:** the hormone produced by the adrenal glands during emotion-arousing situations; increases muscular strength and endurance; prepares the individual for "fight or flight."
**advanced medical directive (AMD):** a legal document which specifies an individual's wishes in regards to end-of-life care.
**affirmation:** a positive statement that fosters a sense of well-being, often used in association with Relaxation or meditation.
**affluent:** having an abundance; wealthy.
**aggression:** a form of behavior that usually indicates hostility; may take the form of verbal attack, physical attack, or refusal to cooperate.
**alcoholism:** physiological dependence on alcohol.
**allopathic:** pertaining to therapy that relies primarily on drugs; as currently used, refers to medical practice in which drug therapy and surgery are the most common forms of treatment.
**alternative therapy:** a nonallopathic therapy; term preferred by most practitioners is *complementary therapy.*
**alternatives:** two available choices.
**altruism:** concern about the well-being of others; may lead one to perform charitable acts.
**ambiguity:** vagueness or lack of clarity.
**AMD:** acronym for *advance medical directive.*
**analgesic:** substance that relieves pain without causing loss of consciousness; less potent than a narcotic.
**anticipatory grief:** grieving experienced during a terminal illness, or before the death of a loved one.
**appraisal:** an evaluation or estimate.
**aptitudes:** natural tendencies, talents, or capabilities. Those who have an aptitude for a specific area (e.g., mathematics) learn material related to that area more easily than someone who does not have that aptitude.
**aspiration:** goal, desire for achievement.
**assume (verb):** to make an assumption, to accept something as true without facts or proof.
**assumption:** acceptance of something as fact without evidence or proof.
**attention deficit disorder (ADD):** a chronic condition characterized by inattention, or difficulty focusing on and completing tasks.
**attention deficit hyperactivity disorder (ADHD):** a chronic condition characterized by inattention and hyperactive or impulsive behavior.
**attitude:** disposition toward something specific; includes feelings, beliefs, and behavior.
**autism:** a developmental disorder which affects communication and social interaction.
**autism spectrum disorder:** one of several related developmental disorders, which include classic autism, Asperger's syndrome, and pervasive development disorder—not otherwise specified (PDD-NOS).

**autonomic nervous system:** the part of the nervous system that controls the activity of vital organs.
**autonomy:** the state of functioning independently, without outside control or direction.
**bereavement:** separation from or loss of someone who is very significant in one's life.
**biorhythm:** the rhythmic or cyclic patterns of various physiological processes and functions.
**blood lactate:** the level of lactic acid in the blood stream.
**brain death:** condition in which cerebral functions, brain stem functions, or both are absent.
**burnout:** a state of physical and mental exhaustion due to cumulative stress.
**capabilities:** unexpressed traits that may be developed under the proper conditions.
**chromosomes:** rod-shaped bodies that carry the genes containing hereditary characteristics; each cell (except the germ cells) has 46 chromosomes in the nucleus.
**circadian rhythms:** intrinsic rhythms with a period of 24 to 25 hours; especially relevant to the sleep cycle.
**clarification:** explanation or qualification of something.
**codependency:** relationship in which the dysfunctional behavior (usually alcoholism or drug addiction) of one person meets certain needs of the other (e.g., a wife receives satisfaction from "rescuing" her alcoholic husband).
**collaborate:** to cooperate with, work together toward a common goal.
**comatose:** in a coma, unconscious.
**compassion:** concern for the suffering or misfortune of another.
**compatible:** able to exist together.
**compensation:** (1) a defense mechanism in which a substitution of some type provides temporary relief from the discomfort of an unmet need, but does not actually satisfy the need; (2) some form of payment or reward.
**complementary therapy:** a nonallopathic therapy.
**condolences:** expressions of sympathy.
**conformity:** tendency to be like others, to observe the conventions of a group.
**congenital:** a condition present at the time of birth.
**consequence:** the result of an action or behavior.
**conservator:** one who has been legally designated to protect the interests of a person who is unable to manage his or her affairs.
**convalescence:** the period of recovery from an illness or accident.
**coping skills:** the skills needed for dealing effectively with various life experiences.
**counterpart:** having the same function or occupying the same level of position.
**covert:** hidden, not observable; opposite of *overt*.
**cremation:** the disposal of a corpse by means of fire or intense heat.
**criterion:** a standard used as a basis for a judgment or decision.
**culpable:** being held responsible for; guilty; being blamed.
**cultural bias:** a misjudgment about a person or group because of his or her cultural background or social class.
**curative:** tending to cure or heal.
**cynicism:** distrustful of human nature or motives.
**debilitating:** weakening; impairing one's strength.
**defense mechanism:** a mental device that helps one avoid uncomfortable feelings or makes one's behavior seem more reasonable.
**dehydration:** condition in which the body lacks adequate water to maintain body functions; if severe, can lead to a life-threatening imbalance of body chemistry.
**denial:** (1) a tendency to avoid recognizing or acknowledging a situation that, if not denied, would cause emotional pain or embarrassment; (2) the usual immediate reaction to an unfavorable diagnosis; (3) the first stage of dying, according to Dr. Kübler-Ross.
**dependency:** reliance on someone or something for support.

**derogatory:** critical or disrespectful.
**desensitize:** to make a person less sensitive to something; to alter reactions to some situation or event.
**desertion reaction:** a form of withdrawal that may occur when a very young child or an elderly person is left in the care of someone other than a family member.
**detachment:** aloofness; withdrawal; usually associated with suppression of feelings.
**developmental disorders:** physical or mental disorders which affect a child's development, often causing the individual to learn or to meet developmental milestones at a slower than typical rate.
**deviation:** a variation from normal or some established standard.
**digital:** using the fingers or toes.
**discrimination:** different treatment of a person because of some specific characteristic, such as age, gender, race, religion, national origin, or economic status.
**disguised behavior:** behavior used by a person to cover up true feelings.
**displacement:** a defense mechanism in which strong feelings (usually anger) about one person are transferred or directed to someone else who did not initially arouse the feelings.
**distress:** a state of discomfort that is due to long-term stress or ineffective ways of managing stress.
**DNA:** acronym for deoxyribonucleic acid, the substance that contains the hereditary makeup of each cell.
**DNR:** acronym for *do not resuscitate*.
**do not resuscitate (DNR):** a legal document that states that an individual should not be resuscitated in the event of cardiac or respiratory arrest.
**dolorology:** a medical specialty concerned with pain management.
**dosha:** in Ayurvedic medicine, refers to classification of body type as kapha, pitta, or vata.
**DPA:** acronym for *durable power of attorney*.
**durable power of attorney (DPA):** a legal document designating an agent to act on one's behalf in the event one becomes incapacitated.
**dynamic:** characterized by ongoing changes; energetic.
**dysfunctional:** faulty or disturbed function.
**dyslexia:** a developmental disorder that affects reading.
**egocentric:** concerned primarily with self.
**emotions:** inner feelings that are responses to life situations, memories, or thoughts.
**empathy:** ability to identify with another person's situation and understand the feelings and reactions of that person.
**empirical:** based on observation and experience, rather than on experimental data.
**empowerment:** becoming stronger and more confident.
**enabler:** one who facilitates another's addictive behavior by helping the addict gain access to the addictive substance.
**enunciation:** the uttering of sounds; may be clear or unclear to the listener.
**ethical:** conforming to standards of conduct established for a specific group or culture.
**ethics:** standards of conduct, a code of behavior for a specific group; medical ethics are the standards of conduct to be observed by health care providers.
**ethnic:** relating to race or nationality; groups of people classed together because of customs, traits, and common beliefs.
**euthanasia:** administration of a lethal substance to a person who is dying and in great pain; also called *mercy killing*.
**excellence:** the quality of being extremely good.
**expectation:** something one thinks will occur.
**external locus of control:** the belief that various factors outside oneself control the events of one's life.

**family dynamics:** the interactions between and among members of a family.
**fantasy:** unrestrained imagination; may be related to a specific aspect of life, such as sexual fantasy.
**FAS:** see *fetal alcohol syndrome*.
**fetal alcohol syndrome (FAS):** a pattern of growth, mental, and physical problems that a child develops as a result of the mother's consumption of alcohol during pregnancy.
**frustration:** any blocking of progress toward a desired goal.
**gene:** unit that carries a hereditary trait.
**genetic:** carried by the genes; pertaining to heredity.
**genome:** the complete set of genes present in a cell or organism.
**genotype:** the specific hereditary makeup of a person.
**grief work:** the process of working through the emotional reaction to loss; generally considered to last at least one year.
**guided imagery:** a meditation in which another person or recorded instructions guide the mental visualization of a particular experience, such as a journey up the mountain.
**habits:** established behavior patterns; series of actions that may occur without conscious effort.
**habituation:** psychological dependence, need, strong desire.
**hallucinogenic:** causing a person to hallucinate, to perceive sights and sounds that are not actually present.
**hassle:** an annoyance.
**herbalism:** the use of herbs for a variety of purposes, including medicinal uses.
**hereditary:** traits inherited from the parents.
**heredity:** the transmission of characteristics from parents to offspring.
**heterosexual:** sexual preference for someone of the opposite sex.
**hierarchy:** arrangement in a specific order or rank from lowest to highest; vertical relationships.
**hindrance:** resistance or obstruction.
**holism:** the belief system that encompasses holistic ideas.
**holistic health care:** perceiving the whole and all of its parts; the philosophy that healing occurs most readily when all aspects of the patient are considered.
**homeostasis:** the balance of chemicals and hormones necessary for normal physiological functioning.
**homosexual:** sexual preference for someone of the same gender.
**horizontal communication:** communication between people on the same level; no one has authority over the others.
**hospice:** facility for the care of terminally ill patients, based on a death-with-dignity philosophy.
**hostility:** anger, either specific or general; may be the basis for aggressive tendencies.
**Human Genome Project:** a scientific research project between 1990 and 2003 that identified all the genes in human DNA.
**humane:** characterized by compassion, sympathy, and consideration.
**hypnosis:** trancelike condition usually induced by another person, in which the subject is receptive to suggestions.
**imminent:** about to occur; may include a sense of threat.
**immortal:** capable of living forever, never dying.
**impending:** to occur soon.
**incapacitated:** incapable of functioning.
**incest:** sexual intercourse between persons whose blood relationship makes it illegal for them to marry; usually involves parent/child, brother/sister, or uncle/niece; may be an aspect of child abuse.
**incompatible:** unable to exist together harmoniously.
**inconsistency:** differing from one occurrence to another.
**individual worth:** right to be valued and respected as a human being, regardless of personal circumstances or qualities.

**institutionalize:** to place someone in an institution such as a hospital, nursing home, or psychiatric facility; may be voluntary or involuntary.
**intention:** a specific purpose (a conscious thought) for a particular action.
**interment:** burial.
**internal locus of control:** the belief that one can utilize inner resources to influence events.
**intervention:** any action performed with the intention of changing what is happening; actions to control or stop a disease process; actions to prevent harm; actions to promote healing.
**invasive:** (1) intrusion into or through body tissues, as by cutting in a surgical procedure or introducing an instrument into an internal organ or body cavity; (2) tending to spread or infiltrate.
**invulnerable:** immune to sickness, injury, or attack.
**kapha:** in Ayurvedic medicine, one of three body types.
**learning:** a change in behavior resulting from acquisition of knowledge and development of a skill.
**lethargy:** abnormal drowsiness, sluggishness.
**litigation:** a lawsuit.
**malingering:** deliberate pretending of illness when there is none.
**manipulative:** using various strategies to influence others in order to obtain something.
**martyr complex:** psychological condition in which a person derives satisfaction from being taken advantage of by another person.
**mastectomy:** surgical removal of a breast.
**mediocre:** performance that is acceptable but not good.
**melatonin:** a hormone that is secreted by the brain as night approaches, creating readiness for sleep.
**menopause:** the period when production of sex hormones decreases.
**meridians:** in Chinese medicine, 12 energy channels that extend through the body on the vertical plane.
**message discrepancy:** difference in meaning between the message sent and the message received; may be due to lack of agreement between the sender's verbal and nonverbal messages.
**metaphysics:** branch of philosophy that is concerned with the nature of being and existence.
**mind-set:** mental readiness to react in a specific way.
**mind-talk:** the stream of thoughts and memories that runs through the mind when it is not focused on a mental task or on an experience that requires attention; may interfere with going to sleep; if uncontrolled, can be a source of stress.
**mortality:** subject to dying.
**narcotic:** addictive type of drug used medically to relieve pain.
**NDE:** acronym for *near-death experience*.
**near-death experience:** being close to death but surviving; some individuals report various transcendent or spiritual experiences.
**necrosis:** death of tissues in a limited area.
**neglect:** failure to pay appropriate attention or, in the case of a child, provide essential needs.
**neurotransmitter:** chemical substances that transmit impulses in the brain and nerves.
**noradrenalin:** hormone produced by the adrenal medulla during emotion-arousing situations.
**nurturing:** providing nourishment and the kind of care that encourages growth and development.
**omnipotent:** unlimited power.
**oppositional defiant disorder:** a behavioral disorder in which the individual defies any type of authority; during childhood, rebellion against the authority of parents and teachers.
**orthodox:** according to established doctrine.
**overt:** obvious, observable; opposite of *covert*.
**palliative:** relieving or controlling symptoms without healing the underlying disease process.
**paradigm:** a model, example, or pattern.
**paraphilia:** diagnostic term for a variety of atypical sexual behaviors.
**paraphrase:** restate; express a meaning in different words.

**passive aggression:** indirect resistance, sometimes while giving the appearance of cooperation; may be due to covert hostility.

**Patient Self-Determination Act:** law passed by Congress in 1990 requiring health care facilities to inform patients about advance health care directives upon admission to the facility.

**patriarchal:** attributing supremacy to the father or a father figure; lineage through the male parent.

**pedophile:** one whose sexual interest is directed toward children.

**pedophilia:** sexual activity between a child under the age of 13 and someone 5 to 10 years older than the child; a type of child abuse.

**perception:** use of the senses to become aware of something.

**perfectionism:** excessive concern about order and what is right; holding *perfect* as the standard of what is acceptable.

**perpetrator:** those who have committed some type of offense or crime.

**phenotype:** an organism's physical type; a set of characteristics that establish physical appearance.

**philosophy:** a theory or set of beliefs held by a person or group that serves as a guide for behavior.

**physiological:** dealing with the functions and vital processes of living organisms; the physical aspect of being, rather than the mental, emotional, or spiritual aspects.

**pitta:** in Ayurvedic medicine, one of three body types.

**placebo:** inactive substance administered instead of a specific therapy.

**placebo effect:** beneficial effect of a placebo, usually reflecting the expectations of the patient, health care provider, or both.

**plateau:** an elevated area or surface.

**posthypnotic:** the period following hypnosis.

**potency:** strength, as in a drug or homeopathic remedy.

**potential:** hidden or undeveloped trait, quality, or talent. (Ability is a quality or talent that has been developed. A characteristic is a trait that has been developed.)

**potentiation:** the increase in potency with each successive dilution of a homeopathic remedy.

**prana:** breath, in Ayurvedic medicine, yoga, and culture of India.

**prejudice:** a preconceived opinion held without regard for the facts; generalized negative feelings toward a person or group because of race, sex, or subculture.

**prepubescent:** child who has not yet experienced the physical changes that accompany puberty.

**probability:** the likelihood that something will occur; stated numerically in science and statistics.

**procrastinate:** to put off doing something until a later time.

**proficient:** skillful.

**prognosis:** predicted course or outcome of a disease or injury.

**prosthesis:** an artificial replacement for a missing body part.

**proxy:** one who has been designated to act on behalf of another person.

**PSDA:** acronym for *Patient Self-Determination Act*.

**psychoanalysis:** method of treating mental/emotional disorders by discovering and analyzing repressed memories, emotional conflicts, and past traumas.

**psychopharmaceutical:** drug that has specific effects on the mind, emotions, or mood, usually by altering brain chemistry.

**psychophysiological illness:** physical disorder due to mental and emotional factors, usually involving an organ or functions controlled by the autonomic nervous system; also known as *psychosomatic illness*.

**psychosomatic:** relating to the interaction of the mind and body.

**psychotherapy:** treatment of mental and emotional illness through one or more psychological techniques.

**psychotic:** mentally ill, out of touch with reality.

**quackery:** the use of ineffective techniques in the pretense of healing, for the purpose of financial gain rather than a desire to help the sick.

**quality control:** a system of checks to ensure that specific standards are maintained.
**quality of life:** the characteristics of one's life situation; may vary from extremely poor to excellent.
**rapport:** a relationship in which there is mutual acceptance, understanding, and respect.
**reflecting:** indicating an awareness of another person's emotional state by "mirroring" his or her feelings.
**regression:** exhibiting behaviors that are appropriate to an earlier stage of development.
**REM:** acronym for *rapid eye movement*.
**REM sleep:** the phase of sleep during which dreaming occurs.
**repertoire:** the complete range of skills possessed by a person; in music, the complete range of musical works a musician is prepared to perform.
**repression:** the storing of unexpressed feelings and the associated painful memories in the unconscious.
**reprimand:** a stern reproof or censure for a fault or mistake.
**resentment:** chronic anger that is not consciously expressed, but may be an unconscious influence on behavior.
**resilience:** the ability to bounce back after a bad experience.
**resuscitation:** the reviving of a person who is apparently dead.
**ritual:** acts that are repeated in a specific form.
**role:** the duties and behaviors expected of a person in a specific situation.
**satisfaction:** an inner feeling of pride or pleasure.
**selective observing:** a tendency to notice certain details of a situation while ignoring or overlooking other details.
**self-concept:** all the things a person believes to be true of himself or herself; may be realistic or unrealistic.
**self-confidence:** believing in oneself as a competent person.
**self-control:** a learned behavior pattern for expressing feelings and dealing with life situations in socially acceptable ways.
**self-deception:** seeing oneself incorrectly; lack of self-awareness.
**self-reliant:** ability to depend upon oneself; confidence in one's own judgment, decisions, abilities, and coping skills.
**separation anxiety:** extreme anxiety that a child may develop when a caregiver is absent or about to leave.
**sexism:** belief or attitude that one sex is inferior to the other; often the basis for discrimination.
**sexual deviation:** often used instead of "perversion" to refer to atypical sexual behavior.
**sexual taboo:** a sexual practice that is forbidden in a specific cultural group.
**sexual variation:** used to refer to any type of sexual deviation.
**sexually transmitted disease (STD):** an infectious disease which is transferred from one individual to another through sexual contact.
**similarity:** a state of resembling something or someone, without being identical; having some of the same characteristics.
**sleep debt:** a state of sleep deprivation.
**sleep deprivation:** loss of sleep; failure to have 6 to 8 hours of sleep every 24 hours.
**social needs:** psychological, emotional, mental, and spiritual needs that can only be satisfied through relationships with other people.
**socioeconomic:** relating to a combination of social and economic factors.
**stance:** a mode of standing or positioning of the body and feet.
**standard:** a level of quality against which something can be measured.
**STD:** acronym for *sexually transmitted disease*.
**stress:** physiological response (internal and adaptive) to extreme or chronic emotional states.
**stressors:** outside influences that arouse some type of emotional response.

**subluxation:** displacement of a vertebra; diagnostic term used by chiropractors.
**subtle:** delicate, refined, not obvious.
**suffocation:** death from lack of oxygen due to the face (nose and mouth) being covered.
**superstition:** a commonly held but unjustified belief.
**suppression:** not expressing, holding in or down.
**survivor guilt:** tendency of a survivor to feel guilty for being alive, especially when someone else did not survive an accident.
**sympathy:** concern for another person, especially one who is experiencing illness, trauma, or crisis.
**synergism:** increased effectiveness or potency of a substance when combined with another substance.
**taboo:** forbidden in a specific culture or circumstance.
**temperament:** the type of emotional state (positive or negative) that characterizes a person.
**teratogens:** any substances that cause abnormalities in a fetus.
**thanatology:** the study of death and dying.
**TLC:** acronym for *tender loving care*.
**trait:** a quality or characteristic.
**transference:** unconsciously directing one's feelings about one person toward another person.
**transformation:** a change in outward appearance, structure, character, or condition.
**unique:** one of a kind.
**vacillate:** waver or hesitate in making a choice, especially between alternatives or among options.
**valid:** true or correct; having legal force.
**value system:** the importance attached to various aspects of living, such as beliefs, ideas, objects, and relationships.
**variable:** a factor that has an influence or ability to bring about change.
**vata:** in Ayurvedic medicine, one of three doshas, or body types.
**verbalize:** express in words; often used to indicate oral expression, rather than written.
**vertical communication:** communication between people at different levels of authority.
**vicious cycle:** recurring behaviors or events that maintain an unsatisfactory situation; will continue unless a change is made to interrupt the cycle.
**visualize:** process of forming a mental image.
**withdrawal:** the shutting off of communication or physical removal of oneself from a situation; may serve as a defense mechanism in a specific situation; indication of emotional or mental illness when there is retreat from reality and refusal to interact with others.
**withdrawal (drug-related):** withholding a substance to which someone is addicted; the group of symptoms that occur as the body reacts to absence of the addictive substance.
**yang:** Chinese conception of the masculine; everything is either yang or yin.
**yin:** Chinese conception of the feminine; harmony results from a perfect balance of yin and yang.

# Index

**A**
AA (Alcoholics Anonymous), 186
Abstinence, 185
Abuse
 child, 53, 106, 160–62
 domestic, 163–68
 elder, 163
 sexual, 53, 160, 161, 162–63
 verbal, 80
Abusers, domestic violence, 163–64
Acceptance, 89–96
 during adolescence, 92–93
 appreciation, 95
 approval from others, 91–92
 belief that others care, 93–94
 conformity, 92–93
 empathy and, 94
 of the illness, 389
 importance of, 89–90
 need for, 89–96
 of patient, 391
 by patients, 240
 as stage in dying process, 347
 sympathy, 94
Accidents, traumatic experience of, 157
ACOA (Adult Children of Alcoholics), 186
Active euthanasia, 316
Acupressure, 420
Acupuncture, 377, 415, 418–19
Adapting behavior to patient, 259–60
ADD (attention deficit disorder), 149
Addiction, 49, 187, 189–90
ADHD (attention deficit hyperactivity disorder), 149
Adjustment, 121–31
 burnout avoidance, 129
 with coping skills, 150–51
 daily hassles and, 125, 126
 to death of family member/friend's, 147
 defense mechanisms and, 190–91
 defined, 121
 to divorce, 146–47
 with effective vs. ineffective behavior, 122–23
 emotions and, 124
 good, 121, 137
 healthy lifestyle and, 128
 helping patients with, 258–60
 improving, 125–31
 inner conflict and, 203–4
 life span, gains and losses in, 305
 to new situations, 130–31
 poor, 122
 reaction to illness and, 229
 to role of health care provider, 131
 role of joy and laughter, 128–29
 after significant loss(es), 305
 after traumatic experience, 170–71
Adjustment, common threats to, 137–51
 during adolescence, 139–40, 142–43
 during adulthood, 140–41, 143–45
 behavior disorders, 150
 change, 138, 145–47
 during childhood, 138–39, 142
 chronic stressors, 147–50
 coping skills, 138, 150–51
 death of family member or friend, 147
 developmental disorders, 149–50
 discrimination, 143
 divorce, 146–47
 family difficulties, 147–48
 financial problems, 147
 illness, 145–46
 learning problems, 148–49
 new experiences, 145
 resilience, 151
 sexism/sexual discrimination, 143–44
 sexual harassment, 144–45
 social stressors, 141–45
 traumatic events, 155
Adolescence
 acceptance during, 92–93
 adjustments during, 139–40, 142–43
 coping with loss during, 302
 death of a parent during, 299–300
 gains and losses in, 302
 inner conflict, 198–99
 sense of self during, 79
 sexual activity/relationships, 139, 142–43
 sexual relationships, 139
 stressors of, 142–43
Adrenalin, 101, 106–7
Adult abuse, 163
Adult Children of Alcoholics (ACOA), 186
Adulthood. *See also* Elderly, the
 adjustment, threat to, 140–41, 143–45
 aggressive behavior in, 248, 251
 coping with loss during, 302–4
 frustration experienced in, 215
 gains and losses during, 302–4
 sexual harassment during, 144–45
 stressors in, 143–45
Advance medical directive (AMD), 321, 322, 324
Affection, 104
Affirmations, 436
Affluence, 23–24
Aggression, patient, 246–48, 251
AIDS, 369
Al-Anon, 186
Alcohol abuse, 184–86, 188–89
Alcoholics Anonymous (AA), 186
Alcoholism, 185
Allopathic, 363
Alpha rhythms, 432
Alternatives, inner conflict and, 197
Alternative therapies, 401–24. *See also* Complementary therapies
 ayurvedic medicine, 415–16
 chiropractic, 408
 defined, 364
 education and credentials for, 402–3
 energy medicine, 407
 homeopathy, 411–14
 legitimate therapy, defined, 402
 naturopathy, 408–9
 osteopathy, 407
 traditional Chinese medicine, 414–15
Altruism, 104
Ambiguity, in communication, 282
American Public Health Association, 317
Amino acids, 380
Analgesic drugs, 199
Anatomy of an Illness as Perceived by the Patient, 128
Ancient Greece, 366
Anger, 100
 dealing with, 112–13, 124
 domestic violence and, 157, 161
 explained, 105–6
 grief and, 332
 as stage of dying, 347
 with traumatic fear and accidents, 157
Annoyance, 105
Anticipatory grief, 331
Antisepsis, 368
Anxiety, 107, 169, 431
Appraisal, 84
Appreciation, need for, 95
Apprehension, 107
Approach-approach conflict, 199–200
Approach-avoidance conflict, 200
Approval from others, 91–92
Approval, self. *See* Self-approval, need for
Aptitudes, 84
Arguing, by patient, 251

455

Aspirations, 211
Assistance to families of dying patient, 339
Assumption, verbal communication, 283, 284–85
AT (autogenic training), 431, 436–37
Attention deficit disorder (ADD), 149
Attention deficit hyperactivity disorder (ADHD), 149
Attitude
　frustration and, 212
　health care worker, 263
Attorney, durable power of, 320–21, 322
Autism spectrum disorders, 149–50
Autogenic training (AT), 431, 436–37
Automobile accidents, 157
Autonomy, 77–78
Avoidance-avoidance conflict, 200–201
Ayurvedic medicine, 415–16

## B
Bargaining, as stage of dying, 347
Bastyr College, 409
Behavior
　effective vs. ineffective, 122–23
　emotions and, 114–16
　as indicator of self-concept, 75–76
　nonverbal, 271–78
　of patients, 245–53
　social needs and, 95
Behavioral effects of grief, 333
Behavioral genetics, 48
Behavior, and problems in living, 135–218
　adjustment, threats to, 137–51
　defense mechanisms, 175–91
　frustration, 209–18
　inner conflict, 197–205
　traumatic events and effects, 155–71
Behavior disorders, 150
Behavior, influences on, 45–61
　assignments, 60–61
　assuming responsibility for behavior, 56
　changing, during one's life, 54–56
　developmental process, 48–49, 52–54
　differences and similarities in people, 45–46
　environmental, 50–54
　heredity, 46–48
　modification of early learnings, 54
　personal interests, 55
　rapport with patient, 57–58
　resources, 58
Behavior, understanding human. See also Self-understanding
　acceptance need, 89–96
　adjustment and, 121–31
　emotions and. See Emotions
　influences. See Behavior, influences on
　physical needs and, 63–69
　self-approval need and, 73–87
　self-understanding and, 37

Beliefs, cultural bias and, 23
Benson, Herbert, 375, 395, 438
Bereavement, 314, 331, 332. See also Grief and bereavement
Berger, Hans, 432
Berk, Lee, 128
Beta rhythms, 432
Bias, cultural, 22–23
Bible, references to healing in, 367
Biofeedback, 376
Biorhythms, 66
Bipolar disorder, 109, 298, 299
Blaming the victim, 156–57
Blood lactate, 431
Borysenko, Joan, 406
Borysenko, Myrin, 406
Brain chemistry, 370–71
Brain wave patterns, 432
Breath-counting meditation, 440–41
Bruyere, Rosalyn, 403
Bullying, 158–59
Burnout, 129
Bush, George W., 319
Bush, Jeb, 319

## C
CAC (certified addiction counselor), 410
Caffeine, 188
Cancer therapy, 372–73
Capabilities, 210
Car accidents, alcohol-related, 185
Carey, Raymond G., 349
Caring communication, 233
Center for Disease Control and Prevention
　on alcohol-related traffic accidents, 185
Certified addiction counselor (CAC), 410
Certified Healing Touch practitioner (CHTP), 418
Certified massage therapist (CMT), 423
Certified rehabilitation counselor (CRC), 410
Challenges of health care providers, 4–5
Change
　life stages and, 138–41
　self-understanding and, 32–35
　as threat to adjustment, 138
Cheerful patients, 250, 252
Chemical dependency, 187
Child abuse, 53, 106, 160–62
Child neglect, 160
Children/childhood
　adjustments in early, 138–39
　adjustments in middle, 139
　aggressive behavior in, 247–48, 251
　with behavior problems, 150
　coping with loss in, 300–302
　death of, 313
　of divorce, 146–47
　formation of emotional patterns in, 108
　frustration experienced in, 215

grief process and, 336
influences on development during, 50–51, 52–54
with learning problems, 148–49
love in, 104
perfectionism and, 215–16
reaction to death of parent, 299
reaction to illness in, 227–28
regression in, 246
role models influencing, 54
self-concept formation during, 76–77
sense of self during, 79
sexual abuse of, 161, 162–63
stressors of, 142
Chinese medicine, traditional, 414–15
Chiropractic techniques, 377, 408
Chopra Center for Well-Being, 416
Chopra, Deepak, 416
Chromosomes, 47
Chronic stressors, 147–50
CHTP (certified Healing Touch practitioner), 418
Cigarette and nicotine addiction, 184
Circadian rhythms, 66
Clarification, 242, 243, 285
CMT (certified massage therapist), 423
Cocaine, 187
Codependency, 189–90
*Coming Home: A Guide to Home Care for the Terminally Ill* (Duda), 350
Communication, 269
　assumptions and, 284–85
　blocks to, 235
　caring, 233
　with co-workers, 261–62
　expectations and, 285
　expressing opinions, 287–88
　gender differences in, 79
　horizontal, 262
　improving skills in, 285–88
　"I talk," 111–12, 144
　listening, 284, 287
　miscommunication, 233–34
　nonverbal behavior, 271–78
　open and honest, 110–12
　with the patient, 232–35
　reasons for ineffective, 234
　techniques for helpful, 242, 243
　tone in, 283–84
　tone of voice, 283–84, 286–87
　verbal, 281–88
　verbal abuse, 80
　vertical, 261–62
　"you talk," 159
Compassion, 104
Compassion and Choices, 317
Compensation
　for physical needs, 67
　for social needs, 74–75
Complaints, by patients, 248, 251
Complementary therapies, 377, 378, 416
　acupressure, 420
　acupuncture, 418–19

defined, 364
Healing Touch, 416–18
health care provider role, 423
psychoneuroimmunology, 406–7
reflexology, 420–21
self-help trend, 423
shiatsu, 420
therapeutic massage, 421–22
Complete *Herbal*, 379
Compliments, hunger for approval and, 91
Condolences, 336
Confidentiality, 243–44
Conflict
inner. *See* Inner conflict
interpersonal, 197
Conformity, 92, 93
Confrontation, 242
Congenital defects, 49
Conscious intention, 391
Consequences (behavior patterns), 68
Conservators, 324
Control
abuser personality and, 163–64, 165
external locus of, 392
of infectious diseases, 369
internal locus of, 392
self-control, 114–15
Controlled Substances Act (1970), 187
Coping skills, adjustment and, 138, 150–51
Coping with loss, 291–357
caring for dying person, 345–57
death, changing attitudes and practices, 311–26
grief and bereavement, 331–39
life span gains and losses, 293–307
Coping with patient behavior. *See* Patient behavior, coping with
Counseling, 409–10
Counterpart, 262
Courts, involved in health care decisions, 323–24
Cousins, Norman, 128
Covert noncooperation, 248
CRC (certified rehabilitation counselor), 410
*The Creation of Health* (Shealy), 390
Crimes
alcohol use and, 185
trauma and, 157
Criticism, by patient, 251
Cruzan, Mary Beth, 320
Crying, by patient, 249–50, 251
Cultural bias, 22–23
Cultural influences
influence on children, 51
influencing pattern of striving, 68
reaction to illness and, 230
suicide and, 297–98
Curative goals, 355
Curie, Irene, 370
Curie, Marie, 370
Curie, Pierre, 370

Curing, healing *vs.*, 390–91
Cyberbullying, 159
Cynicism, 100

**D**
Dacher, Elliott, 407, 430
Daily hassles, 125, 126
Dark Ages, 367
Daydreaming, 179–80
D.C. (doctor of chiropractic), 408, 412
Death. *See also* Dying person, caring for; Grief and bereavement
accepting finality of, 335
adjustment to family member/friend's, 147
changing attitudes and practices, 311–26, 312–13
current attitudes and practices, 313–14
defining, 318
with dignity, 315
do not resuscitate (DNR) orders, 319–20
dying as a growth process, 348–50
dying at home, 315
through euthanasia, 315–16
impact of, on survivor, 295–96
life support technology and, 318–20
living will, 321–22
meaning of, 314–15
of a parent, 299–300
past attitudes and practices, 312
right-to-die, 316–17, 320–24
thanatology, 304
Death with Dignity Act (1997), 317
Debilitating treatments, 205
Decision-making, empowerment and, 10–11
Deep relaxation, 436
Defense mechanisms, 175–91
adjustment and, 190–91
codependency, 189–90
daydreaming, 179–80
defined, 175
displacement, 179
escape into illness, 181–82
projection, 178
purpose of, 175–76
rationalization, 176–77
repression, 182–83
substance dependency, 184–89
withdrawal, 183
Dehydration, 65
Denial, as stage of dying, 346–47
Dependency
on alcohol, 184–85
autonomy *vs.*, 77–78
reaction to illness and, 229–30
self-reliance *vs.*, 68–69
Depression
as reaction to trauma, 169–70
as stage of dying, 347
suicide and, 298–99

Derogatory self-concept, 76
Derogatory statements, 80
Desertion reaction, 227
"Designated agent," 352–53
Detachment, 301
Developmental disorders, 149–50, 163
Developmental process
aspects of development, 49
changing influences during life, 54–56
learning independence, 77–78
prenatal influences, 48–49
preschool influences, 52
school years, influences during, 52
social influences, 52–54
Diagnosis
from holistic perspective, 395–96
Diet, nutrition and, 380–81
Digital skills, 200
Dignity, death with, 315, 317
Disappointment, 107
Discrimination, 141, 143–44
Disguised behavior, 226
Displaced anger, 112, 157
Displacement
death of parent and, 300
as defense mechanism, 179
Divorce, adjustment to, 146–47
DNA (deoxyribonucleic acid), 46, 388–89
DNA testing, 48
D.O. (doctor of osteopathy), 407
Doctor of chiropractic (D.C.), 408, 412
Doctor of naturopathy (N.D.), 409, 412
Doctor of oriental medicine (O.M.D.), 414
Doctor of osteopathy (D.O.), 407
Doctor of veterinary medicine (D.V.M.), 412
Dolorology, 373–74
Domestic violence, 106, 163–68
abuser personality, 163–64
cycle of, 166
effects on victim of, 164–65
escaping, 166–67
hopeful signs in response to, 167–68
Do not resuscitate (DNR) orders, 319–20, 324
Dosha, in ayurvedic medicine, 415, 416
Dossey, Larry, 378
Double-blind study, 364
Double helix, 46
Dread, 107
Drug abuse, 187–89
Drug dependency, 187
Drug misuse, 187
Drugs, as adolescent stressor, 142
Duda, Deborah, 350
Durable power of attorney (DPA), 320–21, 322
D.V.M. (doctor of veterinary medicine), 412

Dying person, caring for, 345–57
   assisting families, 339
   growth process and, 348–50
   guidelines for, 356–57
   home care and, 350–51
   hospice care, 351–52
   medical issues related to, 353–54
   palliative care, 352–53
   personal and family issues related to, 350
   rights of dying person, 354–55
   roles of health care providers, 355–56
   stages of dying, 346–47
   terminal illness diagnosis and, 345–46
Dying, stages of, 346–47, 355
Dynamic, health field as, 265
Dysfunctional family dynamics, 190
Dyslexia, 149

## E

Early childhood
   adjustments during, 138–39
Echoing, 242
Effective listening, 284
Effective vs. ineffective behavior, 122–23
Egocentrism, 245, 251
Elderly, the
   abuse of, 163
   losses of, 304–5
   reaction to illness, 228–29
Emotional support
   during grieving process, 334–35
   for patient, 260
Emotions, 112–13. See also Anger; Defense mechanisms; Fear; Grief and bereavement
   adjustment and, 124
   associated with crimes and accidents, 157
   and behavior, 114–16
   constructive use of, 110–14
   dealing with, 112–14
   defined, 99
   effects of illness, 226
   gender differences in, 110
   grief, 107, 114
   guilt, 107
   importance of, 100
   individual differences in, 108–9
   intensity and frequency of, 109
   involved in inner conflicts, 202
   love, 104–5
   meaning of, 99–100
   mood swings, 109
   negative, 105–7
   nonverbal behavior and, 271–72, 273, 274–75
   open and honest communication of, 110–12
   of others, handling, 116
   pattern formations, 108
   physiological effects of, 101
   positive, 103–5
   self-control and, 114–15
   sensitivity to patient's, 244
   stress, 102–3
   suppressed, 114
   temperament, 109
   with war and terrorism, 158
Empathy, 94
Empirical evidence, 365
Empowerment, 10–11
Enabler, 190
End of life choices, 317
Energy medicine, 407
Enunciation, 283
Environmental influences
   family, and bullying, 159
   heredity and, 50
   home, 52–53
   neighborhood, 54
   physical, 50–51
   preschool years, 52
   during school years, 52
   social, 51, 52–54
   as source of frustration, 211–12
Ethical issues
   confidentiality, 243–44, 353
   of health field, 35
Ethics committees, 325–26
Ethnic culture, 53
Euthanasia, 315–16, 316–17
Euthanasia Research & Guidance Organization (ERGO), 316
Evans, Patricia, 80
Excellence, 4, 5
Expectations
   communication and, 285
   failure, 80, 81
   success, 82
Experiences, learning from, 34
External locus of control, 392

## F

Failure expectation, 80, 81
Families
   bullying and, 159
   care of the dying, 350
   codependency and, 189–90
   difficulties with, as stressor, 147–48
   of dying patient, assisting, 339
   life support and rights of, 319
   participating in dying process, 313–14
Family dynamics, 148
Fantasy, daydreaming and, 180
Fear
   dealing with, 113
   explained, 106–7
   influence on adjustment, 124
   with traumatic crimes and accidents, 157
Feelings. See Emotions
Fetal alcohol syndrome (FAS), 186
Fetal position, 183
"Fight or flight" arousal, 102
Final Exit, 317
*The Final Stage of Growth* (Kübler-Ross), 311, 348
First Freedom First, 317
Food and Drug Administration (FDA), 378
Food, need for, 65
Forgiveness, 107, 112–13
Freud, Sigmund, 370
Friendliness, 252–53
Friendships, 90
Frustration, 209–18
   coping with, 216–18
   cumulative effects of, 210
   defined, 209
   degrees of, 209–10
   effects of, 214
   learned behavior patterns and, 214–15
   perfectionism and, 215–16
   preventing, 217–18
   sources of, 210–13

## G

Gang activity, 142
Gender differences, 79, 110
General adaptation syndrome, 102
Gene therapy, 47
Genetic disorders, 47
Genetics, 46, 47, 48, 372. See also Heredity and behavior
Genetic testing, 47–48
Germ theory, 368
Goal setting, 217–18
Good adjustment, 121, 137
Good judgment, 260
Gordon, Thomas, 106, 110, 111–12
Greece, healing in, 366–67
Green, Elmer, 403
Grief and bereavement, 107
   assisting families of dying patient, 339
   dealing with, 114
   effects of, 332–33
   grief work, 331, 336–38
   health care provider role, 338–39
   importance of grief process, 333–34
   influences on grief process, 334–35
   reactions to, 332
   used as a growth experience, 305–6
Group standards, 93
Guided-imagery meditation, 441–42
Guilt, 107

## H

H1N1 virus, 369
Habits
   modifying, 83–84
   work, 33
Habituation, 187
Hahnemann, Samuel, 411
Hallucinogens, 188
Happiness, positive emotions and, 104
Hassles, 125, 126
Hate, 105
Healing and healers, 387–97
   causes of disease, 389–90
   characteristics of survivors, 391–92

curing vs., 390–91
future health care systems, 396–97
holistic health care, 392–96
immune system, 388
intention and, 391
mind/body system, 388–89
power of love and, 390
psychic, 403
Healing Touch, 416–18
Health agency, introducing a patient to, 259
Health care provider issues. *See also* Human relations with health care provider
adapting to role of, 131
advance medical directives and, 324
alternative therapies and, 403
attitudes and interests for studying, 10
care for dying patient, 324–26
challenges of, 4–5
coping with patient behavior, 239–53
cultural bias and, 22–23
with defense mechanisms, 191
empowerment, 10–11
human relations and, 257–65
illness, behavioral effects, 225–35
inner conflict in, 204–5
preparation for death-and-dying situations, 324–25
relating to the patient, 231–32
resources, 12
responsibilities of, 6–7
satisfactions of, 4
social needs, awareness of, 96
staying informed, 382
stress management for, 429–30
study habits and achievement, 8–9
Health care provider role
care of the dying, 355–56
complementary therapies and, 424
in grief and bereavement process, 338–39
in health care trends, 376
with person who suffered traumatic experience, 171
providing a therapeutic environment, 390
Health care system. *See also* Historical view of health care
accessibility and cost, 382
future, 396–97
innovations in, 376
new therapies and roles in, 377
technological advances, 377
Health care trends, 361
alternative therapies, 401–24
healing and healers, 387–97
historical view, 363–82
stress management, 429–42
Health Insurance and Portability and Accountability Act (HIPAA), 243
Healthful eating, 380–81
Healthy lifestyle, adjustment and, 128

Hemlock Society, 317
Herbalism, 379–80
Hereditary traits, 46
Heredity and behavior, 46–48
environmental influences and, 50
genetic testing, 47–48
health implications, 47
individuality and, 46–47
physiology of, 46
Heterosexuality, sexual abuse of girls and, 160
Hierarchy of needs (Maslow), 63–64
Hindrance, 83
Hinton, John, 353
Hippocrates, 366
Historical view of health care, 363–82
complementary therapies, 377, 378
current health care system, 376–77
early civilizations, 366–67
evolution of modern health care, 367–71
health care issues, 378–82
holistic medicine, 371–72
innovations, 364–66
terminology, 363–64
Holism, 414
Holistic health care, 364, 371–72
basic philosophical assumptions, 395
characteristics of, 394–95, 406
diagnosis and therapy, 395–96
lifestyle choices and, 392–93
mind/body connection and, 393–94
patient responsibility and, 403–5
theoretical basis for, 404
Home care, 350–51
Home environment, 52–53
Homeopathic medicine, 377
*Homeopathic Pharmacopoeia of the United States*, 412
Homeopathy, 411–14
Homeostasis, 409
Homosexuality, sexual abuse of boys and, 160
Honorable suicide, 297–98
Horizontal communication, 262
Hospice care, 315, 351–52
Hostility, 100, 105–6, 248–49, 251
Hudson, Larry, 122
Human care, 356
Human genome, 47
Human Genome Project, 47
Human potential movement, 409
Human relations for health care provider, 257–65
adapting behavior to patient, 259–60
adjustment to illness, 258–60
attitudes, 263
becoming member of health team, 260–64
challenges of, 265
communicating within organizational structure, 261–62
compensation and, 264
effective patient relations, 264–65

good relationship maintenance, 261
health care provider role, 261
identifying patient needs, 259
job satisfaction, standards, and self-respect, 263
providing emotional support, 260
setting the stage for practicing, 275
Humphrey, Derek, 316
Hypertension, management of, 375–76
Hypnosis, 183

I
Identical twins, 46
Illness
acceptance of, 389
adjustment to, 145–46
escape into, as defense mechanism, 181–82
helping patients adjust to, 258–60
influences on patient's reaction to, 227–31
mental, 370–71
reaction to diagnosis of terminal, 345–46
as source of frustration, 213
Illness, effects of, 225–35
emotional, 226
health care communication and, 232–35
physical, 226
with a serious illness, 226–27
Imara, Mwalinu, 348
Imminent defeat, 183
Immortality, 313
Immune system, 388
Incapacitation, 229
Incest, 160
Incompatible needs/goals, 197
Inconsistency, in messages, 283
Independence, learning, 77
Individual differences in emotional patterns, 108–9
Individual worth, philosophy of, 21–29
affluence and, 23–24
cultural bias and, 22–24
daily practice of, 25–26
implications for providers, 25
meaning of, 21–22
poverty and, 23
provider expectations, 24
resources, 26
Individuality, genetic basis for, 46–47
Infants
coping with loss, 300–301
frustration in, 214–15
Infectious diseases, history of controlling, 369
Influenza virus, 369
Inhalants, 187, 188
Inner conflict, 197–205
adjustment and, 203–4
approach-approach conflict, 199–200
approach-avoidance conflict, 200
avoidance-avoidance conflict, 200–201

Inner conflict (*continued*)
  conflict between means, 199
  conflict between needs, 198–99
  dealing with, 201–3
  health care provider and, 204–5
  meaning of, 197–98
  patient and, 205
  types of, 199–201
Inner dialogue, 439
Inner satisfaction of health care providers, 4
Institute of Noetic Sciences, 372
Intention, 391
Internal locus of control, 392
International Institute of Reflexology, 421
International Society for the Study of Subtle Energies and Energy Medicine (ISSSEEM), 367, 407
Internet, the, 159, 160–61
Interpersonal conflict, 197
Interpersonal relations. *See* Human relations for health care providers
Intuitive diagnosis, 374–75
Invasive procedure, 418
Invulnerability, 305
"I talk," 111–12, 144

## J
Jacobson, Edmund, 431, 435
Jamison, Kay Redfield, 298, 299
Janssen, Zacharias, 368
Jenner, Edward, 369
Joy, benefits of, 128
Judeo-Christian period, 366–67

## K
Kabat-Zinn, J., 430
Kapha, in ayurvedic medicine, 415, 416
Koch, Robert, 368
Koop, Everett, 405
Kübler-Ross, Elisabeth, 294, 311, 314, 315, 348, 355

## L
Language barriers, reactions to illness and, 230
Laughter, benefit of, 128–29
LCSW (licensed clinical social worker), 409
Learning
  defined, 32
  experiences and, 34
  as a health care provider, 6
  memorizing *vs.*, 32
Learning problems, as a stressor, 148–49
Learning skills, developing, 32
Legal issues. *See* Rights
Lethargy, 226
Licensed clinical psychologist, 409
Licensed clinical social worker (LCSW), 409
Licensed marriage and family therapist (LMFT), 409–10

Life roles, 35–36
Life span, gains and losses in, 293–306
  adjustment and, 305
  in adolescence, 302
  in adulthood, 302–4
  during childhood, 300–302
  coping with loss, 294
  death as loss, 295–97
  death of a parent, 399–400
  in infancy and early childhood, 300–301
  life changes as, 293–94
  loss as growth experience, 305–6
  during senescence, 304–5
  significance of loss, 294–95
  suicide and, 297–99
Life support, impact of loss and, 296–97
Lindemann, Erich, 348
Listening, 241, 242, 284, 287
Lister, Joseph, 368
Living will, 320–22
LMFT (licensed marriage and family therapist), 409–10
Loaded statements, 242
Locus of control, 392
*London Dispensary*, 379
Loneliness, grief work and, 337
Loss(es). *See also* Coping with loss; Death
  due to death, 295–97
  learning to cope with, 294
  reactions to, 332
  significance, 294–95
  suicide and, 297–99
  used as a growth experience, 305–6
Love
  defined, 104
  learning to, 104
  power of, 390
  self, 104–5
  types of, 104
  unconditional, 105
LSD, 188

## M
Malingering, 181
Manipulative skills, 200
Marijuana, 188
Martyr complex, 90
Maslow, Abraham, 63–64
Maslow's Hierarchy of Needs, 63–64
Massage, 421–22
M.D. (medical doctor), 412
Medical doctor (M.D.), 412
Medication, patient refusing, 250
Mediocre (health care provider), 11
Meditation, 373, 376
  advantages and disadvantages of, 432–33
  background, 431
  breath-counting, 440–41
  guided-imagery, 441–42
  methods and procedures, 438–42
  physical and psychological effects of, 432

principles, 439
types of, 439–40
Melatonin, 66
Memories, repressed, 182–83
Mengten, Janet, 416
Mental illness, 370–71, 409
Mental imagery, 438–39
Mental retardation, 149
Mental skills, developing, 32
Methamphetamines, 187
Middle adulthood, adjustments during, 140
Middle Ages, healing in, 367
Middle childhood, adjustments during, 139
*Mind as Healer, Mind as Slavery* (Pelletier), 393
Mind/body healing system, 388–89, 393–94
Mindfulness, 407, 430–31
Mind-set, 230
Mind-talk, 102–3, 107, 430
Minerals, 380
Minorities, prejudice and, 213
Mirroring, 242
Modern medicine, 372–76
Mood swings, 109
Mortality, 300, 313
Mourning, 312. *See also* Grief and bereavement
Murders, 296

## N
Narcotic drugs, 199
National Center for Children in Poverty (NCCP), 51
National Center for Homeopathy, 412
National Domestic Violence Hotline, 163
Natural disasters, 157–58
Naturopathy, 408–9
N.D. (doctor of naturopathy), 409, 412
Near-death experiences (NDEs), 315
Necrosis, 64
Needs. *See also* Physical needs; Self-approval, need for; Social needs
  for acceptance, 89–96
  for appreciation, 95
  identifying a patient's, 259
  Maslow's Hierarchy of, 63–64
Negative emotions, 100, 105–7
  gender differences in, 110
  temperament and, 109
Neglect, child, 160
Neurotransmitters, 370–71
*New England Journal of Medicine*, 405
Nicotine addiction, 184
Nicotine, as a drug, 188
Noncooperation, 248, 250
Nonverbal behavior, 241, 271–78
Nonviolent behavior, 167
Noradrenalin, 101
Nurturing, 51
Nutrition, 56, 380–81
Nutritional supplements, 380, 381–82

## O

Observation
    of nonverbal behavior, 272–75, 276–78
    of patient, 241
Office of Civil Rights, 243
Older adulthood, adjustments during, 141. *See also* Elderly, the
Omnipotence, 305
Opinions, expressing, 287–88
Opportunity cost, 202–3
Optimism, 109
Oregon Department of Human Services (ODHS), 317
Organic foods, 380
Osteopathy, 407
Overly cheerful patient, 250, 252
Overly friendly patient, 252–53
Over-the-counter drugs, 187
Overt noncooperation, 248
Oxygen, physical need for, 64

## P

Pain management, 373–74
Palliative care, 352–53
Palliative goals, 355
Panic, 106
Panic attacks, 113
Panic disorder, 169
Paraphrase, 284
Parent, death of a, 399–400
Parenting
    need for appreciation and, 95
    unconditional love and, 105
Passive aggression, 248
Passive euthanasia, 316
Pasteur, Louis, 369
Patient behavior, coping with, 239–53
    accepting the patient, 240
    aggression, 246–48
    appropriate communication techniques, 242, 243
    common behavior patterns, 245–53
    confidentiality and, 243–44
    crying, 249–50
    egocentrism, 245
    hostility, 248–49
    identifying patient needs, 244–45
    noncooperation, 250
    observation and listening to patients, 241
    overly cheerful patient, 250, 252
    recognizing significant behavior, 241–42
    regression, 245–46
    sensitivity to feeling behind behavior and, 239–40
    sensitivity to patient's feelings, 244
    showing interest and concern, 240–41
    strategies, 251–52
    unfriendly behavior, 246
    willingness to serve patients, 245
Patients
    acceptance of, 240
    adjusting to illness, helping with, 258–60
    common behavior patterns of, 245–53
    defense mechanisms of, 190
    effects of illness on, 225–27
    establishing rapport with, 57–58
    factors influencing reaction to illness, 227–31
    identifying needs of, 244–45
    inner conflict in, 205
    meeting needs of, 5
    safety and excellence in care of, 5
Patient Self-Determination Act (PSDA), 320, 322–23
PCP (angel dust), 188
Pedophilia, 160
Peer pressure, 142
Pelletier, Kenneth, 393, 406
People, as source of frustration, 212–13
Perception, distorted, 191
Perfectionism, 215–16
Perpetrators, 156
Personal growth, striving for, 37–38
Pervasive developmental disorder otherwise specified (PDD-NOS), 149
Pessimism, temperament and, 109
Pharmaceutical drugs, 378–79
Phenotype, 46
Philosophy of individual worth. *See* individual worth, philosophy of
Phobias, 113, 169
Physical abuse, 53
Physical aggression, 246, 247
Physical effects
    of emotions, 100
    of grief, 333
    of illness, 226
    of relaxation and meditation, 431–32
Physical environment, 50–51
Physical needs, 63–71
    assignments, 71
    comfort and safety, 67–68
    cultural influences on pattern of striving, 68
    essential, 64–66
    food, 65
    oxygen, 64
    protection, 65–66
    resources on, 69
    review on, 70
    satisfaction of, 67
    self-reliance *vs.* dependency, 68–69
    sexual, 68
    sleep, 66–67
    understanding human behavior in terms of, 69
    water, 65
Physiological effects
    of emotions, 101
    of relaxation and meditation, 431
    of stress, 102
Pitta, in ayurvedic medicine, 415
Placebo effect, 387–88, 393–94
Poliomyelitis, 369
Poor adjustment, 122
Positive affirmation, 442
Positive emotions, 103–5, 109, 110
Post-traumatic stress disorder (PTSD), 113, 169
Potential, developing your, 32
Potentiation, homeopathic, 411
Poverty, 23, 29
Power, domestic abuse and, 164, 165
Prana, in ayurvedic medicine, 415–16
Pregnancy, 186
Prejudice, 25, 213
Prenatal influences on development, 48–49
Prenatal testing, 47–48
Preschool influences on development, 52
Prescription drugs, 378–79
Problem-solving skills, 94
Procrastinate, 33
Proficient, 200
Prognosis, 205
Progressive relaxation, 431, 435–36
Projection, as defense mechanism, 178
Prostheses, 200
Protection, need for, 65–66
Proxy, 321–22
Psychiatry, 370
Psychic healers, 374–75, 403
Psychoanalysis, 183, 370
Psychological effects, of meditation and relaxation, 432
Psychoneuroimmunology, 406–7
Psychopharmaceuticals, 371
Psychophysiological medicine, 370
Psychosomatic illness, 103, 393
Psychosomatic medicine, 370
Psychotherapy, 183, 409–10

## Q

*Quantum Healing: Exploring the Frontiers of Mind/Body Medicine* (Chopra), 416
Questioning, 242, 243
Quinlan, Karen Ann, 325

## R

Radiation, 370
Rage, 105
Rape, 156–57, 162
Rapid eye movement (REM), 432
Rapport, 57–58
Rational approach to inner conflict, 202
Rationalization, as defense mechanism, 176–77
Realistic self-concept, 76, 78
Recreational drugs, 187
Reflecting, 242
Reflection, 243
Reflexology, 420–21
Regression, 245–46, 251
Relationships
    healthy, 167
    role as an influence on, 35
    sexual, during adolescence, 139
    teacher-student, 35

Relaxation, 430
    advantages and disadvantages of, 432–33
    autogenic training, 436–37
    background, 431
    methods, 435–38
    physical and psychological effects of, 431–32
    preparation, 434–35
    principles, 433–34
    progressive, 435–36
    self-directed, 437–38
REM (rapid eye movement), 66–67
Renaissance, healing in the, 367
Repertoire of human relations skills, 36
Repressed emotions, 108–9
Repression, as defense mechanism, 182–83
Reprimands, 285
Resentment, 100, 106
Resilience, 151
Resources
    behavior, influences on, 58
    individual worth, philosophy of, 26
    physical needs, 69
    self-approval, 85–86
    self-understanding, 38
Rights
    of dying person, 353, 354–55
    of patients and their families, 319
    right-to-die, 316–24
Right-to-die movement, 316–17
Roentgen, Konrad, 370
Role models, influence on children, 54
Roles. See also Health care provider role
    life roles, 35–36
    self-understanding and, 31, 34–35
    survivor, 170
Rolfing, 422
Rome, healing in, 366–67
Rubin, Sue, 149
Rucker, Henry, 374–75

## S

Sadness, 107, 124
Salaries, 263
Salk, Jonas, 369
Satisfaction
    of health care providers, 3
    job, 263
    of physical needs, 67
Schiavo, Terri, 319
School violence, 142
School years, 52
Schultz, J. H., 431, 436
Scientific model, 364–65
Seasonal affective disorder (SAD), 371
Selective observing, 272
Self-approval, need for, 73–87
    effects of success and failure, 80–82
    influence of others on, 79–80
    resources, 85–86
    review, 86–87
    self-concept, 75–78
    self-esteem, 78
    setting goals for, 83–84
    social needs, 73–75
    striving for, 83–85
    success, 82–83
Self, as source of frustration, 210–11
Self-concept, 75–78, 84, 105
Self-confidence, 4
Self-control of emotions, 114–15
Self-deception
    in health care provider, 191
    projection as, 178
    rationalization as form of, 177
Self-directed relaxation, 437–38
Self-esteem, 78
Self-forgiveness, 113
Self-help trend, 423
Self-love, 104–5
Self-reliance, 10, 77–78
    adjustment to illness and, 146
    dependency vs., 68–69
Self-study, 32–33, 36–37
Self-understanding, 31–41
    change and, 32–35
    developing potential, 32
    guidelines for growth, 36–38
    learning from experience, 34
    learning vs. memorizing, 32
    life roles and, 35–36
    personal growth guidelines, 37–38
    resources, 38
    review, 38–39
    role and role perception, 31, 34–35
    self-evaluation, 32–35
    as student, 31–32
    use of time and, 37
Selye, Hans, 102
Semmelweis, Ignaz Philipp, 368
Senescence. See Elderly, the
Separation anxiety, 138–39, 227, 301
Sexism, 143
Sexual abuse, 53, 160, 161
Sexual activity/relationships, 67, 139, 142–43
Sexual discrimination, 144
Sexual harassment, 144–45
Sexually transmitted disease (STD), 161
Sexual needs, 68
Shealy, C. Norman, 124, 373–74, 375, 379, 390, 395–96, 403, 405, 438
Shiatsu, 420
Shock, as reaction to loss, 332
Siebert, Al, 392
Siegel, Bernie, 390
Similarities (role), 35
Simonton, O. Carl, 372–73, 376, 395, 433, 438
Simonton, Stephanie, 372
Sleep
    brain wave patterns during, 432
    cycle of, 66–67
    effects of deprivation, 67
    human behavior influenced by, 56
    physical need for, 66
Sleep debt, 67
Smallpox, 369
Smoking, 184
Social environment, 51
    influences on childhood development, 52–54
Social needs, 73–75
    behavior and, 95
    compensation for, 74–75
    friendships and, 90
    need for acceptance, 89–96
    types of, 74
Socioeconomic class, 29
    cultural bias and, 22, 23–24
    influencing child's early learning, 51
    standards of behavior and, 56
Spontaneous Healing (Weil), 388–89
Stages of dying, 346–47, 355
Stalking, 162–63
Stance, 273
Standards
    of behavior, 56
    for health care provider performance, 4–5, 8
STDs (sexually transmitted diseases), 161
"Street drugs," 187
Strengths, understanding your, 33
Stress
    chronic, 394
    lifestyle choices and, 393
    mind-talk and, 102, 430
    overview, 102–3
Stress management, 429–42
    hypertension and, 375
    meditation, 431–33, 438–42
    mindfulness, 430–31
    positive affirmations, 442
    relaxation and, 430, 431–33, 433–38
Stressors
    of adolescence, 142–43
    of childhood, 142
    chronic, 147–50
    defined, 102
    mind-talk, 430
Students, health-care provider as, 83
Study plan, 16
Study skills, 10–11
Subluxation of vertebra, 408
Substance dependency
    alcohol use, 184–86
    codependency and, 189–90
    as defense mechanism, 184–89
    drug abuse, 187–89
    nicotine addiction, 184
Subtle prejudices, 213
Success, 82–83
Success expectation, 82
Suffocation, 64
Suicide, 297–99

Superstitions, cultural, 23
Suppressed emotions, 114
Suppression, 106
Survivor guilt, 296
*The Survivor Personality* (Siebert), 391
Survivor role, 170
Swedish massage, 421, 422
Sympathy, acceptance and, 94
Synergism, 380

## T
TCM (traditional Chinese medicine), 414–15
Teacher-student relationship, 35
Technological advances, 377
Temperament, 109
Tender loving care (TLC), 104
Teratogens, 49
Terminal illness diagnosis, 345–46
Terror, 106
Terrorism, trauma and, 158
Thanatology, 314
Therapeutic massage, 421–22
Therapy, holistic perspective, 395–96
Theta rhythms, 432
Time, understanding your use of, 37
Tobacco addiction, 184
Toddlers, frustration in, 215
Tone of voice, 283–84
Traditional Acupuncture Institute, 419
Traditional Chinese medicine (TCM), 414–15
Traffic accidents, alcohol use and, 185
Traits, appraisal of personal, 33
Transcendental Meditation, 376
Transcutaneous electrical nerve stimulator (TENS), 373–74
Transference, 300
Transformation through dying, 348
Trauma, defined, 156
Trauma, reactions to, 168–70
    anxiety, 169
    depression, 169–70
    individual differences in, 168
    panic disorder, 169
    phobias, 169
    post-traumatic stress disorder, 169
    recovering from traumatic event, 168
Traumatic experiences and effects, 155–71
    adjustment following, 170–71
    adult abuse, 163
    blaming the victims, 156–57
    bullying, 158–59
    child abuse and neglect, 160–62
    crimes and accidents, 157
    domestic abuse, 163–68
    health care provider role and, 155–56, 161, 171
    natural disasters, 157–58
    perpetrators, 156
    rape, 162
    repression and, 182–83
    sexual abuse, 161, 162–63
    stalking, 162–63
    survivor role, 170
    war and terrorism, 158
Treatment, drug dependency, 189
Trends in health care.
    *See* Health care trends
Twelve Step program, 186

## U
Unconditional love, 105
Uncooperative patient, 252
Understanding.
    *See* Self-understanding
Unfriendly behavior (patient), 246, 251
Unipolar disorder, 298
University of New Hampshire Crimes Against Children Research Center, 160
U.S. Department of Health and Human Services, 161
U.S. Department of Justice, 162

## V
Vaccines, 369
Vacillation, 200
Validation, 242, 243
Value system, 23, 55
Van Leeuwenhoek, Anton, 368
Variables, 364
Vata, in ayurvedic medicine, 415
Verbal abuse, 80
Verbal aggression, 248
Verbal assault, 251
Verbal communication, 281–88
    ambiguity in, 282
    assumptions in, 284–85
    discrepancies in a message, 283
    effective listening, 284, 287
    expectations and, 285
    expressing an opinion, 287–88
    improving, 285–86
    tone of voice, 283–84, 286–87
Verbalizing feelings, 226
Vertical communication, 261–62
Vesalius, 368
Vicious cycle, 122
Victims
    blaming, 156–57
    of bullying, 159
    of domestic violence, 164–65
    reaction to trauma by, 168–70
    of sexual abuse, 160
Violence
    domestic, 163–68
    school, 142
Violence Against Women Act (VAWA) (1995), 167
Visualization, 438–39, 441
Vitamins, 380, 381–82
Voice, tone of, 283–84, 286–87
Voluntary euthanasia, 316

## W
War, traumatic experience of, 158
Washington Death with Dignity Act (2008), 317
Water, need for, 65
Weaknesses, self-understanding and, 33
Weil, Andrew, 388–89
Withdrawal
    from alcohol, 185, 188–89
    caffeine, 188
    as defense mechanism, 183
    from drug dependency, 187
    nicotine, 188
    from tobacco use, 184
World Federation of Right to Die Societies, 317
Worrall, Olga, 374, 403
Worry, 107
Wright, Jonathan, 381

## X
X-rays, 370

## Y
Yin/yang theory, 414
"You talk," 159
Young adulthood, adjustments during, 140